INDICATIONS FOR HEART VALVE REPLACEMENT BY AGE GROUP

INDICATIONS FOR HEART VALVE REPLACEMENT BY AGE GROUP

EDITED BY
CARLOS GOMEZ-DURAN
AND
GEORGE J. REUL, JR.

KLUWER ACADEMIC PUBLISHERS
BOSTON   DORDRECHT   LONDON

Distributors for North America:
Kluwer Academic Publishers
101 Philip Drive
Assinippi Park
Norwell, Massachusetts 02061 USA

Distributors for the UK and Ireland:
Kluwer Academic Publishers
Falcon House, Queen Square
Lancaster LA1 1RN, UNITED KINGDON

Distributors for all other countries:
Kluwer Academic Publishers Group
Distribution Centre
Post Office Box 322
3300 AH Dordrecht, THE NETHERLANDS

Library of Congress Cataloging-in-Publication Data

International Symposium on Heart Valves (5th: 1987: Fort Lauderdale, Fla.)
    Indications for heart valve replacement by age group: proceedings
of the Fifth International Symposium on Heart Valves/moderated by
Carlos Gomez-Duran and George J. Reul, Jr., April 1–4, 1987,
Bonaventure Hotel and Resort, Fort Lauderdale, Florida; sponsored
by St. Jude Medical, Inc.
        p.   cm.
    Includes bibliographies and index.
    ISBN 0-89838-393-5
    1. Heart—Valves—Surgery—Congresses.   2. Heart valve prosthesis-
Congresses.   3. Surgical indications—Congresses.   I. Gomez-Duran,
Carlos.   II. Reul, George J.   III. St. Jude Medical, Inc.
IV. Title.
    [DNLM: 1. Age Factors—congresses.   2. Heart Valve Prothesis-
congresses.   3. Heart Valves—surgery—congresses.   W3 IN918PC 5th
1987i/WG 169 I6025 1987i]
RD598.35.H42I57 1987
617'.412—dc19
DNLM/DLC
for Library of Congress   88-12963
                                                                                 CIP

Printed in the United States of America

CONTENTS

MODERATORS AND CONTRIBUTING AUTHORS

Anthony J. Acinapura, M.D.
St. Vincent's Hospital &
Medical Center of New York
153 West 11th Street
New York, NY 10011

Kit V. Arom, M.D.
920 East 28th Street
Suite 420
Minneapolis, MN 55407

Professor Eugene M. Baudet
Department of Cardiovascular
  Surgery
Avenue de Magellan
F-33604 Bordeaux FRANCE

Andrzej Biederman, M.D.
National Cardiology Center Anin
UL. ALPEJSKA 52
Warsaw
POLAND

A. Michael Borkon, M.D.
Mid-America Heart Institute
4320 Wornall Road
Suite II-50
Kansas City, MO 64111

Dieter Burckhardt, M.D.
Kantonsspital
Spitalstrasse 21
CH-4031 Basel
SWITZERLAND

Professor Christian Cabrol
Hopital de la Pitié
47–83 Bd de l'Hopital
F-75634 Paris
FRANCE

David Campbell, M.D.
University of Colorado
Health Sciences Center
4200 East 9th Avenue, #C-310
Denver, CO 80262

J. Cleland, M.D.
Cardiac Surgical Unit
Royal Victoria Hospital
Grosvenor Road
Belfast B2 6BA
NORTH IRELAND

Denton A. Cooley, M.D.
Texas Heart Institute
P.O. Box 20345
Houston, TX 77225

Stephanus L. Cronjé, M.D.
Department of Cardiothoracic
  Surgery
Medical University of Southern
  Africa
P.O. Medunsa 0204
REPUBLIC OF SOUTH AFRICA

Gregorio de Rábago, M.D.
Fundacion Jiminez Diaz
Clinica Nuestra Señora de la
  Concepcion
Avda. Reyes Católicos, 2 (Ciudad
  Universitaria)
28040 Madrid SPAIN

Philip B. Deverall, M.D.
Guy's Hospital
St. Thomas' Street
London SE1 9RT
ENGLAND

Address for correspondence:
21 Upper Wimpole Street
London W1M 7TA
ENGLAND

Professor E. Rainer de Vivie
Robert-Koch Str. 40
3400 Goettingen
WEST GERMANY

Diego Figuera, M.D.
Cirugia Cardiovascular
Clinical Puerta de Hierro
28035 Madrid SPAIN

Professor Carlos Gomez-Duran,
    M.D., Ph.D.
Hospital Nacional Marques de
    Valdecilla
Universidal de Cantabria
39008 Santander SPAIN

Lorenzo Gonzalez-Lavin, M.D.
Department of Thoracic and
Cardiovascular Surgery
Deborah Heart & Lung Center
Browns Mills, NJ 08015

Richard J. Gray, M.D.
Cedars-Sinai Medical Center
8700 Beverly Boulevard
Los Angeles, CA 90048

Dominique Grunenwald, M.D.
Hopital Laennec
42 rue de Sevres
F-75007 Paris FRANCE

Renee S. Hartz, M.D.
Division of Cardiothoracic Surgery
Northwestern University Medical
    School
303 East Chicago Avenue
Ward 9–105
Chicago, IL 60611

J. Michael Hasenkam, M.D.
Department of Thoracic and
Cardiovascular Surgery
Skejby University Hospital
8200 Aarhus N
DENMARK

Dieter Horstkotte, M.D.
Department of Medicine B

University of Düsseldorf
Moorenstrasse 5
D-4000 Düsseldorf 1
WEST GERMANY

Kohei Kawazoe, M.D.
National Cardiovascular Center
5-7-1 Fujishiro-dai
Suita City
Osaka 565 JAPAN

Hyoung Mook Kim, M.D.
Korea University Medical College
4, 2-Ka, Myungryun-Dong,
Chongno-Ku
Seoul 110 KOREA

Professor Rainer Körfer
Klinik für Thorax–und
Kardiovaskularchirurgie
Herzzentrum NRW
Geogstrasse, 11
D-4970 Bad Oeynhausen
WEST GERMANY

Professor Yves Logeais
C.H.U. / Hôpital Pontchaillou
Université Rennes
Rue Henri le Guillaux
F-35011 Rennes
FRANCE

Christopher T. Maloney, M.D.
Catholic Medical Center
100 McGregor
Manchester, NH 03102

Ph. Mikaeloff, M.D.
Hospices Civils de Lyon
Hôpital Cardio-Vasculaire et
Pneumologique Louis Pradel
BP Lyon Montchat
69394 Lyon Cedex 03
FRANCE

Eldred D. Mundth, M.D.
Bryn Mawr Cardiac Surgery
    Association
Bryn Mawr Medical Building North

830 Old Lancaster Road
Bryn Mawr, PA 19010

Hugh O'Kane, M.D.
Royal Victoria Hospital
Grosvenor Road
Belfast
NORTH IRELAND

Roque Pifarre, M.D.
Department of Thoracic and
Cardiovascular Surgery
2160 South First Avenue
Maywood, IL 60153

Antonio Pucci, M.D.
Divisione di Cardiochirurgia
Camillo Hospital
Ospedale S. Camile
Circonvallazione Gianicolenze
Roma, ITALY

Dennis F. Pupello, M.D.
2727 West Buffalo Avenue
Tampa, FL 33607

George J. Reul, Jr., M.D.
Texas Heart Institute
P.O. Box 20345
Houston, TX 77225

Robert M. Sade, M.D.
The Medical University of South
  Carolina
Division of Cardiothoracic Surgery
171 Ashley Avenue
Charleston, SC 29425

Professor Volker Schlosser
55 Hugstetterstrasse
D-7800 Freiburg
WEST GERMANY

Craig R. Smith, M.D.
Columbia Presbyterian Medical
  Center
622 West 168th Street
New York, NY 10032

Larry W. Stephenson, M.D.
Hospital of the University of
  Pennsylvania
3400 Spruce Street
Philadelphia, PA 19104

(Armenti F., Stephenson L.W., Edmunds
  L.H., Jr.:Simultaneous implantation of
  St. Jude Medical aortic and mitral
  protheses. J. Thorac Cardiovasc Surg
  1987; 94:733–739.)

Lars I. Thulin, M.D.
Department of Thoracic and
Cardiovascular Surgery
Univesity Hospital
S-221 85 Lund
SWEDEN

Professor Marko Turina
University Hospital
Chirurgische Klinik A
Ramistrasse 100
8091 Zurich
SWITZERLAND

Francis Wellens, M.D.
Department of Cardiac Surgery
University Libre Bruxelles
O.L. Vrouwziekenhuis
Moorselbaan
9300 Aalst BELGIUM

Andre Wessels, M.D.
Division of Cardiothoracic Surgery
Johannesburg Hospital Medical
  School
7 York Road
Parktown 2193 SOUTH AFRICA

REGISTERED TRADEMARKS USED IN THIS BOOK

BIOIMPLANT™—St. Jude Medical, Inc.
BJÖRK-SHILEY®—Shiley Corporation
CARPENTIER-EDWARDS®—American Edwards Laboratories
COUMADIN®—E.I duPont de Nemours and Company, Inc.
DACRON®—E.I duPont de Nemours and Company, Inc.
DELRIN®—E.I duPont de Nemours and Company, Inc.
EDWARDS-DUROMEDICS™—American Edwards Laboratories
HANCOCK®—Medtronic, Inc.
IONESCU-SHILEY®—Shiley Corporation
KAY-SHILEY®—American Edwards Laboratories
LILLEHEI-KASTER®—Medical Incorporated
MEDTRONIC HALL™—Medtronic, Inc.
MITROFLOW®—Mitral Medical of Canada, Inc.
OMNICARBON®—Medical Incorporated
OMNISCIENCE®—Medical Incorporated
PERSANTINE®—Boehringer Ingelheim
PROLENE®—Ethicon, Inc.
ST. JUDE MEDICAL®—St. Jude Medical, Inc.
SMELOFF-CUTTER®—Sutter Biomedical, Inc.
STARR-EDWARDS®—American Edwards Laboratories
TEFLON®—E.I duPont de Nemours and Company, Inc.

INTRODUCTION

The papers presented at the Fifth International Symposium on Heart Valves and published in this volume discuss clinical experience with heart valve replacement in pediatric patients, in adults (age 65 and younger), and in the elderly (age 66 and older). Special considerations in heart valve replacement, such as valve selection, reoperation, results of double valve implantation, quality of life, and the use of valved conduits are also included. Finally, long-term clinical follow-up with the ST. JUDE MEDICAL® heart valve, giving 7- and 8-year data is discussed.

HEART VALVE REPLACEMENT IN PEDIATRIC PATIENTS

Anticoagulation

Anticoagulation in children is a difficult and interesting problem. Three principal considerations in the use of anticoagulants are patient education, timing, and anticoagulating substance. Additional considerations are patient tolerance and compliance.

Generally, the findings indicate, if pediatric patients receive anticoagulation following mechanical valve replacement, it is well accepted and results in few complications. If children are not anticoagulated, complications arise. Conflicting results regarding the efficacy of PERSANTINE® and the use of aspirin vs. COUMADIN® were reported.

Doctor Sade's data address some of these questions.* After a 5-year study in

---

* See J Thorac Cardiovasc Surgery 1988; 95:533–561.

children utilizing only aspirin, he has returned to the use of anticoagulants. In addition, while we think of thrombosis and thromboembolism occurring at a linearized rate, Sade's data show a sudden increase in thromboembolism at 5 years.★ This could indicate that in the early period following valve replacement we do not have to anticoagulate patients, but in the latter years it becomes necessary.

Enlargement

A second consideration in valve replacement in children is enlargement of the aortic root. Papers presented show varying use of these procedures, from only a few cases to two out of every three patients. We conclude that most surgeons are willing to accept a small (19 mm) ST. JUDE MEDICAL® heart valve in the aortic position, especially for aortic insufficiency. Perhaps, in the mitral position, this small size valve would have to be replaced as the child grows.

HEART VALVE REPLACEMENT IN ADULTS AGE 65 AND YOUNGER

A surprising aspect of the data presented was the excellent results of the IONESCU-SHILEY® valve vs. the ST. JUDE MEDICAL valve. In most of these studies, patients were followed only to 5 years. However, Dr. Cooley's data showed a precipitous drop in survival, with a high complication rate, at 6 years. Perhaps the mean follow-up of 5 years is not as high as it should be to demonstrate these problems. In addition, Doctor Kawazoe's paper showed a higher rate of complications with the low profile IONESCU-SHILEY valve than with the standard valve.

VALVE REPLACEMENT IN THE ELDERLY (AGE 66 AND OLDER)

The papers presented in this section demonstrate that it is possible to operate on older patients. However, the risk of complications is higher and their long-term survival is not very good. Neurological complications in these patients varied from 4% to 30%. It is especially high in combined procedures, such as coronary artery bypass plus mitral valve replacement (CAB + MVR). These patients should be screened for arteriosclerosis before surgery. An interesting aspect of the study by Professor Logeais is that the average French male lives 10 years longer than 70 years. This additional life expectancy can be a factor in valve choice.

CONSIDERATIONS IN HEART VALVE REPLACEMENT

Surgical procedures

One of the most disturbing slides, presented by Doctor Schlosser, showed a leaflet of a ST. JUDE MEDICAL valve broken into small pieces. This demonstrates how brittle the valve is and how carefully it must be handled at the time of surgery.

★ Sade RM, Crawford FA, Fyte DA, Stroud MP. Valve prothesis in children: a reassessment of anticoagulation. J Thorac Cardiovasc Surg 1988, 95:553–561.

Valve orientation is important and probably should be in an antianatomical position, that is, perpendicular to the septum in both the aortic and mitral positions. In addition, one must be aware of the pathology present. These precautions may solve some of the sudden death problems and high thrombosis rates that we have observed.

Velocity field flow studies by Doctor Hasenkam showed areas of potential stagnation. This can help us understand how to better orient the valve in the flow field, especially with respect to coronary orifices.

Valve selection

The site of valve replacement is also an important consideration when selecting a mechanical or biological valve for implantation. Doctor Wellen's paper discusses a prevalent indication for the use of a bioprosthesis in the tricuspid position. Mitral valve repair has been meeting with some success and is obviously preferable over mitral valve replacement if it is possible. There was not enough time to adequately discuss the use of porcine versus pericardial valves.

Follow-up

The noninvasive analysis of the ST. JUDE MEDICAL valve by Doctor Hartz using fluoroscopy data was impressive. The ease of this procedure should compel us to follow all patients in this manner. In addition, this may be a way to prevent sudden death and high thrombosis rates. For example, if visualization shows that a leaflet does not move, perhaps the patient should have a stricter COUMADIN regimen.

Quality of life following heart valve replacement is a key consideration. Ninety-seven percent of the patients in Doctor Thulin's study tolerated anticoagulation well, without complaint. In the Texas Heart Institute study, 90% of the patients were well anticoagulated, and there was only a 3.2% per patient-year incidence of bleeding and a 1.0% per patient-year thromboembolic problem. These results point out the need for standardization in anticoagulation care in order to keep complications low.

Differences in follow-up procedures probably account for the variations in reported data. The number of unknown deaths reported—from 13% to 30% —is a prime example and a key concern. Whether these deaths are valve-related or patient-related, the cause should be known. Some uniformity in data reporting has already been achieved, in the use of actuarial curves and incidences per patient-year, but the need for consistency and quality in follow-up remains absolutely essential.

Complications

Mortality due to reoperation following heart valve replacement ranged from 6% to 14%, which is quite high. Most of these reoperations were the result of tissue valve failures. The three greatest variables were age, emergency of operation, and endocarditis, especially aortic valve endocarditis.

Thromboembolic events appear to be more patient-related than valve-related at the present time. With modern prostheses, whether of one type or another, the patient's underlying symptoms or compliance with the anti-coagulation regimen affects the incidence of thromboembolism more than the type of valve implanted.

The rate of hemorrhagic events reported varies from 0.8% to 3.0% per patient-year, which is equal to, if not higher than, the incidence of thrombo-embolic events reported. Are we overanticoagulating these patients? Obviously, incidents of thrombosis are caused by underanticoagulation. Balancing anticoagulation and thromboembolic events remains challenging.

Survival

Survival rates reported are similar at 5, 8, or 10 years, whatever prosthesis is implanted. It would be easy to select one valve type over another if there were a large difference in survival between them. However, the decision must be based on other factors, such as the quality of life vs. reoperation.

LONG-TERM FOLLOW-UP WITH THE ST. JUDE MEDICAL VALVE

The papers presented here give us an opportunity to compare the ST. JUDE MEDICAL valve to other valves. The early and late follow-up of the ST. JUDE MEDICAL valve correlates well with that of all other valves presented in actuarial tables.

These papers discuss a variety of anticoagulant regimens, and the incidence of thromboembolic events varies accordingly. Differences arise regarding when to start anticoagulation, what dosage to give, response to anticoagulation treatment, rates of anticoagulant-related complications, and reoperation due to valve failure. If we closely follow anticoagulation treatment, understanding the level of anticoagulation per patient, we will see a difference in the ST. JUDE MEDICAL valve vs. tissue valves.

Valve design

The bileaflet design of the ST. JUDE MEDICAL valve remains a tremendous advantage in patient safety. The lack of mechanical failure is very encouraging. Only one incidence of a broken, escaped leaflet was reported by Doctor Burckhardt.

An unexplained problem with the ST. JUDE MEDICAL valve is the instances of sudden deaths where the causes are unknown. This also happens with tissue valves.

It is very encouraging to see all the reports indicating that the ST. JUDE MEDICAL valve is equal to, if not superior to other valves. The hemodynamic data are excellent, and the long-term follow-up data now confirm our belief that it is the valve of choice.

George J. Reul, Jr.

PREFACE

Dr. Reul, in his Introduction, has made a number of comments with which I agree. However, after listening to the presentations of these papers, I have some remarks which are necessarily personal.

STANDARDIZATION OF DATA

In relation to the need for standardization, I can say that a lot has already been achieved. Everyone prefers actuarial curves and linearized incidences, but we still have a long way to go. For instance, a very interesting statement was made about the incidence of thromboembolism according to whether the patients were seen every six months, every year, or every two years. The closer the follow-up, the higher the incidence. Quality in follow-up is absolutely necessary, and I am sure that differences in quality of follow-up explains some of the differences in data found among the papers. I am also concerned about the high number of unknown deaths reported. In the presentations, the incidence was between 13% and 14%, although in some cases it reached 30% with the Bjork-Shiley valve. Whether these deaths are valve-related or patient-related is important. One can dream that one day we will standardize data so well that after feeding data into a computer, we can have a coffee and come back to find which valve is best for a particular patient. I am convinced it will come.

ANTICOAGULATION

Although we only report that our patients were anticoagulated, there seems to be a wide variety of anticoagulation regimens. Because of this, it is not surprising that the reported rates vary so widely. However, there is enough evidence supporting the principle that every patient with a mechanical valve should be anticoagulated, even with a ST. JUDE MEDICAL® valve. Personally, I do not feel brave enough to start having my patients go without anticoagulatio1, even children with that valve in the aortic position. On the other hand, I see series of patients with bioprostheses in the mitral position who are anticoagulated, in which case, I do not understand why a mechanical valve was not implanted. I have a strong feeling that many of the thromboembolic events in the mitral position are more patient related than valve related.

The rate of hemorrhagic events reported varies between 0.8% and 3% for 100 patient-years which is equal to, if not higher than, the embolic incidence. It seems that these incidents are secondary to over-anticoagulation. How do we find a balance?

LONG-TERM SURVIVAL

Another area to consider is long-term patient survival. There does not seem to be much difference between valves and, therefore, at the present time, while waiting for the perfect valve, we have to look for the best quality of life for our patients. In my opinion, quality of life is primarily related to anticoagulation, secondarily to mechanical valve implantation and reoperation after a bio-prosthetic replacement. I was impressed by the acceptance of anticoagulation by the people of Norway. Again, compliance to an anticoagulation regimen was surprisingly high and certainly not my experience. I was also surprised to hear that 30% of the patients were aware of the noise of their prosthetic valves that stresses the difficulty in selecting the appropriate valve for each patient.

IMPLANTATION SITE

Site of implantation is obviously an important factor. It has been stated that repair of the atrioventricular valve is better than replacement, but this is not always possible. In the tricuspid position, a bioprosthetic valve is to be favored, but, if not possible, a ST. JUDE MEDICAL valve seems to be the alternative.

VALVE SELECTION

There was not enough time to discuss the question of the porcine *vs.* pericardial bioprostheses. Our personal impression with the available evidence is that the porcine bioprosthesis is superior to the bovine, particularly if we use the information obtained in the very young age group.

I am very impressed by the results presented with the ST. JUDE MEDICAL valve. I think that the fact of its being bileaflet represents a thromboembolic advantage for the safety of the patient particularly when, at present, the movement of each leaflet can be observed noninvasively, and early action is, therefore, possible. Although balloon valvuloplasty is attracting a lot of attention, I am sure cardiologists will keep sending patients for valve replacement and, with present-day prostheses, the results will continue to encourage an earlier, more aggressive attitude.

I must end by taking the opportunity to thank, in the name of us all, St. Jude Medical, Inc. and their staff for their kindness and ability to organize this very informative and enjoyable meeting.

Carlos G. Duran

I. EXPERIENCE WITH HEART VALVE REPLACEMENT IN PEDIATRIC PATIENTS

1. THE DURABILITY OF THE ST. JUDE MEDICAL® VALVE IN CHILDREN

D. GRUNENWALD, P. R. VOUHE, W. KHOURY, J. Y. NEVEUX

Abstract. *Between 1979 and 1986, 69 children, 1 to 15 years of age, underwent cardiac valve replacement with a ST. JUDE MEDICAL® prosthesis (SJM). Seventy-eight SJM valves were implanted during 73 operations. Forty-two children had mitral valve replacement, 20 had aortic valve replacement, and 6 had tricuspid valve replacement. Double valve replacement (mitral and aortic) was performed with ST. JUDE MEDICAL valves in 5 patients. Forty-eight children had undergone a prior operation (70%). The overall early mortality was 8.2%. Of the 78 patients who had SJM valves implanted, 2 needed a reoperation for valve replacement. The authors analyzed 7 years of experience and conclude that the ST. JUDE MEDICAL valve allows definitive cardiac valve replacement in children, particularly in the aortic position.*

INTRODUCTION

Cardiac valvular replacement in the child yields a double problem: 1) the possibility of long survival requires a durable prosthesis with low incidence of valve-related morbidity and 2) these small valves must have optimal hemo-dynamic performance, adaptable to the growth of the child. The present retrospective study reviews our experience with the ST. JUDE MEDICAL valve in 69 infants and children over the past 7 years.

PATIENTS AND METHODS

Between 1979 and 1985, 69 children, 1 to 15 years of age, underwent cardiac valve replacement with the ST. JUDE MEDICAL prosthesis in our institution. Nineteen patients were less than 5 years old. Seventy-eight ST. JUDE MEDICAL valves were implanted during 73 operations. Twenty children underwent aortic valve replacement, 42 had mitral valve replacement, and 6 had tricuspid valve replacement. Double valve replacement (mitral and aortic) was used in 5 patients (table 1-1).

The following were indications for surgery: 42 operations concerned congenital valve malformations; 28 were for rheumatic valve disease; infective endocarditis was found in 2 patients; and prosthetic valve failures required 22 operations. Forty-eight patients had undergone previous cardiac valvular operations (figure 1-1). Of these, 30 were congenital malformations; others were due to rheumatic disease or prosthetic valve failure.

The size of ST. JUDE MEDICAL valves implanted range from 19 mm to 31 mm. Sixteen patients, 11 of whom were more than 5 years of age, required insertion of a 19 mm valve (table 1-2). Two children, less than 2 years of age, received 19 mm ST. JUDE MEDICAL aortic valves, but the other 11 aortic valves (19 mm) were implanted in children more than 5 years of age. Three children, ages 1, 2, and 5, received 19 mm mitral valves.

At operation, 65% of the patients were in New York Heart Association (NYHA) Functional Class IV. Concomitant procedures were performed in 27 children (table 1-3).

Follow-up data were obtained by written or telephone contact with the patient's family or primary physician. It is noteworthy that many patients came from foreign countries, particularly Algeria and Italy. Eight patients could not be traced, yielding an 84.1% follow-up for the hospital survivors. The average follow-up was 4.1 years; the cumulative follow-up interval was 227 patient-years.

RESULTS

There were 6 hospital deaths. All were in patients with severe congenital disease who had undergone a prior operation. Four patients died of low cardiac output; 2 had tricuspid replacements, and 2 had mitral replacements. Another

Table 1-1. Clinical data

	MVR	AVR	TVR	DVR	Total
Interventions	42	20	6	5	73
Age range (years)	1–15	1–15	3–13	9–15	1–15
Mean age (years)	8.03	9.81	5.33	12.60	8.77
Previous valvular operations (%)	75	35	83	80	69
Associated procedures (%)	39	55	33	20	36
Operative mortality (%)	9.52	0	33.33	0	8.20

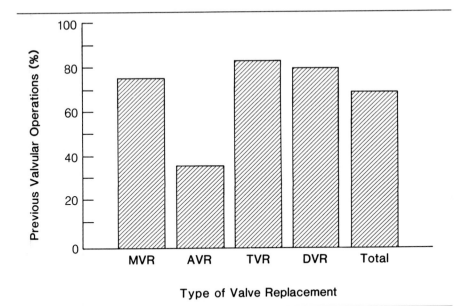

Figure 1-1. Previous valvular operations in patients undergoing valve replacement. MVR = mitral valve replacement; AVR = aortic valve replacement; TVR = tricuspid valve replacement; DVR = double valve replacement.

Table 1-2. Implantation of 19 mm SJM prostheses

	Aortic	Mitral	Total
Patients ≤ 5 years	2	3	5
Patients > 5 years	11	0	11
Total	13	3	16

Table 1-3. Concomitant procedures

	Number of patients
Tricuspid annuloplasty	6
VSD closure	6
Mitral valve annuloplasty	4
Patch enlargement of ascending aorta	3
Excision of subvalvular aortic stenosis	1
Enlargement of aortic anulus	3
ASD closure	1
Ebstein's disease repair	2
Coarctation of aorta	1
Total	27

VSD = ventricular septal defect; ASD = atrial septal defect

child, less than 1 year of age, died of ventricular fibrillation 2 days after operation. A 7-year-old girl, requiring mitral valve replacement for prosthetic failure, died of myocardial infarction.

Every child was given permanent anticoagulation. During the follow-up period, 90.5% of the patients were maintained on systemic anticoagulation with warfarin sodium and 6% received antiplatelet therapy.

There were 2 late deaths. One occurred after aortic valve replacement, from mesenteric embolus without anticoagulation. The other happened suddenly, 4 years after mitral valve replacement.

Nonfatal valve-related complications occurred in 7 patients (table 1-4). Three thromboembolic events were noted. Two children each had a nonfatal hemorrhagic episode. Reoperation for replacement of the ST. JUDE MEDICAL prosthesis was required twice. In 1 of these cases, the size of an aortic prosthesis was inadequate. In the other, a mitral prosthesis was changed due to paravalvular leak. At 6 years, 90.4% of the mitral valve patients and 80% of aortic valve recipients remained free of major complications.

The overall actuarial probability of survival at 6 years, including operative mortality, was 73%. For patients with isolated mitral valve replacement, it was 80% and for aortic valve replacement, 87.5%. Event-free survival without dyspnea has been excellent in 62% of the patients; with effort dyspnea but normal activity in 13%; and with effort dyspnea and disability in 25% of the patients.

Operative mortality and mean patient age are shown in figure 1-2. Intermediate and long-term results of aortic valve replacement are good. There was no hospital mortality in this group. Aortic valvular replacement usually can be delayed until an adult-size valve can be implanted. The mean age of our patients receiving ST. JUDE MEDICAL aortic valves was 10 years. In younger children or in the presence of annular hypoplasia, the anulus can be enlarged to accommodate an adult-sized prosthesis.

The low risk of complications with mechanical valves, together with the alarming occurrence of tissue valve degeneration in children, led us to a clear conclusion: In the aortic position the ST. JUDE MEDICAL valve should be used and satisfactory long-term results can be anticipated.

In the mitral position, however, the early mortality of 9.5% is an important factor. The mean age (8 years) of these patients was slightly lower. There was a high incidence (54.5%) of major congenital disease. Even though the theoretical risk of a thromboembolic event is high in the mitral position, we prefer to implant a pyrolytic carbon bileaflet prosthesis rather than a tissue

Table 1-4. Complications

Thromboembolus	3
Hemorrhage	2
Reoperation	2

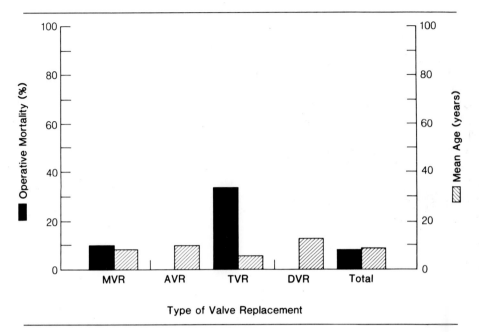

Figure 1-2. Mean patient age and operative mortality following valve replacement.

valve, because the probability of malfunction of a pericardial bioprosthesis at 5 years was as high as 80% in another of our series. Due to the technical impossibility of mitral anulus enlargement in these children, we used small-sized ST. JUDE MEDICAL prostheses, delaying definitive valve replacement until an adult size valve could be used.

Our results in the tricuspid position are poor. The high hospital mortality (33.33%) is obviously related to severe congenital disease. Nevertheless, we believe that the ST. JUDE MEDICAL valve has optimal hemodynamic properties for tricuspid valve replacement in children.

In conclusion, the ST. JUDE MEDICAL prosthesis is our choice for both mitral and aortic valve replacement in children.

REFERENCES

1. Borkon AM, Soule L, Reitz BA, Gott VL, Gardner TJ. Five year follow-up after valve replacement with the St. Jude Medical valve in infants and children. Circulation 1986; 74(I):I-110.
2. Milano A, Vouhe PR, Baillot-Vernant F, Donzeau-Gouge P, Trinquet F, Roux PM, Leca F, Neveux JY. Late results after left-sided cardiac valve replacement in children. J Thorac Cardiovasc Surg 1986; 92:218–225.
3. Lillehei CW. Worldwide experience with the St. Jude Medical valve prosthesis: Clinical and hemodynamic results. Contemp Surg 1982; 20:17–32.

2. A SEVEN-YEAR EXPERIENCE WITH THE ST. JUDE MEDICAL® HEART VALVE

H. O'KANE, D. GLADSTONE, L. HAMILTON, I. GALVIN, I. CLELAND

Abstract. From May 1979 to October 1986, 442 ST. JUDE MEDICAL® valves (175 aortic, 142 mitral, and 61 multiple valve replacements) were inserted in 378 patients, ages 5 to 82 years. The operative mortality rates (30-day) were 1.1% aortic, 4.2% mitral, and 8.2% multiple valve replacement; and the late mortality was 6.8% aortic, 6.3% mitral, and 1.6% multiple valve replacement. All patients were anticoagulated. Three hundred seventy-eight patients have been followed for a total of 912 patient-years. During that time we have not recorded a single occurrence of primary structural failure or significant hemolysis in any patient. One aortic valve patient stopped taking her anticoagulant and the valve thrombosed; it was successfully replaced. In another patient, the mitral valve thrombosed after she switched from warfarin to subcutaneous heparin when she became pregnant; this valve was also successfully replaced. Twenty-four patients experienced isolated thromboembolic episodes (13 major, 11 minor)—an incidence of 2.7% per patient-year (2.6% aortic, 2.8% mitral, and 2.3% multiple). Included in the group were 9 children aged 5 to 16 years, 7 with mitral valve implants and 2 with aortic valve implants. One 9-year-old child who had an aortic valve implant for acute bacterial endocarditis died 2 months postoperatively with multiple organ failure. The remaining 8 patients, all on anticoagulation, continue to make excellent progress, 1 to 6 years later.

INTRODUCTION

Since the time of its first use in our unit in May 1979, until October 1986, we have had extended experience with the ST. JUDE MEDICAL valve in

9

children and adults. Its low profile (especially in the mitral area) and large
effective orifice are particularly important.

METHODS

We inserted 442 ST. JUDE MEDICAL valves in 378 patients (ages 5 to 82
years). There were 175 patients with aortic valve replacement, 142 patients
with mitral valve replacement, and 61 patients with multiple valve replacements. In the latter group, 56 patients had aortic and mitral valve replacements;
3 patients had triple valve replacement; 1 patient had mitral and tricuspid
replacement; and 1 had aortic and tricuspid replacement. The sex ratio, shown
in table 2-1, reflects that commonly seen in valvular lesions. The lower mean
age in the aortic and mitral groups is due to the fact that a number of children
have been included in each group. The valve sizes used are depicted in figure
2-1 and demonstrate that the aortic 23 mm and the mitral 31 mm valves were
the most commonly used sizes. In both the aortic and mitral position, the

Table 2-1. Replacements with the St. Jude Medical heart valve,
May 1979–October 1986

Valve replacement	Patients	Male/Female	Age (mean)
Aortic	175	1.8/1.0	9–82 (55)
Mitral	142	1.0/3.5	5–78 (45)
Multiple	61	1.0/3.9	42–70 (54)
Total	378		

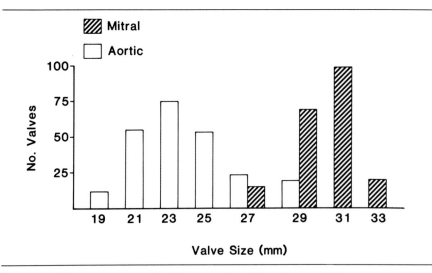

Figure 2-1. Valve sizes implanted in 378 patients, May 1979 to October 1986.

valves were inserted using a continuous suture of 2-0 PROLENE® with standard cardiopulmonary bypass, moderate hypothermia (28°C) and multi-dose cardioplegia. Each valve had its sewing ring soaked in a 0.5% neomycin sulphate solution prior to insertion.

RESULTS AND DISCUSSION

There were 2 early deaths in the aortic valve series, as shown in table 2-2. Both patients had a fulminant endocarditis on the aortic valve, and they died in the early postoperative period with widespread systemic infection. At the time of postmortem, the valve was functioning normally.

Similarly, the 11 early deaths (6 in the mitral and 5 in the multiple valve series) were related to the poor hemodynamic condition of the heart or technical problems at the time of surgery. Postmortem examination confirmed that all the prosthetic valves were functioning satisfactorily.

The late mortality in each group is also shown in table 2-2, with 6.8% mortality in the aortic group, 6.3% in the mitral, and 1.6% for the multiple valve replacements. Of 22 late deaths listed in table 2-3, there were 13 cases (8 aortic, 4 mitral, and 1 multiple valve replacement) in which the cause of death was accurately recorded. The evaluation of the valve up to the time of death and postmortem records showed no incidence of prosthetic dysfunction. In the 9 cases (4 aortic and 5 mitral) where the cause of death was unknown, there were no recent premortem evaluations or postmortem examinations, so we cannot definitely say that there was no recorded incidence of prosthetic valve dysfunction.

Table 2-2. Mortality among 378 patients undergoing heart valve replacement

Valve replacement	≤ 30 days	> 30 days
Aortic	2 (1.1%)	12 (6.8%)
Mitral	6 (4.2%)	9 (6.3%)
Multiple	5 (8.2%)	1 (1.6%)

Table 2-3. Late deaths following heart valve replacement in 378 patients

Valve replacement	Number of deaths	Cause of death
Aortic	12	4 unknown 8 known
Mitral	9	5 unknown 4 known
Multiple	1	1 known

A definition of thromboembolic events and anticoagulant-related hemorrhage is required before presenting the results of these complications. A *thromboembolic event* (TE) is defined as any new focal deficit, either transient (minor) or permanent (major), not including patients who awoke postoperatively with neurological deficits. *Anticoagulant-related hemorrhage* (ACH) is any internal or external hemorrhage necessitating medical intervention. All patients were anticoagulated using oral COUMADIN® (warfarin) to maintain an International Normalized Ratio (INR) from 2 to 4.

Table 2-4 lists complications. The follow-up for survivors was 466 patient-years (aortic), 317 patient-years (mitral), and 129 patient-years (multiple valve). As mentioned previously, there were no recorded cases of mechanical failure. There was 1 thrombosis of an aortic valve in a patient who stopped taking her anticoagulant. She came to emergency surgery and had a successful replacement of the thrombosed valve. Another patient was switched from oral COUMADIN to subcutaneous heparin when she became pregnant and, again, had emergency surgery during which her thrombosed mitral valve was successfully replaced with a tissue valve. The incidence of thromboembolism was 5 major and 7 minor events in the aortic series, 6 major and 3 minor in the mitral series, and 2 major and 1 minor in the multiple valve series, to give a rate of 2.6% per patient-year, 2.8% per patient-year, and 2.3% per patient-year, respectively.

Anticoagulant-related hemorrhage occurred in 4 aortic, 2 mitral, and 2 multiple valve cases, to give an incidence of 0.9% per patient-year (aortic), 0.6% per patient-year (mitral), and 1.5% per patient-year (multiple valve). There were no recorded cases of endocarditis arising *de novo* with the prosthetic valve, nor were there any cases of prosthetic hemolysis severe enough to require valve replacement. Two patients with aortic valves and 3 with mitral valves required further surgery to repair severe paravalvular leaks.

Table 2-4. Complications following replacement with the St. Jude Medical heart valve

	Aortic	Mitral	Multiple
	175 patients	142 patients	61 patients
Total patient-years	466	317	129
Mechanical failure	0	0	0
Valve thrombosis	1	1	0
TE events	5M/7m	6M/3m	2M/1m
% per patient-year	2.6%	2.8%	2.3%
ACH events	4	2	2
% per patient-year	0.9%	0.6%	1.5%
Endocarditis	0	0	0
Hemolysis	0	0	0
Reoperation	2	3	0

ACH = anticoagulant-related hemorrhage; M = major; m = minor

The survival curves show 90% survival at 7 years for the aortic valve group (figure 2-2), 78% survival in the mitral valve group at 7 years (figure 2-3), and for the multiple valve replacement group, 92% at 7 years (figure 2-4).

An interesting subgroup within this series is one of 9 children who had ST. JUDE MEDICAL valves inserted for a variety of reasons between the ages of 5 and 16 years. Seven had mitral valve replacements and 2 had aortic valve replacements, as shown in table 2-5. One reason for replacement was severe mitral regurgitation in a child with an acute rheumatic period. The next child had a severely dysfunctioning calcified HANCOCK® valve replaced; having previously had a mitral valve repair, followed by a fascia lata valve over the previous 16 years. Two more children had corrected transposition of the great

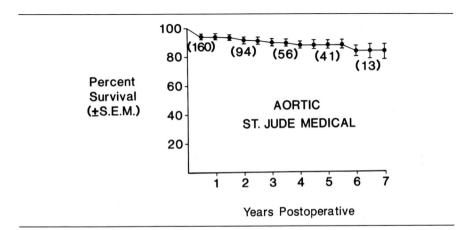

Figure 2-2. Actuarial survival following aortic valve replacement.

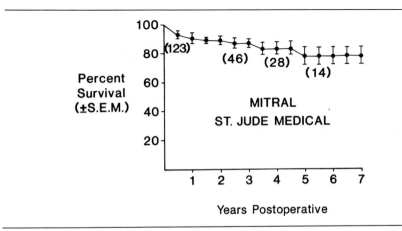

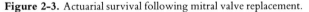

Figure 2-3. Actuarial survival following mitral valve replacement.

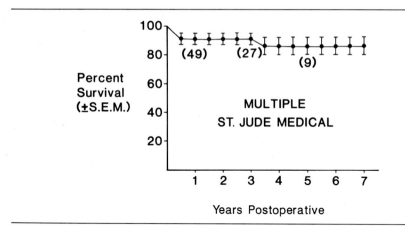

Figure 2-4. Actuarial survival following multiple valve replacement.

arteries and had severely regurgitant left atrioventricular valves replaced. Another was a case of a partial atrioventricular canal with a regurgitant mitral valve; the next was a primary case of mitral regurgitation. Another child had severe mitral stenosis due to a dysplastic valve and associated subaortic stenosis. The next child, who had severe bacterial endocarditis, had a bicuspid aortic valve and died 2 months after surgery from a disseminated infection with multi-organ failure. The final case involved aortic valve replacement for severe aortic incompetence.

The 8 survivors have been followed from 1 to 6 years and are progressing excellently with normal growth patterns; 1 of the older girls is attending a university. We believe that all cases, even children, should be maintained on

Table 2-5. Children receiving St. Jude Medical valves

Age	Sex	Diagnosis	Valve size/ position	Follow-up
10 years	F	Acute RF	29M	6 years
16 years	F	Ca⁺⁺ HNK	29M	6 years
11½ years	M	CTGA	31M	3 years
5 years	F	CTGA	27M	3 years
7 years	M	PAVC	27M	2 years
8 years	M	MR	29M	1½ years
14 years	F	MS	31M	1 years
9 years	F	BE	19A	0
14½ years	M	AI	27A	1½ years

All patients received warfarin.
RF = rheumatic fever; Ca⁺⁺ HNK = Calcified Hancock valve; CTGA = corrected transposition of the great arteries; PAVC = partial atrioventricular canal; MR = mitral regurgitation; MS = mitral stenosis; BE = bacterial endocarditis; AI = aortic incompetence

anticoagulants. These patients were all maintained on the warfarin routine of the INR with values maintained from 2 to 4. To date, there have been no thromboembolic episodes nor anticoagulant hemorrhages.

Our extended clinical experience with the ST. JUDE MEDICAL valve, with its low profile (especially in the mitral area) and large effective orifice, make it our prosthetic valve of choice, especially in children.

3. ST. JUDE MEDICAL® CARDIAC VALVE EXPERIENCE IN INFANTS AND CHILDREN

D. N. CAMPBELL, C. MADIGAN, D. R. CLARKE

Abstract. *During the last 7 years, 44 ST. JUDE MEDICAL® cardiac valves have been placed in 43 children. Nine patients were less than 1 year of age and 1 child had a double valve replacement. Twenty-four valves were placed in the aortic position. Seven of these patients underwent valve replacement only, while 16 patients had concomitant aortoventriculoplasties, and 1 patient had a Manouguian procedure. There were 2 early and no late deaths. Both deaths occurred in critically ill children who underwent emergency operations. Twenty valves were placed in the mitral position (12 annular and 8 supra-annular). There were no deaths with annular replacements and 7 deaths (2 early and 5 late) when supra-annular placement was used. Four of the 5 late deaths had marked preoperative left ventricular dysfunction. Mean patient follow-up is 43 months in 34 long-term survivors. Anticoagulation was achieved with warfarin, often in combination with sulfinpyrazone or dipyridamole. There have been 3 episodes of thromboembolism, all occurring in patients with suboptimal anticoagulation. We conclude that: 1) results from ST. JUDE MEDICAL cardiac valve replacement in the aortic position or in the mitral position with annular placement in children are excellent, 2) anticoagulation with warfarin is warranted, and 3) morbidity and mortality are often related to the underlying disease (mitral annular hypoplasia or left ventricular dysfunction) rather than to valve malfunction or technical problems at operation.*

INTRODUCTION

The ideal valve for mitral or aortic replacement in infants and children has yet to be developed. Many centers became disenchanted with bioprostheses in children in the late 1970s because of accelerated calcification, degeneration, and failure [1–4]. In addition, the mechanical valves that were then available did not allow low morbidity and mortality replacement in small children and infants because of high-profile design or poor hemodynamic performance of the smaller valve sizes. In 1978, implantation of the ST. JUDE MEDICAL cardiac valve was initiated under clinical protocol at the University of Colorado Health Sciences Center. It soon became clear that this low-profile valve had excellent hemodynamic characteristics, particularly in the smaller sizes. These qualities, plus its low thrombogenicity, made it an attractive choice for valve replacement in children. This manuscript details our experience with this valve in infants and children over the last 7 years.

METHODS AND MATERIALS

Patients

Since 1980, 43 children have undergone mitral or aortic valve replacement at the University of Colorado Health Sciences Center and the Children's Hospital in Denver, Colorado. The youngest patient was 6 weeks old and the oldest child was 17 years of age. Nine of the patients (21%) were less than 1 year of age. Twenty-three children had isolated aortic valve replacement; most of these patients were male (74%). Nineteen children had isolated mitral valve replacements and the male/female ratio was nearly equal (47%) males. One child had severe rheumatic aortic and mitral insufficiency and required a double valve replacement.

Diagnoses and indications for operation

In the aortic valve replacement group, the most common diagnosis was congenital aortic stenosis (table 3-1). Many of these children had aortic insufficiency as well, secondary to previous valvulotomies or progressive disease. In children with aortic stenosis, indications for valve replacement were similar to those for standard aortic valve replacement and included: 1) symptoms, 2) progressive cardiomegaly, and 3) a gradient greater than 60 mm Hg. Indications for aortoventriculoplasty were present in two thirds of this group and included: 1) aortic stenosis and/or aortic insufficiency requiring aortic valve replacement where the anulus would not accept an adult-sized valve, i.e.,

Table 3-1. Diagnostic categories for aortic valve replacement

Category	No. of patients
Congenital aortic stenosis	15
Primary aortic insufficiency	5
Subaortic tunnel obstruction	3

19 mm or greater, 2) replacement of a small valve prosthesis, or 3) recurrent tunnel subaortic stenosis. Our technique for aortoventriculoplasty has been previously described [5].

In the mitral group, the most common reasons for replacement were mitral regurgitation secondary to atrioventricular septal defect (AV septal defect) and congenital mitral stenosis (table 3-2). Mitral valve replacement was performed when there was failure of medical management to control congestive heart failure, failure to thrive, or respiratory disease. Supra-annular placement of the valve was performed when the anulus was too small to accept a 19-mm prosthesis.

Previous operations

All but 6 of the children who required aortic valve replacement had undergone at least one prior open heart procedure. Aortic valvotomy was the most common antecedent operation (13 procedures). Resection of a subaortic membrane with or without a Morrow procedure was carried out as a separate procedure in 3 patients. Five patients had bioprostheses placed 2 to 6 years prior to the current replacement. Two of the children also had previous coarctation repair.

In the mitral group, 8 of the 19 (42%) patients had undergone previous operations. AV septal defect repair was the most common. In contrast to the aortic group, only 1 child had received a previous replacement with a bioprosthesis. Additionally, 4 of the 19 had required prior coarctation repair.

Procedures

In the aortic group 7 children required only valve replacement, 16 required an aortoventriculoplasty, and 1 required a Manouguian procedure. Valves implanted ranged in size from 19 mm to 27 mm. Fifteen of the 24 valves were 21 mm or 23 mm (table 3-3).

In the mitral group 12 annular placements were carried out, but 8 children required supra-annular placement. In the annular position, 3 valves were 19 mm, 2 valves were 21 mm, and the remaining 7 were 27 mm or larger. In the supra-annular position, all valves were 19 mm (table 3-4).

Table 3-2. Diagnostic categories for mitral valve replacement

Category	No. of patients
Mitral insufficiency secondary to AV septal defect and/or repair	8
Congenital mitral stenosis	8
Isolated mitral insufficiency	4

Table 3-3. Aortic valve procedures

Type of operation performed	7 valve replacements 16 aortoventriculoplasties 1 Manouguian procedure
Number and sizes of valves placed	3–19 mm 8–21 mm 7–23 mm 5–25 mm 1–27 mm

Table 3-4. Mitral valve procedures

Type of operation performed	12 annular placements 8 supra-annular placements	
Number and sizes of valves placed	Annular	3–19 mm 2–21 mm 2–27 mm 4–29 mm 1–31 mm
	Supra-annular	8–19 mm

RESULTS

Early results

In the aortic valve group, there were 2 operative deaths. Both of these children had undergone emergency operation, and neither one was able to be weaned from bypass successfully. Preoperatively, severe myocardial dysfunction was present in both, and the deaths were unrelated to valve placement or function. One late death occurred in a child who underwent aortoventriculoplasty at age 5 months and required a second operation for residual ventricular septal defect (VSD) approximately 1 month later. The patient did well for about a year and then developed acquired immune deficiency syndrome. Death occurred secondary to fungal prosthetic valve endocarditis.

Following mitral replacement there were no early or late deaths in the annular placement group. However, there were 2 early and 5 late deaths in the supra-annular position group. In 1 of the 2 early deaths, technical problems, including partial obstruction of the left pulmonary veins secondary to the placement of the valve in a very small atrium, was responsible for the poor outcome. Four of the 5 late deaths had marked left ventricular dysfunction preoperatively that did not resolve following operation. Thrombosed valves, secondary to inadequate anticoagulation, were the primary cause of death in 2 patients.

Table 3-5. Operative complications

Placement	Complication	No. of patients
AVR	Residual VSD requiring closure	2
	Mediastinitis	1
	3° heart block	1
MVR	3° heart block	1
	Mild paravalvular leak	1

Major complications following operation are listed in table 3-5. In the aortic valve replacement group, there were 2 instances of residual VSD requiring closure, 1 case of mediastinitis treated successfully with open drainage and irrigation, and 1 episode of third-degree heart block requiring permanent pacemaker placement. The latter was the only complication in a patient with a simple valve replacement. In the mitral group, 1 patient developed a third-degree heart block, which required permanent pacemaker placement, and 1 child developed a mild paravalvular leak, which did not require further operation.

Late results

Thirty-three survivors have been followed for an average of 43 months, and all are asymptomatic. All children have been anticoagulated postoperatively, following removal of their chest tubes and toleration of an oral diet. The anticoagulation regimen primarily utilizes warfarin, often in association with sulfinpyrazone or dipyridamole. The prothrombin time is maintained in the range of 16 to 18 seconds for the aortic valve patients and in the range of 18 to 22 seconds for the mitral valve patients.

The long-term results of valve replacement and anticoagulation have been excellent. In the aortic valve group there has been only 1 episode of thromboembolism, which was transient and secondary to poor parental compliance with medications. At the time of the complication, the child's prothrombin time had returned to normal because the parents had discontinued warfarin. There have been no hemorrhagic complications.

In the mitral group when the valve was placed in the annular position, there have been no episodes of thromboembolism and no hemorrhagic complications. In the supra-annular position group, although there were no hemorrhagic complications, there were 2 thrombosed valves. Both patients were poorly anticoagulated secondary to poor parental compliance, and both of these children died.

Overall, in 123 patient-years of follow-up, there have been 3 major thromboembolic complications (2.4% per patient-year) with 2 deaths and no hemorrhagic complications.

DISCUSSION

Although the evidence is clear that use of bioprostheses in the systemic circulation of the pediatric population is contraindicated, the ideal mechanical valve has not yet been developed. Our results with the ST. JUDE MEDICAL cardiac valve prosthesis have been excellent, but there are still problems to be addressed. Significant differences in results remain between aortic valve replacement and mitral valve replacement in small children, particularly infants.

The results of aortic valve replacement in all ages have been excellent, and for this reason our group has been very aggressive in replacing aortic valves when definite, although not necessarily compelling, indications are present. Our experience in the past, when a less aggressive approach was taken, often resulted in marked left ventricular dysfunction, which did not always resolve postoperatively. Early valve replacement effectively preserves left ventricular function. Our experience includes a significant number of aortoventriculoplasties. This procedure is well tolerated, although more technically demanding, and allows the placement of an *adult*-sized valve in most children. We hope that this will prevent a series of reoperations to change the valve as the child grows and will better preserve ventricular myocardium. Follow-up is too short to establish this fact, but the experience is encouraging. No valves have required replacement so far. We, therefore, continue to enthusiastically support the use of left ventricular outflow tract enlargement.

In children who require mitral valve replacement, we have found that the position of the valve within the anulus has been critical to the outcome. If the valve was seated in the true anulus, mortality was nonexistent and morbidity was small. All children undergoing annular mitral valve replacement in this series are currently asymptomatic. The results of mitral valve replacement in the supra-annular position have been discouraging, yielding only 1 long-term survivor. Eighty percent of the children in this group had left ventricular hypoplasia with ongoing moderate-to-severe left ventricular dysfunction. For this reason, we have become much more conservative when considering mitral valve replacement in small children and infants, where a valve will likely have to be sewn into the supra-annular position. Medical management of these children should be continued until annular size is adequate (as determined by echocardiography) or it is absolutely no longer possible to control their congestive heart failure.

The issue of anticoagulation in the pediatric patient population after implantation of the ST. JUDE MEDICAL valve is complex. Sade et al. [6] have recommended no anticoagulation for several years, but their long-term follow-up results suggest higher thromboembolic rates than may be acceptable. Ebert et al. [7], have recommended that anticoagulation with antiplatelet drugs alone is adequate, at least in the aortic position. Both groups, as well as others [8], have been concerned about major hemorrhagic complications with warfarin as the main drug for anticoagulation. Our hemorrhagic complication rate is extremely low, perhaps due to the fact that we follow the children on warfarin anticoagulation very closely. Our clinical nurse specialist monitors the prothrombin time every 2 to 4 weeks. Approximately 8 to 10 hours per week are invested in following and regulating our patients' anticoagulation. The tests are performed in the outpatient laboratory by a finger prick, manual tilt-tube technique. For the children who do not live in the immediate area, our coagulation lab has been able to help local facilities establish the finger prick technique. Warfarin is usually taken with dinner or at bedtime, and the children and parents are counseled often about not participating in vigorous jumping activities or contact sports.

Perhaps the answer lies somewhere in the middle. Increasing evidence indicates that many of the thromboembolic events are primarily related to platelet deposition soon after the time of valve replacement. In high-flow positions, as with aortic valve replacement, when cardiac outputs are good, antiplatelet therapy alone may be adequate. In fact, antiplatelet agents may prove to be the therapy of choice. We have added antiplatelet therapy to many of our patients' anticoagulation routine but have not yet given up warfarin for all patients. In time, we are likely to drop the warfarin as we become more comfortable with the results of antiplatelet therapy alone.

Mitral valve replacement, however, is a different problem. In many of our patients, a low-flow state with stasis, large left atrium, non-sinus rhythm, and left ventricular dysfunction exist. In these patients we believe that both warfarin and antiplatelet drugs are essential to prevent thromboembolic events. Unfortunately, even this regimen may not be adequate long-term because of the chronic, low-flow state. Thromboembolic rates after mitral valve replacement are likely to always be higher than for aortic valve patients. It is not easy to anticoagulate children, and their prothrombin times do vary more than the adult population. In this group of patients, with mitral valve replacement and left ventricular dysfunction, even small changes in anti-coagulation can lead to progressive thrombosis of the valve. We have seen this twice without survival.

Durability of a prosthetic valve is particularly important in the pediatric population. Our short- and intermediate-term results, along with in vitro data, suggest that the ST. JUDE MEDICAL valve prosthesis will meet or exceed the durability requirements of children. However, much longer follow-up is necessary to establish this as true.

In conclusion, results with ST. JUDE MEDICAL cardiac valve replacement in children in the aortic position or in the annular mitral position have been excellent. Anticoagulation with warfarin is warranted, particularly in those patients who have mitral valve replacements or who have decreased left ventricular function. In the aortic position, anticoagulation with antiplatelet drugs alone may be adequate. Finally, morbidity and mortality are strongly related to the underlying disease (mitral annular hypoplasia or left ventricular dysfunction) rather than to valve malfunction or technical problems at operation.

REFERENCES

1. Dunn JM. Porcine valve durability in children. Ann Thorac Surg 1981; 32:357–368.
2. Walker WE, Duncan JM, Frazier OH Jr, Livesay JJ, Ott DA, Reul GJ, Cooley DA. Early experience with the Ionescu-Shiley pericardial xenograft valve. Accelerated calcification in children. J Thorac Cardiovasc Surg 1983; 86:570–575.
3. Williams DB, Danielson GK, McGoon DC, Puga FJ, Mair DD, Edwards WD. Porcine heterograft valve replacement in children. J Thorac Cardiovasc Surg 1982; 84:446–450.
4. Sanders SP, Levy RJ, Freed MD, Norwood WI, Castaneda AR. Use of Hancock porcine xenografts in children and adolescents. Am J Cardiol 1980; 46:429–438.
5. Schaffer MS, Campbell DN, Clarke DR, Wiggins JW Jr, Wolfe RR. Aortoventriculoplasty in children. J Thorac Cardiovasc Surg 1986; 92:391–395.
6. Pass HI, Sade RM, Crawford FA, Hohn AR. Cardiac valve prostheses in children without anticoagulation. J Thorac Cardiovasc Surg 1984; 87:832–835.
7. Verrier ED, Tranbaugh RF, Soifer SJ, Yee ES, Turley K, Ebert PA. Aspirin anticoagulation in children with mechanical aortic valves. J Thorac Cardiovasc Surg 1986; 92:1013–1020.
8. Bradley LM, Midgley FM, Watson DC, Getson PR, Scott LP III. Anticoagulation therapy in children with mechanical prosthetic cardiac valves. Am J Cardiol 1985; 56:533–535.

4. THROMBOEMBOLIC COMPLICATIONS IN PEDIATRIC PATIENTS UNDERGOING VALVE REPLACEMENT WITH THE ST. JUDE MEDICAL® PROSTHESIS

P. B. DEVERALL

Abstract. *Our experience over a 16-year period of valve replacements in the pediatric age group totals 61 patients. Initially, bioprosthetic valves were used, but a high incidence of early degeneration of porcine and calf pericardial valves necessitated a change. With the evolution of low-profile prosthetic valves of better hydraulic performance, early mortality and morbidity have fallen significantly. Seventeen valve replacements have been performed over the last 5 years in patients under 16 years of age. Eleven were in the mitral position, 2 in the tricuspid position, and 3 in the aortic position. Early in the series, an elective decision was made to not routinely use anticoagulants. However, 3 patients have suffered major thromboembolic complications: 1 thrombosed valve in the tricuspid position in a 7-year-old child, 1 major cerebral embolus in a 15-year-old child with a mitral prosthesis, and a thrombosed mitral prosthesis in a 2-year-old child who survived emergency reoperation. There were 2 further instances of thromboembolism in 2 other children. This experience determined a change in policy, reinstituting the use of anticoagulants.*

INTRODUCTION

Our 16-year experience with valve replacement in the pediatric age group totals 61 patients. Initially we implanted bioprostheses, but a high incidence of early degeneration of both bovine pericardial and porcine valves in this age group necessitated a change.

Over the last 5 years, we have performed 17 valve replacements in 20 patients under 16 years of age, using the ST. JUDE MEDICAL® prosthetic heart valve. Three implants were in the aortic position, 11 in the mitral, and 2 in the tricuspid.

COMPLICATIONS

Early in the series, we elected to not routinely use anticoagulants with these patients. However, 4 patients experienced valve thrombosis (1 death), and 1 suffered a major thromboembolic complication (table 4-1).

A 13-year-old female with Epstein's anamoly had acute thrombosis of the tricuspid valve 8 months after insertion. She had been placed on PERSAN-TINE® and aspirin because she had concomitant mild liver dysfunction. She did very well, but she had an enlarged heart and poor cardiac output. She died suddenly, at home, in the eighth postoperative month. Autopsy revealed complete thrombosis of the ST. JUDE MEDICAL valve.

Another patient, age 9, received double valve replacement for rheumatic aortic and mitral valve disease. This child was not taking medication as prescribed, and his mitral valve occluded 7 months after insertion. He survived emergency reoperation.

Two other incidents occurred: The tricuspid valve of a 7-year-old child thrombosed, and a 2-year-old survived emergency reoperation for a thrombosed mitral prosthesis.

A 15-year-old boy on PERSANTINE and aspirin had an acute thromboembolic episode, which was permanent (left hemiplegia), 4 years after operation. The incident followed a sporting event at school in which he was participating. The boy had a feverish illness associated with gastroenteritis, which often upsets the control of anticoagulants, resulting in thrombogenesis.

It has been shown in our pediatric experience that, perhaps, those patients with instability of rhythm and fluid balance or inadequate cardiac performance and flow are most at risk for thromboembolic events and should be placed on anticoagulants, even though they are active.

In our series, there was also 1 episode of severe intravascular hemolytic anemia associated with paravalvular leak.

Table 4-1. Complications following St. Jude Medical valve replacement in patients without anticoagulation

Complication	Incidents	Position	Age	Results
Thrombosis	1	Tricuspid	13	Death
Thrombosis	1	Mitral	9	Reoperation
Thrombosis	1	Tricuspid	7	Death
Thrombosis	1	Mitral	2	Reoperation
Major thromboembolism	1	Mitral	15	Permanent left hemiplegia

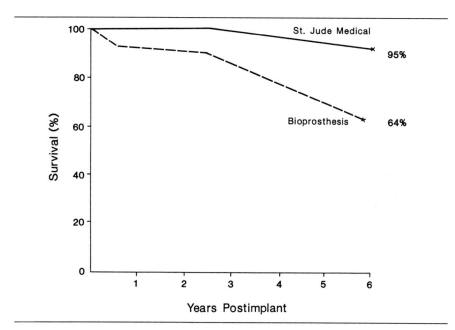

Figure 4-1. Actuarial probability of survival following prosthetic valve replacement in children with St. Jude Medical or bioprosthetic valves.

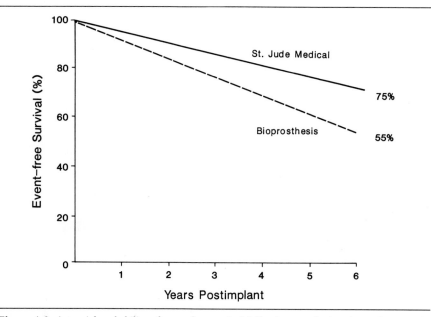

Figure 4-2. Actuarial probability of event-free survival following prosthetic valve replacement in children with St. Jude Medical or bioprosthetic valves.

SURVIVAL

Actuarial probability of survival following implantation with the ST. JUDE MEDICAL valve in children is shown in figure 4-1. There was no operative mortality in this series. With 1 death, survival at 6 years is 95%. The dotted line represents a similar, earlier series when we implanted bioprostheses. The 75% actuarial probability of event-free survival in figure 4-2 reflects the 4 incidents of major thromboembolism in our group of 20 patients. In our earlier series with bioprostheses, 55% were event-free at 6 years.

CONCLUSION

The ST. JUDE MEDICAL heart valve is our current choice for valve substitution. The valve design contributes to a low operative mortality. The probability of event-free survival at 5 years is greater than that for tissue valves, but thromboembolic complications remain a hazard.

5. LONG-TERM RESULTS OF VALVULAR REPLACEMENT IN PEDIATRIC PATIENTS

I. REYES, A. JUFFE, G. PRADAS, R. BURGOS, L. PULPÓN, G. TELLEZ,
R. VARGAS, D. FIGUERA

Abstract. This study presents the long-term results of 52 children who had 52 valvular substitutions between 1971 and 1984. Ages were between 5 and 16 years (mean 10.7 years) with 22 females and 30 males. The etiology was congenital in 35% and rheumatic in 65% of these cases. Eighteen patients underwent aortic valve replacement, 23 underwent mitral valve replacement, 10 patients had double valve replacement (aortic and mitral), and 1 patient had tricuspid valve replacement. Thirty-two BJÖRK-SHILEY®, 7 ST. JUDE MEDICAL®, 7 HANCOCK®, and 6 dura mater valves were used. Hospital mortality due to elective surgery was 6.6%. Six patients required reoperation. The actuarial survival rate after 8 years of follow-up was 77.3%. All patients are postoperatively in New York Heart Association (NYHA) Functional Class I except 1 patient who is in Class II. No thromboembolic complications have appeared. After 8 years, 90.2% of the patients are free of complications due to anticoagulants. There are no significant differences in survival between biological and mechanical prostheses. We conclude that valvular replacement in children does not offer greater risks or complications than in adults. Owing to accelerated deterioration of biological prostheses in this type of patient and the few complications related to anticoagulation we have found, we think that replacement with mechanical prostheses is appropriate in children, except when anticoagulation is contraindicated.

INTRODUCTION

For the purpose of observing the results of valve replacement in children and comparing the complications with respect to those occurring in adults, we have analyzed the experience in Clínica Puerta de Hierro from 1971 to 1984.

PATIENTS AND METHODS

Between 1971 and 1984, 52 children underwent valve replacement; 22 were female, 30 were male. Ages were 5 to 16 years (mean 10.7 years). Thirty-five percent of the lesions were congenital and 65% rheumatic.

The degree of preoperative cardiac insufficiency according to the Classification of the New York Heart Association (NYHA) was: Class I (subjects with associated congenital cardiopathy) in 5 cases; Class II in 8 cases; Class III in 34 cases; and Class IV in 5 cases. Nineteen patients presented with associated pathologies, which constituted the principal disorder in 5 of them (table 5-1). The preoperative cardiothoracic index was Grade III (0.55–0.65) in 32 patients and Grade IV in 9 cases (table 5-2).

Prior surgery had been performed on 5 subjects: 2 resections of aortic coarctation, 1 mitral and aortic STARR-EDWARDS® implant, 1 ductus closure, and, in the remaining patient, aortic commissurotomy.

The interventions were carried out by median sternotomy and cannulation of ascending aorta and both venae cavae. Other features were hypothermia of 20–28°C, continuous perfusion with cold pericardial fluid, and, beginning in 1978, cardioplegia. From 1980 onward, myocardial temperature has also been monitored to maintain it below 15°C.

Table 5-1. Associated congenital pathology

	No. of patients
Coarctation of aorta	5
Intraventricular communication	3
Intraventricular communication + aortic insufficiency	2
Mitral insufficiency (degenerative)	2
Intra-atrial communication	2
Subaortic stenosis	2
CIA + CIV	1
Ductus	1
Fallot Tetralogy	1

CIA = ASD, atrial septal defect; CIV = VSD, ventricular septal defect

Table 5-2. Preoperative cardiothoracic index

		No. of patients	Percent
Grade I	> 0.45	0	
Grade II	0.45–0.55	11	21.2
Grade III	0.55–0.65	32	61.5
Grade IV	< 0.65	9	17.3

The aortic valve was replaced in 18 patients using 10 BJÖRK-SHILEY, 3 ST. JUDE MEDICAL, 3 HANCOCK and 2 dura mater valves (table 5-3). The mitral valve was replaced in 23 cases with 14 BJÖRK-SHILEY, 3 ST. JUDE MEDICAL, 2 HANCOCK, and 4 dura mater valves. In 10 subjects, both mitral and aortic valves were substituted: 8 patients with BJÖRK-SHILEY prostheses and 1 case in which both were HANCOCK valves. The remaining patient received a BJÖRK-SHILEY aortic prosthesis and a HANCOCK mitral prosthesis. In 1 patient, the tricuspid valve was replaced with a ST. JUDE MEDICAL prosthesis. The types and sizes of implants can be seen in tables 5-3 and 5-4.

RESULTS

Clinical mortality was 15.4%, including 3 patients operated on under emergency conditions, 1 with a severe degree of mitral insufficiency with marked deterioration of ventricular function, another with bacterial endocarditis, and the third upon cardiac arrest. Elective surgery resulted in a mortality of 6.6%. The causes of death are shown in table 5-5.

The immediate postoperative complications were respiratory insufficiency requiring tracheotomy in 2 cases and 1 case each of left hemiplegia and atrial flutter requiring electric cardioversion.

Six patients were subjected to reoperation: 2 HANCOCK prostheses presenting calcifications 5 and 6 years after implantation, respectively; 1 case of paravalvular leakage in a BJÖRK-SHILEY valve after 2 years; and 3 dura mater valves removed 5, 6, and 7 years after implantation, respectively. The complications produced by anticoagulants were: 1 case of hemarthrosis, 1 late

Table 5-3. Type of prosthesis implanted

	Aortic	Mitral	Mitral/Aortic	Tricuspid	Total
Björk-Shiley	10	14	8	–	32
St. Jude Medical	3	3	–	1	7
Hancock	3	2	2	–	7
Dura mater	2	4	–	–	6
				1	
Total	18	23	10		52

Table 5-4. Size of prosthesis implanted

	Size							
	19	21	23	25	27	29	31	Mean
Aortic	2	6	13	6	1	–	–	22.8
Mitral	–	–	1	9	12	10	1	27.0
Tricuspid	–	–	–	–	1	–	–	

Table 5-5. Hospital mortality

	No. of patients
Postoperative low output	3
Endocarditis (1 preoperative)	2
Respiratory insufficiency	1
Hypokalemia; cardiac arrest	1
Post-extracorporeal circulation neurological damage	1
Total	8 (15.4%)

Table 5-6. Complications secondary to anticoagulants

No. of patients	34
Interval	12 years
Mean	8.02 years/patient
Total	34 × 8.02 = 273 years/patient

	Number	Probability. %. year
Hemorrhage	3	3/273.100 = 1.1
Embolism	1	1/273.100 = 0.37
Thrombosis	0	
Total	4	4/273.100 = 1.46

death due to brain hemorrhage, 1 case of severe epistaxis (occluded), and 1 episode of systemic embolism. Considering the 34 survivals, the probability of these complications is 1.46% per year (273 years per patient) (table 5-6). After 8 years, 90.2% of the patients were free of complications due to anticoagulants (figure 5-1).

Actuarial survival of the patients after leaving the hospital was 77.3% at 8 years (figures 5-2 and 5-3). Mortality occurred fundamentally in the first year postsurgery. There are no significant differences in survival between biological and mechanical prostheses. The Kaplan-Meier analysis was used [1].

The postoperative functional class was excellent (NYHA Class I) except in 1 case in which it was Class II.

DISCUSSION

In spite of the fact that conservative methods are preferred in the treatment of cardiac valve disease, rheumatic heart disease produces irreversible valve damage. For this reason, together with the malposition of the subvalvular apparatus for the mitral valve (frequent in congenital cardiopathies), valve replacement with a prosthesis is the only therapeutic alternative.

Surgery is postponed for various factors in valve replacement in children.

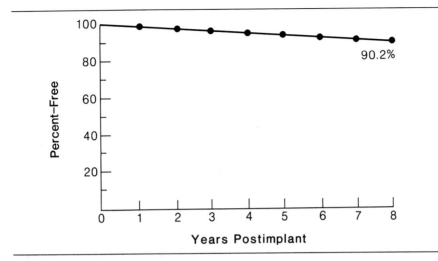

Figure 5-1. Percentage of patients free of complications due to anticoagulants.

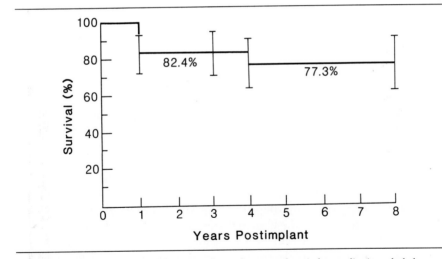

Figure 5-2. Actuarial survival following valve replacement; hospital mortality is excluded.

These include: 1) incidence of thromboembolic complications and the need for anticoagulants for the rest of life; 2) incidence of endocarditis; 3) reintervention due to valve failure, dysfunction, and durability of the biological prostheses; 4) problems caused by repeated medical controls; 5) future pregnancy; 6) implant of prosthesis of a fixed size in a child still developing; 7) changing anticoagulant doses due to growth; 8) possibility of frequent traumatisms; and

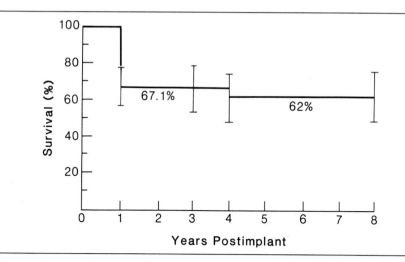

Figure 5-3. Actuarial survival following valve replacement; hospital mortality is included.

9) psychological trauma resulting from the different examinations necessary for control.

The valve therapy must be conservative, with realization of aortic and mitral commissurotomy or valvuloplasty over atrioventricular valves.

The surgical decision in patients with severe mitral or aortic valvulopathy is based on the presence of: 1) NYHA Functional Class III or IV; 2) resting trans-aortic gradient of more than 60 mm Hg; 3) left heart insufficiency crises; 4) progression of cardiomegaly or cardiothoracic index greater than 60%, 5) pulmonary hypertension of more than 50 mm Hg; 6) telediastolic elevation of the left or right ventricle or both; 7) resting venocapillary hypertension of more than 20 mm Hg; 8) episodes of congestive cardiac insufficiency of difficult control; and 9) angiographic evidence of severe mitral or aortic insufficiency with deterioration of ventricular function in asymptomatic patients.

The greater incidence of rheumatic valve disorder found in our series coincides with the experience of groups in Latin America, Africa, and Israel [2, 3] but disagrees with series in the United States [4, 5], in which the most frequent etiology of prosthetic replacement is congenital.

With respect to valve replacement in growing children and the need for future prosthetic valve substitution, we should take into account the following: Friedberg [6] considers that an aortic area of 1 cm^2 and a mitral area of 1.5 cm^2 should not produce significant obstruction in an adult; the aortic ring normally continues to grow until 20 years of age; at 15 years, its size is 16–18 mm [7, 8].

We know from catheterization data that a size 19 mm tissue anulus BJÖRK-SHILEY or ST. JUDE MEDICAL aortic prosthesis is hemodynamically satisfactory (although this depends on the patient's body surface). On the other hand, children who require valve replacement due to rheumatic heart disease or Marfan's syndrome frequently present insufficiency with anulus dilation. In our experience, the size of the prostheses utilized does not differ from that of adults (table 5-4) [9, 10]. We have established the normal relationship between the body surface and the anulus size in our patients (table 5-7) and, although the theoretical size is small, because of cardiac dilation it is always possible to implant an adult-size prosthesis.

Generally in aortic stenosis in children, the treatment of choice is commissurotomy. Patients with bicuspid aortic valves and severe aortic stenosis occasionally present slight or null commissural fusion; the orifice is anatomically adequate but functionally obstructive. In these cases aortic replacement is mandatory, given that commissurotomy does not solve the problem [11].

In a review of 424 children in whom aortic commissurotomy was performed, 60% of the late deaths were due to stenosis, and all patients who developed severe aortic insufficiency after commissurotomy expired within the first year [11].

When the type of prosthesis to be employed is smaller than a 19 mm prosthesis, it is advisable to widen the patient's tissue anulus. We prefer widening towards the noncoronary sinus and reconstruction with precoagulated DACRON® of a width varying between 1.5 cm and 3 cm.

W. G. Williams [12] widened the ring in 36% of the children requiring prostheses. We reserve the Konno aortoplasty for cases in which extreme hypoplasia of the aorta and/or the outflow point of the left ventricle exists, given the high index of surgical mortality [13].

At the level of the tricuspid valve, we have performed valvular substitution in only 1 case; in 2 cases a de Vega annuloplasty was carried out in association with mitral replacement.

Table 5-7. Theoretical and actual valve sizes with respect to body surface

	Mean	Maximum	Minimum
Body surface (m²)	1.10 ± 0.33	1.43 m²	0.77 m²

Theoretical Anulus Size		
Body surface (m²)	Mitral (mm)	Aortic (mm)
0.80	18.8	13.0
1.40	22.3	15.5

Mean Size of Prosthesis Employed	
Mitral (mm)	Aortic (mm)
27.1	22.8

With respect to thromboembolic and hemorrhagic complications and mortality, the incidences are similar to those in adults [14–18].

The probability of valvular dysfunction in mechanical prostheses is low; this is not the case with biological prostheses. With respect to porcine prostheses, numerous authors [19–23] report early and rapid deterioration toward valve degeneration and calcification, an initial symptom being severe venocapillary hypertension [14]. It is important to stress that onset of dysfunction is frequently brusque and the need for valve replacement may require emergency surgery. Absence of auscultatory evidence is frequent [23]. Echocardiography may be useful in early diagnosis, prior to appearance of symptoms.

For all these reasons, we feel that the porcine or pericardial prosthesis should not be employed in valve replacement in children. Although follow-up of the dura mater prosthesis has been shorter, and our experience is limited, it is reasonable to expect similar complications.

The causes invoked as favoring dysfunction of biological prostheses are: 1) continuous change in the calcium metabolism; 2) acceleration of valve "rejection" in growing children; 3) utilization of small valves producing increased fatigue, transvalvular gradients, and greater turbulence; and 4) incremental traumatism at the valvular level due to greater heart rate. Gardner [15] finds a dysfunction in 37% of biological valves followed for 6 years.

Our clinical mortality in elective surgery was 6.6%. That found in the literature varies between 0% and 33% [12, 16–18, 24–31]. Williams and Freed [12, 17] report lower mortality in aortic replacement than in mitral procedures. We found no significant difference in mortality between biological and mechanical prostheses, depending on the etiology. Gardner [15] reports greater mortality in valve replacement in congenital cardiopathies.

The causes that most frequently motivate reoperation in childhood are: 1) dysfunction due to valve deterioration (the most frequent); 2) endocarditis; 3) paravalvular leak; 4) tissue overgrowth and subsequent prosthetic obstruction; and 5) undersized prosthesis with respect to the growth of the child (rare). Williams [12] subjected 21 out of 92 patients to reoperation (33%); the size of the valve employed in the second operation was 2 mm to 6 mm larger than in the first.

The number of reinterventions owing to tissue overgrowth, which frequently obstructs the subvalvular area, seems to be greater in children than in adults [12, 15].

Actuarial survival in our series, 8 years after replacement, was 77.3%. Mata [24] reports 92.7% survival at 8 years.

Improvement is not limited only to the NYHA Functional Class (Class I in the majority of cases) but is reflected in the decrease of ventricular growth potential as shown by electrocardiograms and in reduction of cardiomegaly as observed radiologically. Patients with atrial fibrillation frequently revert to sinus rhythm after surgery, with quinidine or cardioversion [30].

One question to keep in mind is the recurrence of rheumatic fever. Mendoza

[32] reports that 70% to 85% of the school-age patients suffer relapses in the first 3 years and 10% in the following 2 years. Duplessis [33], in a series of 34 children with mitral valve replacement followed for 8 years, discovered 8 episodes, 1 of them fatal. This data justifies the use of prophylaxis with benzyl-penicillin to diminish the incidence of recurrence [24].

With respect to the selection of the prosthesis to be used, we should take into account the following: It is a well-known fact that biological prostheses have a greater incidence of calcification and that small sizes, especially in porcine pros-theses, are obstructive. On the other hand, BJÖRK-SHILEY and, especially, ST. JUDE MEDICAL valves present acceptable gradients in the smaller sizes [15]. On the other hand, because of cardiomegaly, children can receive pros-theses of greater size than that which would correspond to their body surface, rendering unnecessary future valve replacement due to patient growth.

In children under age 4, the use of biological prostheses is advisable, given the difficulties arising from anticoagulant control produced by growth and the psychological trauma derived from the frequent controls necessary for their proper anticoagulation.

In adolescent women, implantation of biological prostheses is preferable since there is less valvular degeneration at that age and, in case of pregnancy, the complications for mother and child are greater in anticoagulated patients [34, 35].

In view of our results, we feel that valvular substitution with the mechanical prosthesis is the most advisable, with the exception of children under age 4, adolescent women, and those patients in whom adequate anticoagulation is not possible. In these cases, we recommend the utilization of biological pros-theses made of pericardium and similar substances.

REFERENCES

1. Kaplan EL, Meier P. Nonparametric estimation from incomplete observations. Am Stat Assoc J 1958; 53:457–481.
2. Pérez-Alvarez JJ, Pérez Traviño C, Reta C, Jiménez A, Cuellar ML. Valvular prosthesis in children. Surgery 1969; 65:688.
3. Van Der Horst RL, Leroux BT, Rogers NMA, Gotsman MS. Mitral valve replacement in childhood. A report of 51 patients. Am Heart J 1973; 85:624.
4. Mathews RA, Zuberbuhler SC, Bahnson HT. Valve replacement in children and adolescents. J Thorac Cardiovasc Surg 1977; 73:872.
5. Smith JM, Cooley DA, Ott DA, Ferreira W, Reul GJ. Aortic valve replacement in preteenage children. Ann Thorac Surg 1980; 29:512.
6. Friedberg CK. Disease of the Heart. WB Saunders, Philadelphia 1966; p 1033.
7. Braunwald NS, Brais M, Castañeda A. Considerations in the development of artificial heart valve substitutes for use in infants and small children. J Thorac Cardiovasc Surg 1976; 72:539.
8. Rowlatt VF, Rimoldi HJA, Lev M. The quantitative anatomy of the normal child's heart. Pediat Clin North Am 1963; 10:499.
9. Figuera D, Zavanella C, Rufilanchas JJ, Téllez G, Agosti J. Heart valve replacement in children with the Björk-Shiley prosthesis. J Cardiovasc Surg 1974; 15:510.
10. Rufilanchas JJ, Juffe A, Miranda AL, Téllez G, Agosti J, Maroñas JM, Figuera D. Cardiac valve replacement with the Björk-Shiley prosthesis in young patients. Scand J Thorac Cardiovasc Surg 1977; 11:11.
11. Wittig J, McConnell D, Buckberg G, Mulder D. Aortic valve replacement in the young child.

Ann Thorac Surg 1975; 19:40.

12. Williams WG, Pollock JC, Geiss OM, Trusler GA, Fowler RS. Experience with aortic and mitral valve replacement in children. J Thorac Cardiovasc Surg 1981; 81:326.

13. Konno S, Imai Y, Iida Y, Nakasima M, Tatsuno K. A new method for prosthetic valve replacement in congenital aortic stenosis associated with hypoplasia of the aorta valve ring. J Thorac Cardiovasc Surg 1976; 70:909.

14. Attie F, Kuri J, Zanoniani C, Rentería V, Martínez Ríos MA. Mitral valve replacement in children with rheumatic heart disease. Circulation 1981; 64:812.

15. Gardner TJ, Roland JMA, Neill CN, Donahoo JS. Valve replacement in children; A fifteen-year perspective. J Thorac Cardiovasc Surg 1982; 83:178.

16. Stansel HC, Nudel DB, Berman MA, Talner NS. Prosthetic valve replacement in children. Arch of Surg 1975; 110:1397.

17. Freed MD, Bernhard WF. Prosthetic valve replacement in children. Prog Cardiovasc Dis 1975; 17:475.

18. Wada J, Yokoyama M, Hashimoto A, Imai Y, Kitamura N, Takao A, Momma K. Long-term follow-up of artificial valves in patients under 15 years old. Ann Thorac Surg 1980; 29:519.

19. Geha AS, Laks H, Stansel HC, Cornhill JF, Buckley MJ, Roberts WC. Late failure of porcine valve heterografts in children. J Thorac Cardiovasc Surg 1979; 78:351.

20. Kutsche LM, Oyer P, Shumway N, Baum D. An important complication of Hancock mitral valve replacement in children. Circulation 1979; 60(I):98.

21. Sanders SP, Levy RI, Freed MD, Norwood WI, Castañeda AR. Use of Hancock porcine xenografts in children and adolescents. Am J Cardiol 1980; 46:429.

22. Silver MM, Pollock J, Silver MD, Williams WG, Trusler GA. Calcification in porcine xenograft valves in children. Am J Cardiol 1980; 45:685.

23. Thandroyen FT, Whitton IN, Pirie D, Rogers MA, Mitha AS. Severe calcification of glutaraldehyde-preserved porcine xenografts in children. Am J Cardiol 1980; 45:690.

24. Mata LA, Carrillo F, Kuri J, Attie F, Baz R, Pliego J, Sandoval M, Martínez Ríos MA. Reemplazo valvular mitral en niños y adolescentes. Arch Inst Cardiol Mex 1975; 45:203.

25. John S, Munsi S, Cherian G. Mitral valve replacement in children and adolescents with rheumatic heart disease. Jpn Heart Journal 1976; 17:570.

26. Sade RM, Ballenger JF, Horn AR, Riopel DA, Taylor AB. Cardiac valve replacement in children. Comparison of tissue with mechanical prostheses. J Thorac Cardiovasc Surg 1979; 78:123.

27. Nonoyama A, Masuda A, Kasahara K, Kotani S, Katsuda H, Nakahashi M. The use of the Björk-Shiley prosthetic valve in children under 10 years of age. Jpn Circ J 1977; 41:401.

28. Nudelman I, Schachner A, Levy MJ. Repeated mitral valve replacement in the growing child with congenital mitral valve disease. J Thorac Cardiovasc Surg 1980; 79:765.

29. Geha AS. Valve replacement in children. Ann Thorac Surg 1980; 29:500.

30. Gotsman MS, Van Der Horst RL. Surgical management of severe mitral valve disease in childhood. Am Heart J 1975; 90:685.

31. Chen SC, Laks H, Fagan L, Terschluse D, Kaiser G, Barner H, William VL. Valve replacement in children. Circulation 1977; 56(II):117.

32. Mendoza F. Fiebre reumática. Su naturaleza. Boletín Médico, Instituto Médico, Seguridad Social (México) 1959; 1:61.

33. Duplessis LD, Chester E. Surgery for severe mitral regurgitation in children. J Thorac Cardiovasc Surg 1969; 58:730.

34. Beadle EM, Leupker RV, Williams PP. Pregnancy in a patient with porcine valve xenografts. Am Heart J 1979; 98:510.

35. Russo R, Bortolotti V, Shivazappa L, Girolami A. Warfarin treatment during pregnancy. A clinical note. Hemostatis 1979; 8:96.

6. PERFORMANCE OF MECHANICAL VALVES IN PEDIATRIC PATIENTS

A. WESSELS, M. ANTUNES

Abstract. Mechanical cardiac valve replacement was performed in 182 patients, age 15 years and younger, from May 1980 to July 1985. All patients belonged to a relatively underdeveloped population group. Twelve patients (6.5%) died in the perioperative period. One hundred forty-seven patients were followed up for 604 patient-years. There were 26 late deaths, of which 5 were known to be valve-related, 7 cardiac non-valve-related, 1 noncardiac, and 12 unknown. The linearized incidences for valve-related complications were: valve failure (valve-related mortality and reoperation) 4.3% per patient-year; thromboembolism 1.7% per patient-year; thrombotic obstruction 1.7% per patient-year; bacterial endocarditis 1.3% per patient-year; bland paravalvular leak 0.8% per patient-year; and anticoagulant-related hemorrhage 0.3% per patient-year. In actuarial analysis, 96% of patients were free of valve-related mortality at 5 years. The corresponding figures were: freedom from valve failure 80%; thrombotic obstruction 91%; thromboembolism 81%; and reoperations 84%. The performance of mechanical valves in children was superior to that of tissue valves but similar to that in adults. Therefore, we believe that mechanical prostheses should be used in these patients whenever the natural valves cannot be preserved.

INTRODUCTION

Mechanical cardiac valve replacement was performed in 182 patients, age 15 years and younger, from May 1980 to July 1985. All patients belonged to a relatively underdeveloped population group.

The indications for surgery were acute rheumatic carditis, chronic rheumatic carditis, and infective endocarditis in patients who had significant hemodynamic lesions. In some of the severe cases of acute rheumatic carditis, we observed a very thickened pericardium and markedly edematous epicardium. Areas of calcification in the anterior mitral leaflet were observed in cases of chronic rheumatic carditis.

PATIENTS AND METHODS

In 147 patients, there were 99 mitral valve replacements, 22 aortic valve replacements, and 59 double valve replacements. Both ST. JUDE MEDICAL® and MEDTRONIC-HALL™ valves were used in these patients. Twelve patients (6.5%) died in the perioperative period; 1 death was valve-related. All patients were maintained on anticoagulants and follow-up extended to 604 patient-years.

RESULTS

There were 26 late deaths, of which 5 were valve-related. The remainder included 7 cardiac non-valve-related deaths, 1 noncardiac death, and 13 deaths due to unknown causes.

The linearized incidence of valve-related failure (valve-related mortality and reoperation) was 4.3% per patient-year; thromboembolism was 1.7% per patient-year; thrombotic obstruction was also 1.7% per patient-year. The remaining complications included bacterial endocarditis of 1.3% per patient-year, bland paravalvular leak of 0.8% per patient-year, and anticoagulant-related hemorrhage of 0.3% per patient-year.

In actuarial analysis, 96% of our patients were free of valve-related mortality at 5 years. Correspondingly, freedom from valve failure was 80%; thrombotic obstruction, 91%; thromboembolism, 81%; and reoperation, 84%.

In conclusion, we believe that mechanical valve performance is superior to that of tissue valves. The protocol in our unit is that where we cannot preserve the natural valve, mechanical valve replacements are performed in children.

PART I. DISCUSSION

A. MICHAEL BORKON, MODERATOR

AORTOVENTRICULOPLASTY

E. RAINER DE VIVIE: The three indications for aortoventriculoplasty are: 1) multi-level stenosis in the subvalvular and supravalvular regions in patients who were previously operated on; 2) the outgrown prosthesis; and 3) rare cases of HOCM reoperations. Dr. Campbell mentioned he uses the double patch technique to prevent bleeding problems. Since we began using fibrin glue with approximately 81 patients, we have not had any bleeding problems. Dr. Campbell, up to what size have you been able to enlarge the anulus using the Manouguian technique? And, what was the function of the mitral valve after this procedure?

DAVID CAMPBELL: In regard to our aortoventriculoplasties, I discussed our two major indications. In subaortic tunnel obstruction, many of the patients had undergone previous multiple operations at different levels. The child with the complex left ventricular outflow tract obstruction is representative of the children we treat. Most have multi-level disease; it's very rare for us to find just one level. For older children who did not require early operations, we were able to do only a valve replacement. The Manouguian procedure was done earlier in our practice, before we ever started doing aortoventriculoplasties, and we abandoned that as well. From what we can tell, the mitral valve after the Manouguian procedure functions fairly well; we have not had a problem with it. We have done the procedure in older patients, where we have not used aortoventriculoplasty as much. We have tried aortoventriculoplasty, but it seems to work better for children than for adults.

TRICUSPID VALVE REPLACEMENT

THOMAS SPRAY: I think there's general agreement that for left-sided AV valve replacement in children with a ST. JUDE MEDICAL mechanical prosthesis, or something similar, is the prosthesis of choice except for, perhaps, homografts in the aortic and pulmonary positions. But I think there still is a great collection of opinion regarding isolated tricuspid valve replacement. None of the series presented today, nor any other major series, talks about isolated tricuspid valve replacement because the number of implants is very small. My patients with a mechanical valve in the tricuspid position have had anticoagulant-related hemorrhage or early thrombosis. Because evidence suggests tissue valves do not degenerate quite as rapidly in the tricuspid position, do the panelists think there is any reason to continue to use a mechanical prosthesis in the tricuspid position?

ANDRE WESSELS: We do not use mechanical valves in the tricuspid position at all. If possible, we will repair the tricuspid valve; failing that, we will replace the tricuspid valve with a tissue prosthesis.

ROBERT SADE: Some surgeons use a tissue prosthesis in the tricuspid position because thrombosis is common in that position. There is also evidence that tissue valves last longer there than they do in the left side of the heart, however I am not sure that is true. We have a small experience, perhaps 5 or 6 patients, with tricuspid valves. I have had to replace one of these tissue valves because of calcification after only 2 years of implantation. So I am not sure that the durability question is really settled. However, the use of streptokinase to treat thrombosis pushes me toward using mechanical valves and not having to worry about calcification and reoperation to replace valves. Thromboembolism, of course, in the tricuspid position is not as big a problem as it is in the mitral or aortic position. Any small thromboemboli will be trapped by the lung and disappear after a short period of time without producing strokes. Thrombosis, on the other hand, does produce valve malfunction. Treated with streptokinase, the clots have been shown to dissolve and completely free the tricuspid valve. We treated one patient this way who responded very well. Other surgeons have reported great success with larger series using streptokinase to treat thrombosis of mechanical valves.

So, I am not as worried as I used to be about malfunction of mechanical valves on the right side of the heart and, although I would prefer to use a tissue valve, I do not hesitate to use a mechanical valve, if needed. Last week, for example, I removed a tricuspid valve from a child who had septic thrombi from an infected aneurysm of the ventricular-septal defect that also totally destroyed her tricuspid valve. I excised her tricuspid valve, closed her ventricular-septal defect, and replaced her tricuspid valve because she had pulmonary-vascular disease, that is, thromboemboli in her pulmonary circulation. Because she was only 3 months old I chose a ST. JUDE MEDICAL valve. I expect that she will eventually need to have that valve replaced because of size. I think that the mechanical valve is going to remain a fairly good option because of the development of streptokinase to treat thrombosis.

PHILIP B. DEVERALL: Just a month ago, I spent 10 days visiting and operating with surgeons in India. For a variety of reasons, mostly economic, these doctors largely use tissue valves. They have been particularly interested in the use of the pericardial valve in both the left and right atrioventricular valve positions and have had a very high incidence of endocarditis affecting the pericardial valve in the right atrioventricular position. I think the specific Achilles heel with the pericardial valve, of course, is that one side of the pericardium is very smooth.

DIEGO FIGUERA: We have had experience with the de Vega annuloplasty for the tricuspid valve in adults and, in 2 cases, in children. In only 1 case was it necessary to remove the tricuspid valve and use a ST. JUDE MEDICAL prosthesis.

ANTICOAGULATION

RICHARD WESTERMAN: Could we quickly poll the panel with regard to their use of anticoagulants? Do they use warfarin alone, antiplatelet agents alone, or both together? Also, do they feel that their choice is adequate for all mechanical prosthetic valves, or do they vary the choice according to the type of mechanical prosthesis?

ROBERT SADE: We use the ST. JUDE MEDICAL valve as the valve of choice for the left side of the heart in children, and we are randomizing PERSANTINE® and aspirin COUMADIN®. We'll know the results of that experience in another 2 or 3 years.

PHILIP B. DEVERALL: We use a combination of warfarin and PERSANTINE. Our dosage of PERSANTINE is 100 mg 3 times a day, and when using warfarin we try to keep the prothrombin index between 35% and 50%.

ROBERT SADE: We use COUMADIN to keep the prothrombin time about 1.5 times control, whether the valve is in the mitral or the aortic position. We use a dosage of 5 mg per kilogram of PERSANTINE 3 times a day and aspirin in a very small dose, one baby aspirin or one adult-size aspirin, depending on the child, per day.

HUGH O'KANE[?]: We use the International Normalized Ratio (INR) and keep the control figure between 2 and 4 using sodium warfarin. In the first 6 months we also add 50 to 100 mg of PERSANTINE per day. After that, the child continues indefinitely on the warfarin alone with the INR kept between 2 and 4.

QUESTION: Dr. O'Kane, could you explain the pregnancy case you mentioned?

HUGH O'KANE: Our cardiologists usually switch pregnant patients from oral anticoagulants, such as warfarin, to heparin because of the chance of COUMADIN crossing the placental barrier. However, you have to weigh the risk of valve thrombosis against the risk of damage to the fetus. We are now switching back to keeping on oral anticoagulants the prosthetic valve patients who become pregnant. Of course, females considering bearing children would be candidates for using a biological valve.

DAVID CAMPBELL: In Denver we are changing our philosophy. We used to give COUMADIN to all children with any kind of valve replacement. Midway into the series, we added either PERSANTINE or sulfinpyrazone. We now feel that children who have ventricular dysfunction or other evidence of low flow, particularly in the mitral position, need to be anticoagulated with COUMADIN. We maintain the prothrombin times in the range of about 22 seconds. Even in these children, we're probably going to see thromboembolic events and thrombosed valves, because anticoagulants, even when taken with antiplatelet drugs, will not prevent thromboembolism in that group. Many other series have shown the same thing, that it has more to do with the function of the ventricle than it does with the valve and that there is no way to completely anticoagulate those children. In aortic valve replacement we still use COUMADIN, but we are backing away from that. Just as the San Francisco group has shown, antiplatelet agents alone are probably adequate because the high flow keeps those valves fairly free of thrombosis.

QUESTION: Dr. Sade, do you have any comments on that or whether, by your experience, anticoagulation is not indicated now in the aortic position in children?

ROBERT SADE: In the 7 episodes of thrombosis and thromboembolism (4 aortic and 3 mitral) in our series, none of these patients were anticoagulated. I think all patients, regardless of the position of the valve, should be treated with anticoagulants or antiplatelet drugs. Because of our experience, we recommend using anticoagulants or antiplatelet agents and use either COUMADIN or aspirin and PERSANTINE.

DAVID CAMPBELL: There is a difference in the way these agents act. Antiplatelet agents have a different job than does sodium warfarin, and, in the aortic position, antiplatelet drugs are generally adequate. We don't use antiplatelet drugs alone, but there are several good examples in the literature that support its sole use. In our series, the evidence against COUMADIN is very low, because our hemorrhagic complications are almost nonexistent. However, that's not true of other series. In each institution it depends on how easily the prothrombin times in the children can be monitored. For a group of patients who are less compliant or more difficult to manage, the use of an antiplatelet agent would be more favorable than COUMADIN. Still, it sounds like your study is going to show something, Dr. Sade. I hope so.

PHILIP B. DEVERALL: I don't think we ought to start separating children and adults, because there are few biological differences. The Brompton Hospital in London has had a dramatic experience trying to dispense with the use of anticoagulants. I think their experience is very important and it's good solid data. I believe that Stuart Lennox of Brompton is in the audience. Perhaps we can persuade him to say a word about what happened.

STUART LENNOX: I'm a little worried about the comments I have heard about anticoagulants. First of all, it's very important that we know what we mean by anticoagulants. We use the International Normalized Ratio as Hugh O'Kane does. The incidence of emboli relates to the INR number. We use an INR of 3.5. This is considerably higher than the 1.5 times ratio reported today, which is unacceptable. Also a patient in sinus rhythm with a small heart will have a lower incidence of thromboembolism than a patient with a large heart in atrial fibrillation. We cannot draw conclusions from small patient cohorts with a low incidence of thromboembolism. In our study we compared TE rates in patients having mitral valve repair with those having mitral valve replacement. Our overall incidence of thromboembolism in the replacement group was only 4 of 117 patients over 17 years. The rate is low because they had good hearts in sinus rhythm. The incidence of thromboembolism in a group with chronic rheumatic heart disease and a big heart in atrial fibrillation will be much higher.

A. MICHAEL BORKON: I'd like to echo some similar thoughts. Since 1979, we have had 40 children undergo valve replacement using the ST. JUDE MEDICAL valve in a variety of positions. We have been impressed with the need for a selective management scheme similar to what has been proposed by the discussants so far. Specifically, patients with low risk factors, such as small hearts in sinus rhythm, valves in the aortic position, or age less than 5 years, are placed on aspirin and then converted to COUMADIN at a later date, unless we feel there is a risk factor that would contraindicate chronic warfarin therapy. Our prothrombin times are maintained in the range of 1.5 to a little less than 2. Our experience has supported the concept of warfarin anticoagulation, no matter what the age, for patients who appear to be at increased risk for thromboembolic complications, as delineated by a large heart, atrial fibrillation, or mitral valve replacement.

QUESTION: I would like to know the panel's opinion about the use of bioprostheses in childbearing-age patients. Secondly, it was stated that when pregnant patients are switched to heparin, they have a higher incidence of problems. Do you switch the patients to heparin only for the first 12 weeks and then back onto COUMADIN until the completion of the pregnancy, or do you keep them on heparin during the entire pregnancy?

HUGH O'KANE: Just from our experience with one pregnant patient who thrombosed her ST. JUDE MEDICAL valve, we would tend to favor the insertion of a biological valve in childbearing years. However, at the British Cardiac Society meeting, Dr. Celia Oakley looked at our case of the thrombosed ST. JUDE MEDICAL valve in the mitral area and said she believed it was wrong to switch from warfarin to heparin. She believes that patients, even pregnant women, will thrombose their mechanical valves if they are treated with heparin because it's hard to control. She based her comments on a large experience.

With regard to anticoagulation, we all may be talking about comparing apples and oranges. Perhaps it is time we all began using a standard control and the International Normalized Ratio, where the substrate is a standard international substrate. This would make our discussions more logical.

GERALD LEMOLE: In 70 children with valve problems, we've implanted approximately 28 valves, both mechanical and tissue. Nine years ago we arbitrarily chose to give aspirin to children below the age of 5 and use anticoagulation with COUMADIN for those above the age of 5. The only thromboembolic event that we have had was a child who, just as he turned age 5, had an embolus and a major thromboembolic event in his brain. At that time, we changed all children from aspirin to COUMADIN. We firmly believe that all children with prostheses should have COUMADIN anticoagulation, unless for some reason, such as in children under age 5, you can't give COUMADIN. In those cases we give aspirin.

DAVID CAMPBELL: Again, we don't feel that age really is important because, if followed closely, children can be anticoagulated at any age. It's just as safe to anticoagulate them under 5 years. You really have to look at the patient's flow and cardiac output. If these are low, then I think the patient needs to be anticoagulated with COUMADIN, no matter what the age.

R. L. BEAUDET: Dr. Sade, you reported 75.3% freedom from anticoagulation-related complications at 5 years in adult patients. When you accumulate all complications in the group, it comes to 40.3%, which is very low. I think there's a big difference between 75% and 40% at 5 years, and I'd like you to expand on this difference, explaining what you included in your complications.

ROBERT SADE: These data were published in the *Annals of Surgery*★ about 2 years ago, and the details, at that time, were presented. The incidence for freedom from thromboembolism in adults went from 75% down to 60%. Freedom from all complications was 40% in the pediatric group and 61% in the adult group. The difference between that 75% and the 61% was due to infective endocarditis and paravalvular leaks, as well as some other complications. However, when you look at all of the complications and deaths, the experience in adults was significantly better than in children. Valve replacement in children is not a happy thing to do. Still, 70% of the children who were alive then, are now alive. Of those, none has neurological deficits or other major problems related to the valve. So the quality of life for the children who do survive, who don't have fatal early or late complications, is really quite good.

★ Crawford FA, Sade RM, Kratz JM, Stroud M, Bartles D. Aortic and mitral valve replacement with the St. Jude Medical prosthesis. Annals of Surgery 1984; 199:753–761.

II. HEART VALVE REPLACEMENT IN ADULTS (AGE 65 AND YOUNGER)

7. PROSPECTIVE RANDOMIZED STUDY OF THE ST. JUDE MEDICAL®, BJÖRK-SHILEY®, AND STARR-EDWARDS® 6120 VALVE PROSTHESES IN THE MITRAL POSITION

PH. MIKAELOFF, O. JEGADEN, M. FERRINI, J. COLL-MAZZEI, J. Y. BONNEFOY, A. RUMOLO

Abstract. During a 5-year period (January 1979 to December 1983), 357 patients received mitral valve replacement. Group A was comprised of 179 patients receiving a ST. JUDE MEDICAL® prosthesis in the mitral position. Group B included 178 patients; initially 113 patients were implanted with a BJÖRK-SHILEY® valve, and later 65 patients received a STARR-EDWARDS® 6120 valve prosthesis in the mitral position. All implants were performed by the same surgeon and the groups were randomized. Analysis of 21 preoperative (clinical and hemodynamic data) and operative variables showed the groups to be well randomized. All patients were anticoagulated postoperatively. A follow-up study was performed each year postoperatively. At the end of 1986, there was a 35-month to 95-month follow-up with a mean of 64.7 months (1596 patient-years of follow-up). Fifteen patients were lost to follow-up. The actuarial survival rate is significantly different (p < 0.05) at 5 years with 87.6 ± 4.5% for Group A vs. 77.4 ± 6% for Group B, and at 7 years with 83.4 ± 6.5% for Group A vs. 73.2 ± 7.2% for Group B. In conclusion, in the mitral position, the ST. JUDE MEDICAL prosthesis gives a significant benefit compared to BJÖRK-SHILEY or STARR-EDWARDS 6120 prostheses.

INTRODUCTION

Late results of mitral valve replacement (MVR) remain unsatisfactory based upon thromboembolic and death rate evaluations at 5- and 10-year follow-up. There is a need to improve both bioprostheses and mechanical valves for

MVR. For the present time, one should try a conservative operation on the mitral valve if possible. If it is not feasible, the patient should be given the best available type of prosthesis, according to the anatomic and hemodynamic conditions. Unfortunately, it has been difficult to objectively choose the optimal mechanical valve for a patient. This is why we conducted a prospective randomized study of mechanical mitral valves.

METHODS

Patients and randomization

During a 5-year period of time, from January 1979 to December 1983, all MVR performed were randomized into two groups. Nineteen patients with selective indications for a bioprosthesis in the mitral position were excluded from the study.

The choice of mitral prosthesis was done the day of operation, at random, with the help of random table numbers. Randomization started between ST. JUDE MEDICAL (SJM) and BJÖRK-SHILEY (B-S) valves, but at the end of the third year, analysis of preliminary results showed a statistical difference in survival rate, with a lower survival rate for the B-S group. We felt obliged, from an ethical point of view, to stop MVR with the B-S valve and replaced it with a STARR-EDWARDS (SE 6120) from January 1982 to the end of the study.

During the first period (January 1979 to December 1981), a total of 116 SJM and 113 B-S valve prostheses were implanted in the mitral position, for a total of 229 operated patients. During the second period (1982 to 1983), 63 SJM and 65 SE 6120 valves were implanted, for a total of 128 operated patients.

Group A was comprised of 179 patients who received a ST. JUDE MEDICAL prosthesis (SJM) in the mitral position. Group B included 178 patients who received a BJÖRK-SHILEY valve (B-S) initially or, later, a STARR-EDWARDS 6120 valve prosthesis (SE 6120).

Main clinical hemodynamic preoperative and operative data were recorded for each patient on a computer registry (Zenith 100). A total of 21 variables were recorded for each patient.

Operative methods

All patients were operated on by the same surgeon (Ph. Mikaeloff). Extracorporeal circulation was used under moderate hypothermia (26–30°C), with a bubble oxygenator and hemodilution. Myocardial protection techniques varied, but by the same proportions in the two groups, according to three methods: topical cooling and cross-clamping of the aorta for single MVR; coronary perfusion with cold diluted blood for associated aortic valve replacement [1]; and, from 1982 onward, oxygenated crystalloid cardioplegia for all cases [2].

The valves in the mitral or aortic position were secured with an interrupted suture technique. As previously advised [3], an SJM valve was placed in the mitral position with an antianatomical orientation (perpendicular to natural leaflets). The largest prosthetic size compatible with good hemodynamic function was inserted (usually size 27 mm to 31 mm). The size of the B-S valve (usually 25 mm to 27 mm) was chosen in order that the large opening was placed toward the posterior wall of the left ventricle, as it has been advised [4], to keep the disc moving freely. From 1979 to March 1981, 78 Standard spherical disc B-S valves were used; afterwards the Convexo-Concave model was inserted in 35 patients.

The size of the SE 6120 was chosen according to the size of the left ventricular cavity (usually size 3 M or 4 M). For all patients necessitating concomitant aortic valve replacement, a BJÖRK-SHILEY prosthesis was used in both groups. At the end of the procedure, special care was taken to prevent systemic and coronary microair emboli with the regular use of our ultrasonic device [5].

Postoperative anticoagulation therapy

The day following operation, intravenous heparin was instituted. Warfarin was started 6 to 8 days postoperatively, and heparin was stopped when the prothrombin rate was below 0.30. Patients were asked to strictly adhere to their anticoagulation regimen and have their prothrombin rate checked at least once a month. Most of these patients live in the city or in the proximity and are closely followed up by their referring doctors and cardiologists.

Collection of follow-up data, definitions

At the end of each year, beginning in 1980, a study of late results was performed by mailing a questionnaire. If the answer was unsatisfactory, direct contact with the cardiologist or referring physician was established. Many patients were seen in the hospital for routine follow-up or restudied when complications occurred.

The following criteria were used to define deaths and complications [6]:

- **Peripheral arterial embolic complications** included any embolic event, even a transient episode of neurologic deficit.
- **Thromboembolic complications** included all peripheral arterial emboli, thrombosis of valves, and sudden death, as it has been suggested [7]. When patients had several thromboembolic events, the first episode was taken into account for actuarial studies.
- **Dysfunction of valve** was limited to mechanical dysfunction.
- **Complications related to prosthesis** included all thromboembolic events, dysfunction, endocarditis, paravalvular leak, reoperation, and anticoagulant-related hemorrhage.
- **Immediate postoperative deaths** were those occurring during the first postoperative month.
- **Deaths** were classified as cardiac, noncardiac, and undetermined.

- **Sudden deaths** included deaths from arrhythmias and deaths occurring after rapid deterioration of clinical situation.
- **Deaths related to prosthesis** included deaths from cardiac and undetermined causes.

Statistical analysis

Computer statistical analysis employed t-test analysis for continuous variables and chi square analysis for categorical analysis. Continuous data are presented as mean ± SEM (standard error of the mean). The statistical cutoff point used for significance is $p < 0.05$. Actuarial methods according to Kaplan-Meier [8] were used and expressed as mean actuarial probability ± SEM [9]. For the comparison of two event-free curves, the log-rank test is given [10]. Postoperative complications are expressed as % per patient-year [11].

RESULTS

Patient population and operative data

Analysis of 21 preoperative clinical, hemodynamic, and operative variables show the two groups to be well randomized. Main preoperative clinical data are summarized in table 7-1. In both groups, most patients were in New York Heart Association (NYHA) Functional Class III, and about two-thirds of them had chronic atrial fibrillation. As usually seen for mitral valve disease

Table 7-1. Comparison of main preoperative clinical data

	Group A (n = 179)		Group B (n = 178)		p value
	n	%	n	%	
Female sex	112	62.6	115	64.6	NS
Mean age (years)	54.1		53.9		NS
	(11.4)		(11.3)		
History of rheumatic disease	113	63.1	125	70.2	NS
Previous cardiac operation	33	18.4	35	19.7	NS
Functional state (NYHA)					
II	22	12.3	13	7.3	
III	134	74.9	144	80.9	NS
IV	23	12.8	21	11.8	
Chronic atrial fibrillation	111	62	126	70.8	NS
Mean cardiothoracic ratio	0.60		0.61		
	(0.08)		(0.08)		NS
Mitral stenosis	42	23.5	30	16.9	
Mitral incompetence	51	28.5	45	25.3	
Mitral stenosis and incompetence	86	48	103	57.8	NS
Associated valvular aortic disease	74	41.3	89	50	
Associated valvular tricuspid disease	21	11.7	20	11.2	NS
Associated coronary artery disease	15	8.4	7	3.9	

in France, the percentage of associated coronary disease is low. Almost half of the patients had an associated aortic valve disease necessitating aortic valve replacement.

Most of the patients submitted to preoperative hemodynamic study. The data, summarized in table 7-2, show no significant difference (NS) for the two groups.

For 94 patients in Group A and 99 in Group B, a concomitant operative procedure was performed (aortic valve replacement, valvular tricuspid annuloplasty, or associated coronary artery bypass surgery), but without significant difference for the two groups.

Mean bypass time was 81.2 min. ($\pm$ 25.4) for Group A and 82.1 min. ($\pm$ 30.4) for Group B (NS).

Follow-up of patients

In November 1986, there was a 35- to 95-month follow-up for the long-term survivors, with a mean of 64.7 months ($\pm$ 16.2). Fifteen patients were lost to follow-up (4.5% of long-term survivors) after a mean postoperative follow-up of 27.1 months. These 15 patients included 4 in Group A and 11 in Group B. There were 148 long-term survivors in Group A, with a total of 798.7 patient-years of follow-up. In Group B, 125 patients were long-term survivors, with a total of 673.4 patient-years of follow-up.

Immediate and late postoperative deaths

In the whole population studied (n = 357) there were 21 immediate postoperative deaths (5.9%) and 48 late deaths (14.3%). Immediate postoperative death was 5.5% for single MVR (n = 164) and 6.2% if a concomitant procedure was performed (n = 193). Statistical comparison of death is summarized in table 7-3, and details about the causes of early and late postoperative deaths are given in table 7-4.

Immediate postoperative death was 3.4% in Group A and 8.4% in Group B ($p < 0.05$). Analysis of cause shows that this difference could be attributed to

Table 7-2. Comparison of hemodynamic data; mean value (SEM)

	Group A (n = 179)	Group B (n = 178)	p value
Number of right heart catheterizations	172	168	NS
Number of left heart catheterizations	134	147	NS
Mean pulmonary artery pressure, mm Hg	29.8 (12.9)	29.7 (12.4)	NS
Mean wedge capillary pressure, mm Hg	19.5 (7.2)	19.2 (6.9)	NS
Mean cardiac index, 1/min	2.2 (0.5)	2.2 (0.5)	NS
Mean left ventricular end diastolic pressure, mm Hg	11.5 (5.8)	11.8 (5.2)	NS
Mean left ventricle ejection fraction, percent	58.8 (12.9)	55.9 (13.5)	NS

Table 7-3. Comparison of early and late postoperative deaths

Deaths	Group A (n = 179)		Group B (n = 178)		p value
	n	%	n	%	
Immediate postoperative (1 month) death	6	3.4	15	8.4	P < 0.05
Late postoperative death	21	12.1	27	16.6	NS
Immediate and late postoperative death	27	15.1	42	23.6	p < 0.05
All deaths related to prosthesis	15	8.4	36	20.2	p < 0.001

Table 7-4. Comparison of causes of immediate and late postoperative deaths

	Group A (n = 179) n	Group B (n = 178) n
Early Deaths		
Thromboembolic cause	2	6
Sudden death	0	3
Valvular dysfunction	0	2
Cardiac failure	1	2
Myocardial infarct	1	0
Noncardiac	2	2
Late deaths		
Thromboembolic cause	2	3
Sudden death	3	15
Cardiac failure	4	3
Endocarditis	2	0
Hemorrhage	0	2
Noncardiac	8	2
Undetermined	2	2

more early deaths from thromboembolic causes, sudden deaths, and valvular dysfunction in Group B. Three sudden early deaths, probably due to valve thrombosis, occurred with B-S valves. Two deaths from immediate dysfunction occurred. In the first case, sudden, complete loss of arterial pressure with an elevated left atrial pressure occurred in the operating room. The patient was reopened and the Convexo-Concave disc was found blocked in closed position, without interfering extrinsic factors. It could be opened only by pushing it firmly and needed to be rotated to move again freely. The second case was identical and occurred in the intensive care unit.

Late postoperative deaths do not differ significantly for the two groups, but there were strikingly more sudden deaths in Group B, mainly in patients with B-S valves. Most of the sudden deaths occurred in peripheral hospitals or at the patient's home. Unfortunately, autopsy was not available. For several patients, it was learned that before death there was a rapid, unexplained de-

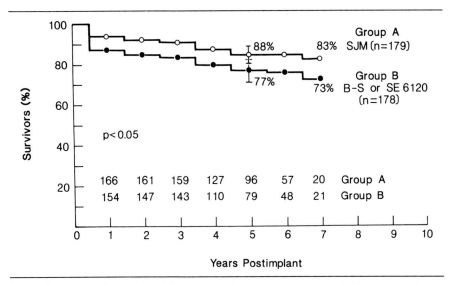

Figure 7-1. Comparison of actuarial survival rate between the two groups (early postoperative mortality included).

terioration of clinical condition with severe cardiac failure. This was probably due to a valve thrombosis.

Comparison of all postoperative deaths shows a significant difference (p < 0.05), with a better survival rate in Group A. There were significantly more sudden deaths (p < 0.001) in Group B.

Comparison of actuarial survival rates, including early postoperative deaths (figure 7-1), shows a significant difference between the two groups (p < 0.05). In Group A, survival rates are 87.6% (± 4.5) at 5 years and 83.4% (± 6.5) at 7 years. Group B survival rates are 77.4% (± 6) at 5 years and 73.2% (± 7.2) at 7 years.

Postoperative complications related to prosthesis

These have been summarized in table 7-5. There are more peripheral embolic complications in Group B (4.3% per patient-year) than in Group A (2.3% per patient-year), but the difference is not statistically significant. Three patients in Group A and 8 in Group B had a recurrent peripheral embolic complication. Comparison of all thromboembolic events, including sudden deaths, shows a highly significant difference (p < 0.001), with a rate of 3.1% per patient-year in Group A and 7.9% per patient-year in Group B. The actuarial probability to be free from all thromboembolic events including sudden deaths (figure 7-2) at 5 years postoperatively is 87.6% (± 4.5) for Group A vs. 73.7% (± 6.5) for Group B and, at 7 years, 83.7% (± 5.7) for Group A vs. 66.3% (± 7.3) for Group B (p < 0.001). The rate of other postoperative complications is not statistically different for the two groups. The same number of reoperations has

Table 7-5. Comparison of postoperative complications related to prosthesis (percent per patient-year)

| Complications | Group A (n = 179) | | Group B (n = 178) | | |
	n	% per pt-yr	n	% per pt-yr	p value
Peripheral arterial embolic complications	18	2.3	29	4.3	NS
All thromboembolic events (sudden deaths included)	26	3.1	53	7.9	p < 0.001
Anticoagulant-related hemorrhage	13	1.6	16	2.4	NS
Endocarditis	2	0.3	6	0.9	NS
Valvular dysfunction	0	—	2	—	—
Paravalvular leak	0	—	1	—	—
Reoperation	6	0.75	6	0.89	NS
All complications and deaths related to prosthesis	43	5.1	87	11.7	p < 0.001

been observed in both groups after a mean postoperative interval of 25.2 months in Group A and 31.5 months in Group B.

The 3 patients with thrombosed valves had a modification of their anticoagulant therapy and were put under subcutaneous heparin because of pregnancy, general surgery, or dental care. In Group A, causes of reoperation were: 3 valve thromboses, 1 case of endocarditis, 1 hemolysis from an un-

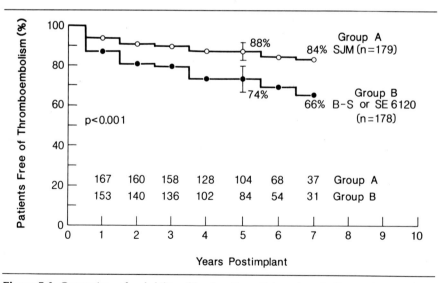

Figure 7-2. Comparison of probability of freedom from all thromboembolic complications (sudden deaths included).

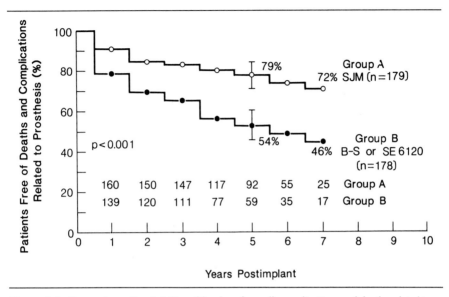

Figure 7-3. Comparison of probability of freedom from all complications and deaths related to prosthesis.

known cause, and 1 end-stage cardiac failure that received a heart transplant. In Group B, causes of reoperation were 3 valve thromboses, 2 cases of endocarditis, and 1 paravalvular leak. The difference in the rate of all complications and deaths related to prosthesis is highly significant ($p < 0.001$) at 5.1% per patient-year in Group A vs. 11.7% in Group B. The actuarial probability to be free from all complications and deaths related to prosthesis (figure 7-3) at 5 years postoperatively is 79% ($\pm$ 6.5) for Group A vs. 54% ($\pm$ 7.5) for Group B and, at 7 years, 72% ($\pm$ 7.5) for Group A vs. 46% ($\pm$ 8.5) for Group B ($p < 0.0001$).

Comparison of subgroups

Comparison of subgroups of patients operated on during the first 3 years of randomization (January 1979 to December 1981) receiving SJM and B-S valves, has been summarized in table 7-6. Table 7-7 compares results of 1982 and 1983 between SJM and SE 6120 valves.

Approximately the same differences appear between these subgroups. However, peripheral arterial embolic complications were more frequent with SE 6120 valves, while there were more early deaths, valve thrombosis, and sudden deaths with the B-S valve.

Functional results of long-term survivors

At the end of November 1986, there were 148 long-term survivors in Group A and 125 in Group B. Functional results of both groups are indicated in table

Table 7-6. Comparison of patients operated on during the first period (January 1979 to December 1981) with randomization between St. Jude Medical and Björk-Shiley prostheses

	St. Jude Medical (n = 116) %	Björk-Shiley (n = 113) %	p value
Immediate postoperative deaths	3.4	10.6	p < 0.05
All postoperative deaths	15.5	26.6	p < 0.05
Deaths related to prosthesis	7.8	23	p < 0.01
Peripheral arterial embolic complications	2.5*	3.2*	NS
All thromboembolic complications (sudden deaths included)	3.2*	8.3*	P < 0.01

* Percent per patient-year

Table 7-7. Comparison of patients operated on during second period (January 1982 to December 1983) with randomization between St. Jude Medical and Starr-Edwards 6120 prostheses

	St. Jude Medical (n = 63) %	Starr-Edwards (n = 65) %	p value
Immediate postoperative deaths	3.2	4.6	NS
All postoperative deaths	15	18.5	NS
Deaths related to prosthesis	9.5	15.4	NS
Peripheral arterial embolic complications	1.5*	5.3*	p < 0.01
All thromboembolic complications (sudden deaths included)	3.4*	7.6*	p < 0.01

* Percent per patient-year

Table 7-8. Functional results of long-term surviving patients of both groups

	Class I (NYHA)	Preoperative (n)	Postoperative (n)
Group A (n = 148)	I	0	91
	II	20	47
	III	111	9
	IV	17	1
		p < 0.001	
Group B (n = 125)	I	0	62
	II	12	51
	III	102	12
	IV	11	0
		p < 0.001	

Table 7-9. Comparison of mean cardiac functional state preoperatively and postoperatively in the 2 groups of long-term surviving patients; mean value (SEM)

State (NYHA)	Group A (n = 148)	Group B (n = 125)	p value
Preoperative	2.98 (0.50)	2.99 (0.43)	NS
Postoperative	1.46 (0.64)	1.60 (0.66)	NS

7-8. Functional improvement is highly significant for both groups (p < 0.001), but, as shown in table 7-9, the mean value of Functional Class is not statistically different for Group A and Group B long-term survivors, preoperatively as well as postoperatively.

DISCUSSION

MVR carries a higher rate of prosthetic complications and deaths, mainly thromboembolic events, compared to aortic valve replacement. If one has decided to implant a mechanical mitral valve in a patient, the problem remains of giving the patient the best available model.

From the literature it is difficult to compare mechanical valves for several reasons:

1. Retrospective studies may compare series of patients operated on at different time intervals. It has been shown that year of operation, with the same type of valve, is a risk factor in the survival [12] and rate of thromboembolic complications [13].
2. Studies comparing results of valves from different institutions may be misleading because of differences in patient populations [14], operative techniques, or anticoagulant therapy protocols [15]. However, interesting nonrandomized comparative studies have been published, with similar groups of patients after MVR [16–18]. Very few randomized studies have been published on MVR [19, 20].

From a practical point of view, we were interested in making a randomized study after MVR comparing two mechanical prostheses, which seemed to be among the best available in 1979.

The BJÖRK-SHILEY tilting disc valve (B-S), with a free-floating disc, was introduced in 1970. Improved hemodynamics were expected and reported with this valve [21]. We have been using the various types of B-S valves in the aortic position (the DELRIN® disc valve, the pyrolytic carbon Standard spherical disc, the Convexo-Concave disc, and the Monostrut model) for more than 15 years, with optimal results (minimal rate of valve dysfunction and thromboembolism), as others have [22, 23]. Therefore, we have not been tempted to change from this type of valve, if a mechanical aortic valve replacement is indicated. No randomized study on aortic mechanical valves was conducted by our team, due to a limited period of time to operate on enough patients with aortic valve disease to produce a statistically significant difference.

We also chose to randomize with the B-S Standard spherical disc mitral valve in 1979 due to publications of good clinical results with a follow-up over 5 years [24, 25].

We selected the ST. JUDE MEDICAL valve (SJM) to be the second valve for this randomization. This low profile, bileaflet central flow, all pyrolytic-carbon prosthesis, was introduced clinically in 1977 [26]. It was a new, attractive type of valve, and despite its lack of late follow-up, we were tempted to use it because of the following advantages: opening of the two leaflets to 85° of the horizontal axis, which provided a central near-laminar flow, small transvalvular pressure gradient, large effective orifice area, and rapid ventricular filling with a low risk of thromboembolism, according to surgeons who started to use it before us [3, 26].

At the end of 1981, after 3 years of randomization, preliminary studies of the results showed a significant difference between the B-S and SJM valves, mainly because of more early deaths, more sudden late deaths or rapidly occurring deaths, probably from valve thrombosis of the B-S. Moreover, in 1981, we replaced the B-S Standard spherical disc with the new B-S Convexo-Concave disc, and we saw 2 deaths from typical valve dysfunction with this model as reported by others [27, 28]. They occurred in the immediate postoperative period and were due to intrinsic occlusion of the valve by the disc in the closed position. This was different from published extrinsic obstructions [29], which we tried to prevent by choosing a size small enough to avoid interference with valve opening by ventricular myocardium and careful excision of chordal remnants.

In fact, more recent publications confirmed our pessimistic results with the B-S valve in the mitral position. A comparative nonrandomized analysis of B-S and SE 6120 valves done by Murphy [17] could not find a difference in survival rates between these valves with a mean follow-up of over 5 years. However, there were more cases of valve failure due to late thrombotic occlusion in the B-S group. Early postoperative mortality was higher in the B-S group, as in our study. In the work reported by Karp [30], the rate of sudden deaths and deaths from B-S valve thrombosis was high after MVR; the incidence of thrombosis at 4 years was 13%. Wright [31] published a study of the B-S prosthesis with an incidence of valve thrombosis of 4% after MVR. The thrombus on the hinge mechanism of the valve immobilizes the disc and causes acute or rapidly progressive left heart failure, leading to sudden death if immediate reoperation is delayed. Thrombotic catastrophe in the patient with multiple B-S prostheses have been reported by Mattingly [32], with an incidence of 26.8% at 6 years, with most of these related to mitral valve thrombosis.

In December 1981, we were obliged to discontinue the use of the B-S valve in the mitral position after 3 years of randomization, because analysis of preliminary results clearly showed a higher rate of mortality and morbidity than that of the SJM group. We replaced it, for the following 2 years of the study, with the SE 6120 prosthesis.

We had previously reported experience with this valve [33] in a series of 302 used in MVR, operated on from 1970–1978, with an actuarial survival rate of 77.4% at 5 years and an incidence of embolic complications of 3.7% per patient-year. Peripheral arterial emboli were our main problem in the late follow-up of this valve.

A randomized study by Horstkotte [19] between B-S, SE 6120, and LILLEHEI-KASTER® mitral prostheses found a similar survival rate at 5 years, but more frequent thromboembolic complications with SE 6120 than the B-S valve.

In our present study, we have seen more peripheral embolic complications with the SE 6120, but sudden death and valve thrombosis were less frequent than with the B-S valve. Altogether, comparison of the SJM valve in the mitral position with the B-S or SE 6120 prostheses shows the SJM valve to be superior, mainly due to a lower incidence of thromboembolic complications.

Comparison of late complications between B-S and SJM valves by Horstkotte [34] in the mitral position leads to the same conclusion: There were more thromboembolic events and more deaths from valve thrombosis with a B-S valve in the mitral position than with SJM. Postoperative event-free curves for all complications were significantly higher for the SJM valve.

Several clinical studies have reported satisfactory results after MVR with the SJM prosthesis, with a low rate of thromboembolic complications and deaths related to prosthesis [3, 26, 34, 35].

Our survival rate of 87.6% at 5 years and 83.4% at 7 years (figure 7-1), including early postoperative mortality, is similar to these reports and has an improved rate compared to late survival with the SE 6120 [12, 15, 33] or B-S prostheses [17–19, 23–25].

We have observed a rate of peripheral arterial embolic complications of 2.3% per patient-year and a rate of all thromboembolic complications, including sudden deaths, of 3.1% per patient-year with the SJM valve in the mitral position. This is significantly better than the results obtained with the B-S or SE 6120 valves.

However, as others report [3, 34, 35], we think that the quality of anticoagulant therapy is very crucial after MVR with the SJM valve. We had 3 cases of valve thrombosis reoperated on because anticoagulant therapy was unsatisfactorily changed and unsatisfactory in the late follow-up.

Overall, we found the probability of freedom from all complications and deaths related to the prosthesis to be 79% at 5 years and 72% at 7 years with the SJM valve (figure 7-3). This is superior to the rate obtained with the SE 6120 or B-S mitral valves.

These improved results are probably due to better antithrombogenic and hemodynamic qualities of the SJM valve as reported by well-documented hemodynamic [26, 37], echocardiographic [38], and in vitro studies [39].

REFERENCES

1. Mikaeloff P, Amouroux C, Boivin J, Loire R, Vial C. Technique de protection myocardique par perfusion en hypothermie profonde (10°C) avec ou sans cardioplegie. Nouvelle Presse Médicale 1979; 8:4105–4108.
2. Bleese N, Doring V, Kalmar P, Pokar H, Polonius MJ, Steiner D, Rodewald G. Intraoperative myocardial protection by cardioplegia in hypothermia. Clinical findings. J Thorac Cardiovasc Surg 1978; 75:405–413.
3. Baudet EM, Oca CC, Roques XF, Laborde MN, Hafez AS, Collot MA, Ghidoni IM. A $5\frac{1}{2}$ year experience with the St. Jude Medical cardiac valve prosthesis. J Thorac Cardiovasc Surg 1985; 90:137–144.
4. Björk VO. Optimal orientation of the 60° and the 70° Björk-Shiley tilting disc valves. Scand J Thor Cardiovasc Surg 1982; 16:113–118.
5. Mikaeloff P, Van Haecke P, Girard C, Tartulier M, DeVolfe C, Guillaud C, Lakestani F, Roche M, Guillerm R, Masurel G. Prevention des microembolies gazeuses en chirurgie cardiaque: controle numerique du debullage des cavites cardiaques par detecteur a ultrasons. Arch Mal Coeur 1984; 77:314–323.
6. Oyer PE, Stinson EG, Griepp RB, Shumway NE. Valve replacement with the Starr-Edwards and Hancock prosthesis. Comparative analysis of late morbidity and mortality. Ann Thorac Surg 1977; 186:301–307.
7. Edmunds LH. Thromboembolic complications of current cardiac valvular prostheses. Ann Thorac Surg 1982; 34:96–106.
8. Kaplan EL, Meier P. Nonparametric estimation from incomplete observations. Am Stat Assoc J 1958; 53:457–481.
9. Grunkemeier GL, Starr A. Actuarial analysis of surgical results: Rationale and method. Ann Thorac Surg 1977; 24:404–408.
10. Mantel N. Evaluation of survival data and two new rank order statistics arising in its consideration. Cancer Chemother Rep 1966; 50:163–171.
11. Bodnar E, Haberman S, Wain WH. Comparative method for actuarial analysis of cardiac valve replacements. Br Heart J 1979; 42:541–552.
12. MacManus Q, Grunkemeier GL, Lambert LE, Teply JF, Harlan BJ, Starr A. Year of operation as a risk factor in the late results of valve replacement. J Thorac Cardiovasc Surg 1980; 80:834–841.
13. Teply JF, Grunkemeier GL, D'Arcy Sutherland H, Lambert LE, Johnson VA, Starr A. The ultimate prognosis after valve replacement: an assessment at twenty years. Ann Thorac Surg 1981; 32:111–119.
14. Mitchell RS, Miller DC, Stinson EB, Oyer PE, Jamieson SW, Baldwin JC, Shumway NE. Significant patient-related determinants of prosthetic valve performance. J Thorac Cardiovasc Surg 1986; 91:807–817.
15. Fuster V, Pumphrey LW, McGoon MD, Chesebro JH, Pluth JR, McGoon DC. Systemic thromboembolism in mitral and aortic Starr-Edwards prostheses: A 10–19 year follow-up. Circulation 1982; 66(Suppl I):157–161.
16. Horstkotte D, Haerten MK, Herzer JA, Seipel L, Bircks W, Loogen F. Preliminary results in mitral valve replacement with the St. Jude Medical prosthesis: Comparison with the Björk-Shiley valve. Circulation 1981; 64(Suppl II):203–208.
17. Murphy DA, Levine FH, Buckley MJ, Swinski L, Daggett WM, Akins LW, Austen WG. Mechanical valves; A comparative analysis of the Starr-Edwards and Björk-Shiley prostheses. J Thorac Cardiovasc Surg 1983; 86:746–752.
18. Perier P, Deloche A, Chauvaud S, Fabiani JN, Rossant P, Bessou JP, Relland J, Bourezak H, Gomez F, Blondeau P, D'Allaines C, Carpentier A. Comparative evaluation of mitral valve repair and replacement with Starr, Björk and porcine valve prostheses. Circulation 1984; 70(Suppl I):187–192.
19. Horstkotte D, Haerten K, Herzer JA, Loogen F, Scheibling R, Schulte HD. Five-year results

after randomized mitral valve replacement with Björk-Shiley, Lillehei-Kaster and Starr-Edwards prostheses. J Thorac Cardiovasc Surg 1983; 31:206–214.

20. Bloomfield P, Kitchin AH, Wheatley DJ, Walbaum PR, Lutz W, Miller MC. A prospective evaluation of the Björk-Shiley, Hancock, and Carpentier-Edwards heart valve prostheses. Circulation 1986; 73:1213–1222.

21. Björk VO, Book K, Cernigliaro C, Holmgren A. The Björk-Shiley tilting disc valve in isolated mitral lesions. Scand J Thorac Cardiovasc Surg 1973; 7:131–143.

22. Cheung D, Flemma RJ, Mullen DC, Lepley D, Anderson AJ, Weirauch E. Ten-year follow-up in aortic valve replacement using the Björk-Shiley prosthesis. Ann Thorac Surg 1981; 32:138–145.

23. Daenen W, Nevelsteen A, VanCauwelaert P, De Maesschalk E, Willems J, Stalpaert G. Nine years' experience with the Björk-Shiley prosthetic valve: Early and late results of 932 valve replacements. Ann Thorac Surg 1983; 35:651–663.

24. Lepley D, Flemma RJ, Mullen PL, Singh M, Chakravarty S. Late evaluation of patients undergoing valve replacement with the Björk-Shiley prosthesis. Ann Thorac Surg 1977; 24:131–139.

25. Björk VO, Henze A. Ten years' experience with the Björk-Shiley tilting disc valve. J Thorac Cardiovasc Surg 1979; 78:331–342.

26. Nicoloff DM, Emery RW, Arom KV, Northaus WF, Jorgensen CR, Wang Y, Lindsay WG. Clinical and hemodynamic results with the St. Jude Medical cardiac valve prosthesis. A three year experience. J Thorac Cardiovasc Surg 1981; 82:674–683.

27. Saunders CR, Rossi NP, Rittenhouse EA. Failure of a Björk-Shiley mitral valve prosthesis to open—clinical recognition. J Cardiovasc Surg (Torino) 1977; 18:571–576.

28. Negre E, Ferriere M, Negre G, Blin B. Blocages immediats des protheses mitrales de Björk-Shiley a disque convexo-concave. Ann Chir Thorac Cardiovasc 1983; 37:160–162.

29. Williams DB, Pluth JR, Orszulak T. Extrinsic obstruction of the Björk-Shiley valve in the mitral position. Ann Thorac Surg 1981; 32:57–62.

30. Karp RB, Cyrus RJ, Blackstone EH, Kirklin JW, Kouchoukos NT, Pacifico AD. The Björk-Shiley valve: Intermediate-term follow-up. J Thorac Cardiovasc Surg 1981; 81:602–614.

31. Wright JO, Hiratzka LF, Brandt B, Doty DB. Thrombosis of the Björk-Shiley prosthesis. Illustrative cases and review of the literature. J Thorac Cardiovasc Surg 1982; 84:138–144.

32. Mattingly WT, O'Connor W, Zeok JV, Todd EP. Thrombotic catastrophe in the patient with multiple Björk-Shiley prostheses. Ann Thorac Surg 1983; 35:253–256.

33. Mikaeloff P, Van Haecke P, Frieh J, Convert G, Biron A, Amouroux C, Boivin J. Facteurs pronostiques après remplacement valvulaire mitral par la prothèse de Starr-Edwards modèle 6120. Arch Mal Coeur 1981; 74:799–807.

34. Horstkotte D, Korfer R, Seipel L, Bircks W, Loogen F. Late complications in patients with Björk-Shiley and St. Jude Medical heart valve replacement. Circulation 1983; 68(Suppl II):175–184.

35. Dupon H, Michaud JLL, Duveau D, Despins P, Train M. Mitral valve replacement with St. Jude Medical prostheses: A 60 month study of 350 cases at Centre Hospitalier Universitair. In Matloff JM (ed): Cardiac Valve Replacement; Martinus Nijhoff, Boston 1985; pp 179–188.

36. Horstkotte D, Haerten K, Seipel L, Körfer R, Budde T, Bircks W, Loogen F. Central hemodynamics at rest and during exercise after mitral valve replacement with different prostheses. Circulation 1983; 68(Suppl II):161–168.

37. Ferrini M, Tartulier M, Boutarin J, Ritz B, Delahaye JP, Delaye J, Deyrieux F, Blum J, Corsini G, Mikaeloff P. Contrôle hémodynamique au repos et à l'effort après remplacement valvulaire mitral par prothèse de St. Jude Médical. Arch Mal Coeur 1985; 78:111–117.

38. Sutton J, Roudaut M, Oldershaw P. Echocardiographic assessment of left ventricular filling characteristics after mitral valve replacement with the St. Jude Medical prosthesis. Br Heart J 1981; 45:365–368.

39. Bruss KM, Rene M, Van Gilse J, Knott E. Pressure drop and velocity fields at four mechanical heart valve prostheses: Björk-Shiley standard, Björk-Shiley convexo-concave, Hall-Kaster, and St. Jude Medical. Life Support Systems 1983; 1:3–22.

8. NINE YEARS EXPERIENCE WITH 1287 CARPENTIER-EDWARDS® PORCINE BIOPROSTHESES

A. J. ACINAPURA, D. M. ROSE, J. N. CUNNINGHAM, JR., I. J. JACOBOWITZ, M. D. KRAMER, Z. ZISBROD

Abstract. The durability and functional results of porcine prosthetic valves remain controversial. In order to assess these parameters, 1287 porcine prosthetic valve insertions from January 1977 through September 1986 were reviewed. There were 523 mitral (MVR), 518 aortic (AVR), 238 combined AVR + MVR, and 8 tricuspid (TVR) implants. The average age was 59 years. The male:female ratio was 68%:32%. The majority of patients were in New York Heart Association (NYHA) Class III or IV preoperatively. Rheumatic or calcific valvulitis was present in 78%, myxomatous degeneration in 10%, and infective endocarditis in 12%. Valve replacement was performed utilizing moderate hypothermia (22 °G) and cold blood cardioplegia (10 °C). The operative mortality for MVR was 2.8% (14/523), for AVR was 1.8% (19/518), for AVR + MVR was 4.8% (11/238), and 0% for TVR (0/8). Thromboembolic events occurred in 7 MVR patients (1.3%), 5 AVR patients (1%), and 4 combined AVR/MVR patients (4%). Primary valve failure occurred in 20 MVR (3%) and 18 AVR cases (2%). Endocarditis has occurred in 15 patients (1.1%). Gated scans (6 to 12 months postoperative) have shown stable or improved left ventricular function. Endocardiograms (1 to 9 years postoperative) demonstrated excellent valve function in 90% of the patients. Survival at 9 years has been 85% from all causes and 92% from cardiac deaths. These results support continued use of the porcine prosthetic valve in valvular heart disease.

INTRODUCTION

Porcine bioprostheses have been widely used for heart valve replacement because of their excellent hemodynamic performance and low incidence of

both early and late complications. Their durability, however, remains controversial, making overall assessment difficult and raising the question of their
long-term effectiveness. Since 1977, porcine bioprostheses have been our first
choice for valve replacement. All prosthetic valves are judged by their functional performance, frequency of clinical complications, and durability. In
order to assess these parameters and possibly reassess our policy for choosing
prosthetic valves, we reviewed our porcine prosthetic valve insertions.

MATERIALS AND METHODS

From January 1977 through September 1986, 1287 patients at St. Vincent's
Hospital and Maimonides Medical Center underwent valve replacement with
CARPENTIER-EDWARDS® bioprostheses. There were 523 mitral (MVR),
518 aortic (AVR), 238 combined aortic and mitral (AVR + MVR), and 8
tricuspid (TVR) valve replacements (table 8-1). The patients ranged in age
from 22 to 81 years (mean 59 years). There were 875 males (68%) and 412
females (32%). The clinical classification ranged from NYHA Class II to IV
(table 8-2). Rheumatic or calcific valvulitis was present in 78%, myxomatous
degeneration in 10%, and infective endocarditis in 12% (table 8-3). All of the
tricuspid valve replacements were for bacterial endocarditis. Preoperative left
ventricular function was assessed by calculating the ejection fraction from
either a ventriculogram or gated pool scans. The majority of our patients
(80%) had diminished left ventricular function (table 8-4). Valve replacement
was performed utilizing moderate systemic hypothermia (22 °C), cold blood

Table 8-1. Valve replacement with Carpentier-Edwards
bioprostheses, 1977–1986

	Number of patients
Mitral (MVR)	523
Aortic (AVR)	518
Combined (AVR + MVR)	238
Tricuspid (TVR)	8
Total	1287

Table 8-2. NYHA Functional Classification

	Number of patients	
NYHA I	—	—
NYHA II	206	(16%)
NYHA III	927	(72%)
NYHA IV	154	(12%)
Total	1287	(100%)

Table 8-3. Etiology of valvular disease

	Number of patients	
Rheumatic	618	(48%)
Calcific	386	(30%)
Myxomatous	129	(10%)
Infective	154	(12%)
Total	1287	(100%)

Table 8-4. Left ventricular function

Ejection fraction	Number of patients	
> 55%	257	(20%)
40–55%	541	(42%)
< 40%	489	(38%)
Total	1287	(100%)

cardioplegia (10 °C), and topical hypothermia. Myocardial temperatures were maintained at 15 °C. When mitral valve replacement was performed, the left atrial appendage was either ligated directly or oversewn from within.

Aortic valve sizes ranged from 23 mm through 29 mm tissue anulus. In only 2% of our patients was a 23 mm valve size used. The majority (94%) received either a 25 mm or 27 mm porcine valve. In the mitral position, valve sizes ranged from 29 mm through 33 mm. Ninety percent of our patients received either a 31 mm or 33 mm porcine prosthesis. In the tricuspid position, only 31 mm or 33 mm valve sizes were utilized.

The operative mortality for mitral valve replacement was 2.8% (14/523); for aortic valve replacement, 1.8% (9/518); for combined aortic and mitral valve replacement, 4.8% (11/238); and for tricuspid valve replacement, 0% (0/8), as shown in table 8-5.

There has been 100% follow-up over the past 9 years, with a mean of 6.2 years. Clinical improvement in the NYHA Classification has occurred in a

Table 8-5. Operative mortality

	Number of patients	
MVR	14/523	(2.8%)
AVR	9/518	(1.8%)
AVR + MVR	11/238	(4.8%)
TVR	0/8	(0.0%)
Total	34/1287	(2.6%)

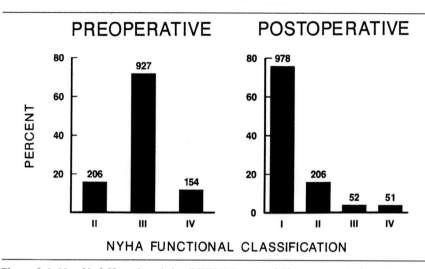

Figure 8-1. New York Heart Association (NYHA) Functional Class preoperatively in 1287 patients and postoperatively in 1253 survivors.

majority of our patients (figure 8-1). Left ventricular function, assessed by gated pool scans, has shown improvement (figure 8-2). All patients have been evaluated at yearly intervals utilizing echo-Doppler evaluation to assess valve stenosis and/or insufficiency. Gradients across the mitral valve of 0 to 4 mmHg with a standard deviation of ± 2.0 were recorded. Echo-Doppler evaluation showed that patients with aortic prosthetic valves had gradients

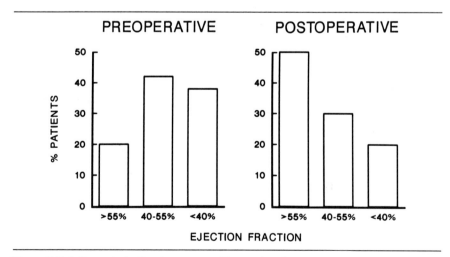

Figure 8-2. Left ventricular function as assessed by gated pool scans.

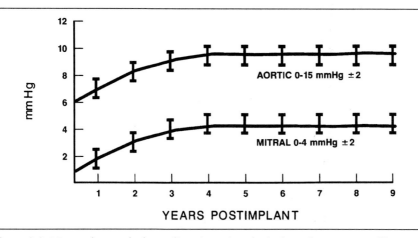

Figure 8-3. Measured transvalvular gradients in aortic and mitral prostheses as assessed by echo-Doppler evaluation.

ranging from 0 to 15 mmHg with a standard deviation of ± 2.0 (figure 8-3).

Thromboembolic episodes occurred in 16 of 1287 patients for an incidence of 1.2% (table 8-6). Anticoagulation was not utilized for aortic prostheses and was maintained for 6 to 8 weeks in patients with mitral valve replacement. Only those patients who were found to have left atrial thrombi at the time of valve replacement were maintained on long-term anticoagulation.

Primary valve failure occurred in 18 of 756 aortic prostheses (2.4%) and in 20 of 761 mitral prostheses (2.6%), as shown in figure 8-4. Tissue wear with disruption of the leaflets was responsible for 28 of the primary valve failures. Calcification of the cusps occurred in 10 of the prosthetic valves. Bacterial endocarditis was responsible for valve destruction in 15 patients (table 8-7).

The actuarial survival at 9 years (108 months) was 80% for patients receiving mitral valve prostheses, 86% for patients with aortic valve replacement, and 65% for patients with combined aortic and mitral valve replacement (figure 8-5).

Table 8-6. Thromboembolic events

	Number of patients	
MVR	7/523	(1.3%)
AVR	5/518	(1.0%)
AVR + MVR	4/238	(1.7%)
TVR	0/8	(0.0%)
Total	16/1287	(1.2%)

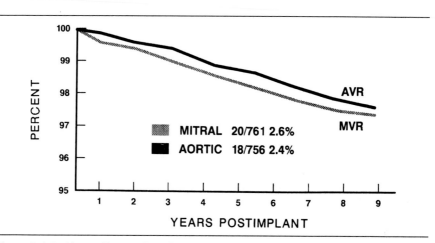

Figure 8-4. Incidence of bioprosthesis failure.

Table 8-7. Etiology of valve failure

	Number of patients	
	Aortic	Mitral
Tissue wear	14	14
Calcification	4	6
Endocarditis	10	5

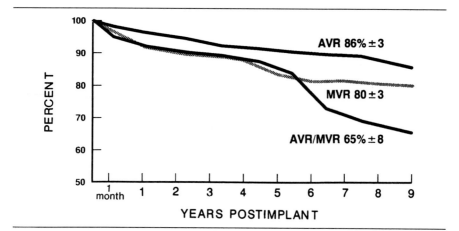

Figure 8-5. Nine-year actuarial survival for patients with mitral, aortic, and combined bioprostheses.

DISCUSSION

As with all prosthetic cardiac valves, the major questions that must be answered for porcine prostheses relate to their hemodynamic performance, durability, and incidence of thromboembolism. Our results are comparable to those reported by other institutions [1–6] and attest to the low thromboembolic rate and excellent hemodynamic qualities of the CARPENTIER-EDWARDS porcine prosthesis.

From the early experience with porcine bioprostheses, it was recognized that the occurrence of thromboembolism was reduced [7–13]. When they occur, thromboembolic episodes are more frequent in the mitral position. Chronic atrial fibrillation, enlarged left atrial cavity, and subsequent stasis of blood, producing left atrial thrombi, appear to be the major etiological factors of thromboembolism occurring in mitral valve replacement. Accordingly, anticoagulation has been recommended in this type of patient. Our current policy involves intraoperative ligation or exclusion of the left atrial appendage by direct suture technique, thereby excluding the primary focus for blood clot formation. Anticoagulation therapy is started on the third postoperative day and continued for 8 weeks. Patients are then placed on antiplatelet substances and COUMADIN® is discontinued, regardless of whether atrial fibrillation or an enlarged left atrium is present. Anticoagulation is continued for patients with mitral valve prostheses only when they were found to have a left atrial thrombus that required extensive endarterectomy of the left atrial wall for its removal. Patients with aortic bioprostheses are placed on antiplatelet substances on the third postoperative day and are not anticoagulated. Our data, utilizing this approach, substantiates the low thromboembolic rate of the CARPENTIER-EDWARDS bioprosthesis.

The functional and hemodynamic characteristics of a prosthetic valve can be determined by multiple objective parameters. With the improvement of non-invasive techniques such as the echo-Doppler, accurate evaluation of recurrent stenosis and/or insufficiency can be obtained. Left ventricular function can be accurately evaluated with gated pool scans, and the clinical status of a patient's progress can be evaluated utilizing the NYHA Clinical Classification.

The echo-Doppler study, in our series, shows low transvalvular gradients both in the aortic and mitral positions. In this regard, we feel that the smallest sized valve in the aortic position should be a 25 mm, and in the mitral position, a 31 mm. Measured gradients across mitral prostheses utilizing this non-invasive technique ranged from 0 to 4 mmHg with a standard deviation of ± 2.0. Recorded gradients across aortic valve prostheses ranged from 0 to 15 mmHg with a standard deviation of ± 2.0. This data, along with the excellent improvement in both the left ventricular function and the improvement in the clinical status, attest to the excellent, long-term hemodynamics of the porcine bioprosthesis.

The durability of the porcine bioprosthesis continues to evoke controversy. Our data show a low primary valve failure rate of 2.6% in the mitral position and 2.4% in the aortic position. Ten of the primary valve failures related to calcification were in patients 22 and 27 years of age. These occurred early in our series and, accordingly, we have not used a porcine bioprosthesis in any patient younger than 35 years of age, unless circumstances prohibit use of anticoagulants. This data, along with the excellent 9-year survivals, certainly suggests the durability of the CARPENTIER-EDWARDS porcine bioprosthesis in both the aortic and mitral positions and supports the continued use of this porcine bioprosthesis for valvular heart disease in patients 45 years of age or older.

REFERENCES

1. Cohn LH, Koster JK, Mee RBB, et al. Long-term follow-up of the Hancock bioprosthetic heart valve: A 6-year review. Circulation 1979; 60:93.
2. Oyer PE, Stinson EB, Reitz BA, et al. Long-term evaluation of the porcine xenograft bioprosthesis. J Thorac Cardiovasc Surg 1979; 78:343.
3. Williams JB, Karp RB, Kirklin JW, et al. Considerations in selection and management of patients undergoing valve replacement with glutaraldehyde-fixed porcine bioprostheses. Ann Thorac Surg 1980; 30:247.
4. Craver JM, Jones EL, McKeown P, et al. Porcine cardiac xenograft valves: Analysis of survival, valve failure, and explanation. Ann Thorac Surg 1982; 34:16.
5. Oyer PE, Stinson EB, Rossiter SJ, et al. Extended experience with the Hancock bioprosthesis. In Sebening F, Klovekorn WP, Meisner H, Struck E (eds): Bioprosthetic Cardiac Valves; Deutsches Herzzentrum, Munich 1979; pp 47–59.
6. Angell WW, Angell JD, Kosek JC. Twelve-year experience with glutaraldehyde-preserved porcine xenografts. J Thorac Cardiovasc Surg 1982; 83:493.
7. Oyer PE, Stinson EB, Griepp RB. Starr-Edwards and Hancock prostheses: Comparative analysis of late morbidity and mortality. Ann Surg 1977; 186:301.
8. Cohn LH, Sanders JG Jr, Collins JJ Jr. Aortic valve replacement with the Hancock porcine xenografts. Ann Thorac Surg 1976; 22:221.
9. Stinson EB, Griepp RB, Oyer PE, et al. Long-term experience with porcine aortic valve xenografts. J Thorac Cardiovasc Surg 1977; 73:54.
10. McIntosh CL, Michaels LL, Morrow AG, et al. Atrioventricular valve replacement with the Hancock porcine xenografts: A five-year clinical experience. Surgery 1975; 78:768.
11. Hannah H, Reis RL. Current status of porcine heterograft prostheses—a 5-year appraisal. Circulation 1976; 54(Suppl III):27.
12. Stinson EB, Griepp RB, Shumway NE. Clinical experience with a porcine aortic valve xenograft for mitral valve replacement. Ann Thorac Surg 1974; 18:391.
13. Cevese PG. Long-term results of 212 xenograft valve replacements. J Cardiovasc Surg (Torino) 1975; 16:639.

9. PRIMARY TISSUE FAILURE IN PORCINE AORTIC AND BOVINE PERICARDIAL BIOPROSTHESES

K. KAWAZOE, T. FUJITA, F. YAMAMOTO, S. TAKEUCHI, N. FUJII, H. MANABE

Abstract. *From October 1977 until December 1984, bioprostheses were routinely used for all cardiac valve replacements at the National Cardiovascular Center in Japan. Through a retrospective comparative study, the clinical consequences, especially of primary tissue failure (PTF), of the HANCOCK® porcine aortic xenograft (HX), the IONESCU-SHILEY® bovine pericardial bioprostheses, the standard model (ISU), and the low-profile model (ISL) were examined. Primary tissue failure occurred in 10 out of 95 patients with HX during 574.5 patient-years of follow-up, in 25 of 349 patients with ISU during 1373.9 patient-years, and in 6 of 131 patients with ISL during 320.7 patient-years. The linearized incidence of PTF was 1.7% per patient-year for the HX group, 1.8% per patient-year for the ISU group, and 1.6% per patient-year for the ISL group. Actuarial freedom from PTF for the HX group was 87.2 ± 4% at 9 years, 90.0 ± 2% for the ISU group at 6.5 years, and 94.2 ± 2% for ISL at 3 years. Intervals from initial valve replacement, intravascular hemolysis in PTF, and cases requiring reoperation will also be discussed. A careful follow-up of patients with the ISX valves and attention to the onset of valve failure is recommended.*

INTRODUCTION

Because of the theoretical superiority, a porcine aortic bioprosthesis had been routinely used for cardiac valve replacement at our institution from 1977 through 1980, when disadvantages with its hemodynamic performance and antithrombogenicity led us to change to the use of a bovine pericardial bioprosthesis.

Table 9-1. Distribution of bioprostheses and follow-up data

	HX	ISU	ISL
Implantation interval	Oct. 1977 to Apr. 1980	Aug. 1979 to Aug. 1983	July 1983 to Dec. 1984
Number of cases	95	349	131
Aortic valve replacement	28	147	50
Mitral valve replacement	54	152	63
Multiple valve replacement	12	42	18
Months of follow-up	51–109	41–81	24–41
(average)	(73.5)	(48.6)	(29.4)
Total follow-up (patient-years)	574.5	1373.9	320.7

HX = Hancock porcine xenograft; ISU = Ionescu-Shiley (standard); ISL = Ionescu-Shiley (low profile)

In recent years, however, it appeared that primary tissue failure in the pericardial series occurred faster and required reoperation earlier than in the porcine series. This study describes clinical consequences of primary tissue failure through a retrospective comparative study between porcine aortic and bovine pericardial bioprostheses.

PATIENT POPULATION

At the National Cardiovascular Center of Japan, the HANCOCK porcine aortic bioprosthesis (HX) was implanted in 95 patients from October 1977 to April 1980, and the IONESCU-SHILEY bovine pericardial bioprosthesis (ISPX) was used in 480 patients from August 1979 to December 1984. In 349 of 480 patients with IONESCU-SHILEY valves, the standard model (ISU) was used, and in the remaining 131 patients the low-profile model (ISL) was used from July 1983 onward.

The distribution of bioprostheses is contained in table 9-1. The cumulative duration of follow-up is 574.5 patient-years in the HX series, 1373.9 patient-years for ISU, and 320.7 patient-years for ISL.

RESULTS

Incidence of primary tissue failure

Primary tissue failure (PTF), which was defined by the findings at reoperation or autopsy, occurred in 10 patients with HX, 25 with ISU, and 6 with ISL.

Reoperations for valve failure were carried out in 39 patients; however, 2 patients with mitral ISU died from severe heart failure soon after the onset of valve failure. The linearized incidence of PTF was 1.7% per patient-year for HX, 1.8% for ISU, and 1.9% for ISL. The probability of being free from

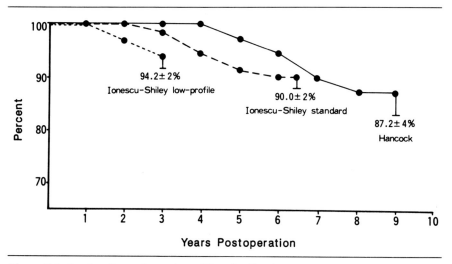

Figure 9-1. Freedom from primary tissue failure for all patients.

valve failure for all patients with HX was 87.2 ± 4% at 9 years, with ISU was 90.0 ± 2% at 6.5 years, and with ISL was 94.2 ± 2% at 3 years (figure 9-1).

Our data seem to show no apparent difference in the incidences of PTF between two types of bioprostheses and also appear to be roughly comparable to other reports [1, 2].

Intervals from initial valve replacement

The average intervals from initial valve replacement to onset of valve failure and to reoperation were 63.8 and 69.7 months in the HANCOCK series, 41.6 and 45.1 months for ISU, and 25.5 and 26.7 months for ISL (figure 9-2).

There were significant differences, not only in mean time to onset or re-operation, but also in each interval between onset and reoperation. These were 6 months in the HANCOCK series, 3.5 months for ISU, and 1 month for ISL.

Intravascular hemolysis in PTF

The increase of serum LDH level is a simple, but sufficient, parameter for chronic intravascular hemolysis in patients with valve malfunction, in comparison to normally functioning prostheses [3].

We found marked elevation of LDH levels after onset of PTF in bioprosthetic valves; significant differences among the three types of bioprostheses are shown in figure 9-3. Therefore, it was suggested that the regurgitation flow in valve failure of ISPX strongly affected red blood cells and that massive hemolysis was a main concern with limited valve durability with ISPX, even if the amount of regurgitation was still small.

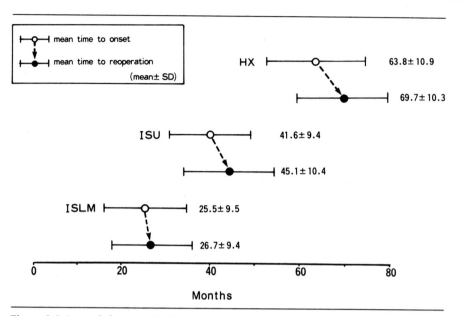

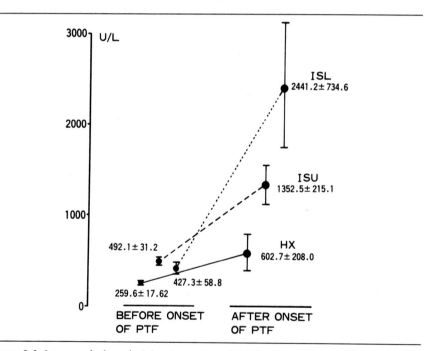

Figure 9-2. Intervals from initial valve replacement to onset of primary tissue failure and to reoperation.

Figure 9-3. Intravascular hemolysis in primary tissue failure by means of serum LDH levels.

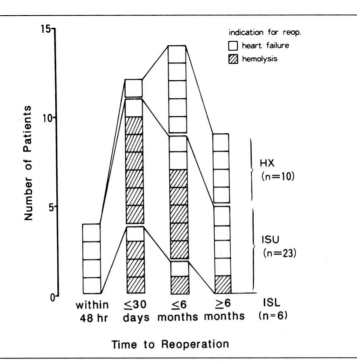

Figure 9-4. Indication for reoperation by interval from onset of valve failure to reoperation.

Indication for reoperation by the interval from onset of valve failure to reoperation

Twelve out of 25 patients with ISU failure and 4 out of 6 patients with ISL failure were forced into reoperation by hemolysis alone. Nine out of 10 ISPX patients with hemolysis have required reoperation within 1 month from onset of valve failure. In contrast to ISPX valves, all reoperations for HX failure were due to heart failure (figure 9-4).

On the other hand, critical heart failure has been recognized at the time of onset of ISU failure in 6 mitral patients. Reoperation was performed within 48 hours in 4 patients, but 2 patients died without chance of reoperation.

CONCLUSION

The important disadvantage of PTF in pericardial bioprostheses is that it appeared to occur early after implantation, resulting in the need for early re-operation because it is catastrophic and is associated with severe hemolysis.

We recommend a close follow-up of patients who received IONESCU-SHILEY valves and careful attention to the onset of valve failure.

REFERENCES

1. Brais MP, Bedard JP, Goldstein W, Kokal A, Keon WJ. Ionescu-Shiley pericardial xenografts: Follow-up of up to 6 years. Ann Thorac Surg. 1985; 39:105.

2. Jamieson WRE, Allen P, Janusz MT, Germann E, Chan F, MacNab J, Munro AI, Miyagishima RT, Gerein AN, Burr LH, Tyers GFO. First-generation porcine bioprostheses: Valve-related complications in the intermediate term. In Bodnar E, Yacoub M (eds): *Biologic and Bioprosthetic Valves.* Yorke Medical Books, New York 1986; p 105.
3. Horstkotte D, Aul C, Seipel L. Influence of valve type and valve function on chronic intravascular hemolysis following mitral and aortic valve replacement using alloprostheses. Z Kardiol 1983; 72:119.

10. MIDTERM FOLLOW-UP OF THE BIOIMPLANT™ (LIOTTA) HEART VALVE

I. GANDJBAKHCH, V. BORS, M. FONTANEL, A. PAVIE, C. CABROL, A. CABROL

Abstract. The use of a low profile bioprosthesis is interesting in particular anatomical conditions. In some patients with mitral stenosis, the left ventricular cavity is not enlarged. The characteristic low profile of this valve avoids obstruction of flow and traumatization of the left ventricular wall. In the tricuspid position, this design is particularly interesting because it leaves the right ventricular cavity totally free. From February 1981 to November 1984, 280 St. Jude Medical, Inc. BIOIMPLANT™ (Liotta) low profile bioprostheses were implanted in 257 patients in our hospital. Eighty-six patients underwent aortic valve replacement (AVR). Preoperatively, 64% of patients were in New York Heart Association (NYHA) Classes III and IV. One hundred thirty-eight patients had mitral valve replacement (MVR), and 11 had tricuspid valve replacement (TVR). Twenty-two patients underwent mitral and aortic valve replacement (DVR). The operative mortality was 8.2% (AVR 5.8%, MVR 10%, DVR 9%). The 236 operative survivors were followed over a period of 3 months to 4 years. Actuarial analysis of late results indicates an expected survival rate at 4 years of 92.2 ± 2.7% for the whole group (AVR 96%, MVR 89.2%, DVR 94.6%). The actuarial rate of patients free of thromboembolism was 98.1 ± 1% (MVR 98.7%, DVR 86.8%); 96.1 ± 2.1% of patients were predicted to be free of infection at 4 years (AVR 97.2%, MVR 94.8%). The actuarial rate of freedom from valve failure was 89.6% (AVR 83.3%, MVR 96%). Postoperatively, 91.2% of patients were in NYHA Classes I or II.*

INTRODUCTION

We have used the Liotta low profile porcine xenograft, now called the BIOIMPLANT heart valve, for the last 6 years. This true low profile device is especially useful for patients with small ventricles and small aortic roots, because it allows unobstructed blood circulation around the prosthesis. We have implanted more than 500 such tissue valves, but we will limit this discussion to our first 4 years of experience with this device.

METHODS

Between February 1981 and November 1984, 280 BIOIMPLANT heart valves were placed in 257 patients. These implantations included 86 isolated aortic replacements, 138 isolated mitral replacements, 11 isolated tricuspid replacements, and 22 double valve replacements (aortic and mitral) in 257 patients, 77 of whom were in New York Heart Association (NYHA) Classes III or IV. Valve sizes were mainly 25 mm and 26 mm outer diameter for aortic valves, 28 mm and 30 mm for mitral prostheses, and 30 mm for tricuspid valves.

Most of the aortic valves were placed in the subannular position, which allowed the use of a larger prosthesis. In some of the mitral replacements involving a heavily calcified anulus or abscess, the valve was placed in an intra-atrial position, with the use of the enlarged cuff prosthesis designed by Professor Gandjbakhch.

Associated lesions required various concomitant procedures. Aortic valve replacements involved 12 coronary artery bypasses, 8 mitral repairs, 1 total replacement of the ascending aorta, and 1 tricuspid repair. Mitral valve replacements included 18 coronary artery bypasses and 18 tricuspid repairs, while double valve replacements (aortic and mitral) required 2 coronary artery bypasses and 1 tricuspid repair.

RESULTS AND DISCUSSION

The early mortality of the first month was 5.8% in cases of isolated aortic valve replacement, 10% for isolated mitral valve replacement, and 9% in double valve replacement, for an overall mortality of 8.2%. There were no early deaths among the isolated tricuspid replacements. Two hundred thirty-six patients (92% of the survivors) were followed over a period of 3 to 48 months with a mean of 17 months, for a total of 347 patient-years.

The actuarial survival rate for all valve patients was 92.2% ± 2.7% at 4 years, including 96% for aortic, 89.2% for mitral, and 94.6% for double valve replacement. Early mortality was excluded from this analysis. There were 12 late deaths; 3 in aortic cases (4%), 8 in mitral procedures (7%), and 1 in double valve replacement.

All patients were treated with anticoagulants for 3 months postoperatively. This was subsequently discontinued, except when circumstances called for anticoagulation therapy. To date, 38% of the aortic patients and half of the other patients are receiving anticoagulation therapy.

No case of valve thrombosis was seen, but 3 cases of regressive thromboemblism have been observed, 1 at 6 months and 2 at 10 months postoperatively. This equals 0.86% per patient-year. Actuarial analysis shows that 98.1 ± 1% of patients are free of any thromboembolism at 4 years (100% for aortic, 98.7% for mitral, and 86.8% for double valve replacement).

Two incidents of valve deterioration were observed. These failures (1 aortic and 1 mitral) occurred at 29 and 44 months after implantation, in a 9-year-old girl and a 20-year-old boy, respectively. This equals 0.57% per patient-year. There were no failures in the tricuspid position. Overall, 89.6% of all patients (83.3% aortic; 96% mitral) were free from deterioration at 4 years.

Three cases of endocarditis were observed; 1 aortic and 2 mitral. A total of 96.1 ± 2.1% of patients have been free of infection at 4 years: 97.2% of aortic patients and 94.8% of mitral cases. Eight patients have been reoperated upon due to 2 valve failures, 3 cases of endocarditis, and 3 paravalvular leaks. In total, 85% of patients did not require any reoperation at 4 years (82% of aortic patients and 90% of mitral cases). Also, 83% of the patients were free of any complication at 4 years: 100% for tricuspid cases, 89% for mitral patients, 81% of aortic procedures, and 79% of double valve replacement patients.

As usual, postoperative functional status of the patients improved markedly. Before operation, 77 of the patients were in NYHA Class III or IV. After operation, 91.2% were in Classes I or II. Postoperatively, 38 patients were catheterized at 1 month, and again 1 year, after surgery. In 20 aortic patients, the average transvalvular aortic gradient was consistently found to be the same at 1 month and at 1 year after surgery: 12.4 mm Hg at rest and 17 mm Hg during exercise. Similarly, the average effective orifice area was 1.6 cm^2 at rest and increased to 2.0 cm^2 during exercise.

During the same period, 18 mitral valve replacements were examined. The average mitral transvalvular gradient was found to be low at rest (6.0 mm Hg); it increased to 12.0 mm Hg during exercise. The average mitral effective orifice was 2.0 cm^2 at rest and 2.9 cm^2 during exercise. Again, early and late results were similar.

In conclusion, this midterm follow-up shows good results, especially in terms of thromboembolism, infection, and valve dysfunction. The St. Jude Medical BIOIMPLANT valve appears to have excellent immediate and midterm results. It is a very good choice, not only for special circumstances that require a low profile valve, but also for routine valve replacement.

11. A COMPARISON OF ST. JUDE MEDICAL® AND CARPENTIER-EDWARDS® XENOGRAFT VALVES IN THE MITRAL POSITION

J. CLELAND, I. GALVIN, L. HAMILTON, D. GLADSTONE, H. O'KANE

Abstract. This study compares the clinical results of patients receiving isolated mitral valve replacement with a ST. JUDE MEDICAL® prosthesis (SJM) or a CARPENTIER-EDWARDS® xenograft (CEX) over a period of 6.5 years. There were 85 patients (66 females and 23 males) with SJM valves, ages 5 to 70 years. Ninety-four patients (63 females and 31 males), ages 29 to 71 years, had CEX valves implanted. Although the groups were not randomized, surgical techniques were comparable and myocardial protection was constant throughout the period. The CEX was used more frequently early in the study and, therefore, has a longer follow-up period (CEX: 301 patient-years; SJM: 207 patient-years). The 30-day mortality rate was 4.3% for CEX and 7% for SJM cases; late mortality was 8.5% in CEX and 5.9% in SJM patients. There were no reported cases of primary structural failure or significant hemolysis in either group. All patients in the SJM group and 80% in the CEX group were anticoagulated. Thromboembolic episodes occurred in 8 CEX patients, totaling 14 events (5 major, 9 minor), with a rate of 4.6% per patient-year. In the SJM group, 6 patients experienced isolated thromboembolic events (1 valve thrombosis, 2 major events, 3 minor), with a rate of 2.9% per patient-year. Thromboembolism resulted in 2 deaths in the CEX group and no deaths in the SJM group. Reoperation for paravalvular leaks was necessary in 5 patients (2 CEX, 3 SJM). While there were no cases of endocarditis in the SJM group, there were 3 (2 Q fever) in the CEX group with 1 death. The results in the two groups were similar in the number of patients alive and event-free at 6 years. Because of the known long-term failure rate

Table 11-1. Patient profiles (1979–1985)

	St. Jude Medical	Carpentier-Edwards Xenograft
Number of patients	85	94
Mean age	52★	55
(Range)	(5–70)	(29–71)
Sex		
Male	23	31
Female	66	63
Follow-up		
Total	207 pt-yrs	301 pt-yrs
Mean (range)	32 (2–73 months)	40 (5–70) months

★ Five patients less than 16-years-old

of tissue valves and the high percentage of tissue valves anticoagulated, our choice for mitral valve replacement is the ST. JUDE MEDICAL valve.

INTRODUCTION

During a 6.5-year period, we compared the results of isolated mitral valve replacement using either the CARPENTIER-EDWARDS xenograft (CEX) or the ST. JUDE MEDICAL (SJM) mitral prosthesis. During that time, the

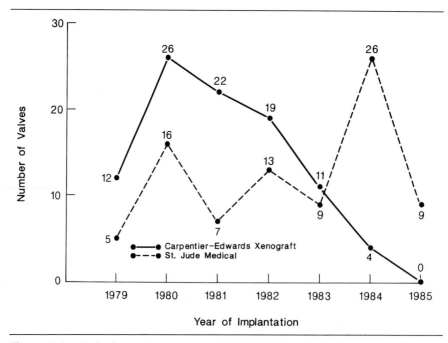

Figure 11-1. Mitral valves implanted between 1979 and 1985.

surgical techniques were comparable and myocardial protection was constant. This was not a prospective randomized study.

METHODS

The patient profiles for the two groups are reasonably comparable (table 11-1). The sex distribution was similar, however, the mean age is lower for the ST. JUDE MEDICAL group than for the CARPENTIER-EDWARDS valve group. This is because 5 children are included in the SJM experience. A total of 85 ST. JUDE MEDICAL and 94 CARPENTIER-EDWARDS prostheses were inserted. The follow-up of 207 patient-years in the ST. JUDE MEDICAL group was shorter than that of the CARPENTIER-EDWARDS patients. The mean follow-up of 32 months was also shorter.

We first started using the ST. JUDE MEDICAL prosthesis in 1979. There were more CARPENTIER-EDWARDS valves used until 1985, when we stopped using that prosthesis. In the same time frame, the number of ST. JUDE MEDICAL prostheses used increased (figure 11-1).

RESULTS AND DISCUSSION

At preoperative diagnosis, there were more patients with mitral stenosis in the SJM group, but there were more patients with mitral regurgitation and mixed mitral lesions in the CEX group. There was high incidence of atrial fibrillation: 74% SJM and 77% CEX (table 11-2).

Sixty-one percent of patients in the SJM group and 58% of CEX patients had previous operations (table 11-3). The majority of these were of closed mitral valve origin, but in the SJM group there were a larger number of patients who had repeat valve replacement. This was usually due to failure of a HANCOCK® prosthesis. Open mitral valve repair was also more common preoperatively in the SJM group.

Associated lesions and operations were followed (table 11-4). In the SJM group there were 22%, and in the CEX group 29%. There were more patients

Table 11-2. Preoperative diagnosis

	St. Jude Medical patients	Carpentier-Edwards Xenograft patients
Total patients	85	94
Mitral stenosis	40 (47%)	38 (40%)
Mitral regurgitation	24 (28%)	30 (32%)
Mixed	21 (25%)	26 (28%)
Normal sinus rhythm	22 (26%)	22 (23%)
Atrial fibrillation	63 (74%)	72 (77%)

Table 11-3. Previous cardiac operations

	St. Jude Medical	Carpentier-Edwards Xenograft
	85 patients	94 patients
Closed mitral valvotomy	38	40
Open mitral valve replacement	9	3
Open mitral valve repair	3	0
Open aortic valve repair	1	6
Open tricuspid valve repair	1	6
Total previously operated patients	52 (61%)	55 (58%)

Table 11-4. Associated lesions

	St. Jude Medical	Carpentier-Edwards Xenograft
	85 patients	94 patients
Saphenous vein grafting	8	4
Aortic repair	3	8
Tricuspid repair	3	11
Atrioventricular canal	1	0
Corrected transposition great vessels	2	0
Atrial septal defect	0	1
Acute bacterial endocarditis	2	4
Total patients with associated lesions	19 (22%)	28 (29%)

who had saphenous vein grafting in the SJM group, but more tricuspid or aortic repairs in the CEX group. Acute bacterial endocarditis was also more common in the CEX group.

The preoperative New York Heart Association (NYHA) Classification was similar in both groups (figure 11-2). There were more Class IV patients in the SJM group and more Class III patients in the CEX group. Again, although this was not a prospective study, the two groups were reasonably comparable.

Mitral valve size was different in both groups (figure 11-3). In the CEX group, the majority were either 31 mm or 33 mm. In the SJM group, the sizes were smaller: 29 mm and 31 mm.

The early mortality for both groups (table 11-5) was 5.6%: 7% SJM and 4.3% CEX. Low cardiac output was the most common cause of death, including 3 deaths in the SJM group and 3 in the CEX group. In each group, there was 1 death from perioperative myocardial infarction and 1 from multiple

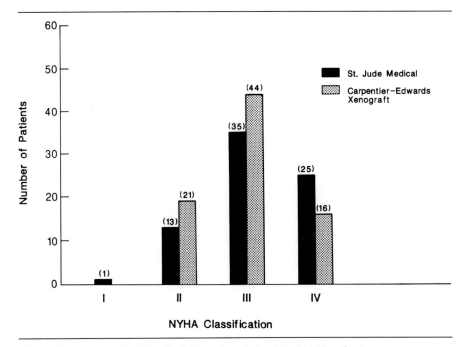

Figure 11-2. Preoperative New York Heart Association (NYHA) Classification.

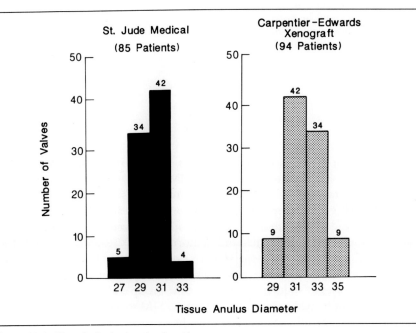

Figure 11-3. Size of mitral valves implanted.

Table 11-5. Early mortality

	St. Jude Medical	Carpentier-Edwards Xenograft
	85 patients	94 patients
Low cardiac output	3	2
Perioperative myocardial infarction	1	1
Respiratory failure	1	0
Multiple organ failure	1	1
Total (5.6%)	6 (7%)	4 (4.3%)

Table 11-6. Late mortality

	St. Jude Medical	Carpentier-Edwards Xenograft
	85 patients	94 patients
Myocardial infarction	1	1
Cerebral embolus	0	2★
Acute bacterial endocarditis	0	1★
Left ventricular failure	1	1
Subarachnoid hemorrhage	0	1★★
Intra-abdominal sepsis	0	1
Hepatorenal failure	1★	0
Sudden	2★★	1★★
Total	5 (5.9%)	8 (8.5%)
★ Valve-related	1	3
★★ Possible valve-related	2	2

organ failure. In the CEX group, there was 1 death from respiratory failure.

There were 5 (5.9%) late deaths in the SJM group and 8 (8.5%) among the CEX patients (table 11-6). Myocardial infarction was the cause of death in 1 patient in each group. Cerebral embolus caused 2 deaths and acute bacterial endocarditis lead to 1 death in the CEX group. Left ventricular failure caused 1 death in each group. Subarachnoid hemorrhage was responsible for 1 death in the CEX group. Hepatorenal failure occurred once in the SJM group, due to a paravalvular leak that caused severe hemolysis prior to the operation. There were 2 cases of sudden death in the SJM group and 1 in the CEX group. There was 1 confirmed valve-related death in SJM group, 3 among the CEX patients, and 2 possible valve-related deaths in each group.

The actuarial survival curve (figure 11-4) shows that at the end of 6 years,

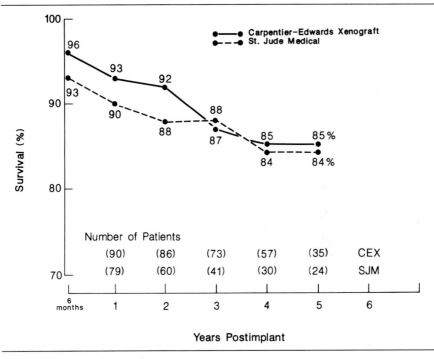

Figure 11-4. Actuarial survival.

85% and 84% of the patients were alive in the CEX and SJM groups, respectively. This includes operative mortality.

The postoperative New York Heart Association (NYHA) Classification is, again, similar in both groups (figure 11-5). More patients in the SJM group were in Class I, while there were more Class II cases in the CEX group. There was 1 CEX patient in Class III and 1 SJM case in Class IV.

As shown in table 11-7, valve thrombosis occurred in 1 patient in the SJM group, (0.5% per patient-year). There were no valve thromboses in the CEX group. There were 6 cases of thromboembolism in the SJM group (2.9% per patient-year), including the single case of valve thrombosis. However, there were 14 cases in the CARPENTIER-EDWARDS group (4.6% per patient-year). This high rate was probably because there were 3 patients who had multiple emboli. There was 1 valve failure in the CEX group, 1 anticoagulant hemorrhage in the SJM group, and 3 in the CEX group, as well as 3 cases of prosthetic valve endocarditis in the CEX group, but none in the SJM group. There were 3 cases of paravalvular leak in the SJM group that required reoperation and 2 in the CEX group. There were no cases of hemolytic anemia that were not related to paravalvular leak. Overall, there were 10 valve-related complications in the SJM group for a rate of 4.8% per

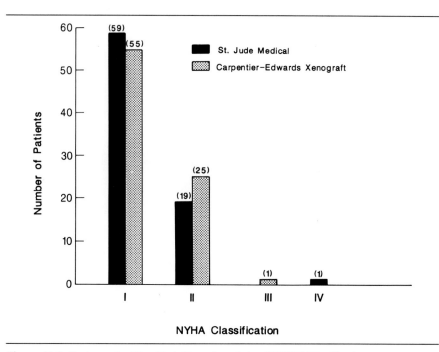

Figure 11-5. Postoperative New York Heart Association (NYHA) Classification.

patient-year and 22 in the CEX group for a rate of 7.6% per patient-year.

There were 2 deaths among CEX patients with emboli, and 1 CEX patient with bacterial endocarditis died. There was also 1 death due to paravalvular leak in the SJM group.

Table 11-7. Valve-related complications

	St. Jude Medical	% per pt-yr	Carpentier-Edwards Xenograft	% per pt-yr
Valve thrombosis	1	(0.5)	0	(0)
Embolism	5	(2.4)	14★	(4.6)
Valve failure	0	(0)	1	(0.33)
Anticoagulant hemorrhage	1	(0.5)	3	(1.0)
Prosthetic valve endocarditis	0	(0)	3★★	(1.0)
Paravalvular leak (re-op)	3★★	(1.5)	2	(0.7)
Hemolytic anemia	0	(0)	0	(0)
Total	10	(4.8)	22	(7.6)

★ Two deaths
★★ One death
CEX anticoagulation is 80%; SJM anticoagulation is 100%.

Table 11-8. Thromboembolism

	St. Jude Medical	Carpentier-Edwards Xenograft
	79 patients	90 patients
No. of patients with TEs	6	7
Valve thrombosis	1	0
Major TE	2	5
Minor TE	3	9
Total TEs	6	14
% per pt-yr	2.9	4.6
Deaths	0	2
Residual defects	1 (mild)	2 (moderate)

All patients in the SJM group and 80% in the CEX group required anti-coagulation. This was due to the very high incidence of postoperative atrial fibrillation.

Thromboembolism was examined separately (table 11-8). There were 6 patients in the SJM group who had thromboembolic events and 7 in the CEX

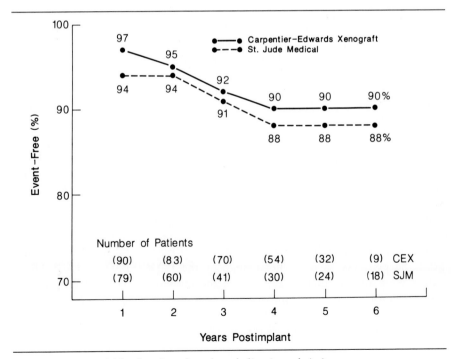

Figure 11-6. Actuarial freedom from thromboembolism (cumulative).

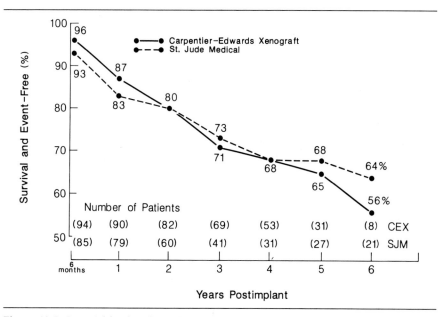

Figure 11-7. Actuarial freedom from all complications (all survivors).

group. There were 2 major and 3 minor thromboembolic episodes in the SJM group, as well as the valve thrombosis case discussed earlier. In the CEX group, there were 5 major and 9 minor incidents. A total of 6 thromboembolic events (2.9% per patient-year) occurred in the SJM group, while there were 14 (4.6% per patient-year) in the CEX group. There were with 2 deaths in the CEX group, 1 mild residual defect in the SJM group, and 2 moderate defects in the CEX group.

At the end of 6 years, the actuarial freedom from thromboembolism rates were 90% in the CEX group and 88% in the SJM group (figure 11-6). There does not appear to be any significant difference between the two groups. Actuarial freedom from complications among survivors at the end of 6 years was 64% for CEX patients and 56% for SJM patients (figure 11-7).

In summary, the results for both groups are similar in survival, thromboembolic events, and complications rates. There were fewer deaths with the ST. JUDE MEDICAL valve than with the CARPENTIER-EDWARDS xenograft. Surprisingly, a large percentage of the CARPENTIER-EDWARDS valves were anticoagulated. Because of the known long-term failure rate of bioprostheses and the high incidence of anticoagulation in this group of patients, we believe that, overall, the ST. JUDE MEDICAL valve was a better long-term choice for these patients.

12. THREE-DIMENSIONAL VISUALIZATION OF VELOCITY FIELDS DOWNSTREAM OF THE ST. JUDE MEDICAL AORTIC VALVE IMPLANTED IN PIGS

J. M. HASENKAM, J. H. ØSTERGAARD, E. M. PEDERSEN, P. K. PAULSEN, B. A. SCHURIZEK, H. STØDKILDE-JØRGENSEN

Abstract. *The study of velocity fields downstream of artificial heart valves is an important part of the evaluation since, for example, hemolysis and thrombus formation are considered to be caused by hemodynamic disturbances. Traditionally, velocity profiles have been visualized in one or two diameters over the cross-sectional area, leaving the major part of the flow field unstudied. Therefore, we have developed a method for a three-dimensional visualization of velocity fields downstream of aortic valves in vivo. Using standard cardiopulmonary bypass, size 25 mm ST. JUDE MEDICAL® valves were implanted in the aortic position of 15 pigs weighing approximately 100 kg each. After a short postcardioplegic recovery, the point blood velocities in the ascending aorta were registered with a 1 mm hot-film anemometer needle probe. By computerized drawing technique, a three-dimensional visualization of velocity profiles was made. Throughout one mean heart cycle (obtained by ensemble averaging of the velocity signals) 100 profiles were made. By successive photography of each profile, an animated film was made, giving a dynamic impression of the velocity profile development downstream of the ST. JUDE MEDICAL valve during one heart cycle. In the acceleration phase of systole, the profiles were flat. At top systole, the characteristics of the valve design were recognized. This showed higher velocities over the major orifices and the central opening between the leaflets and low velocities in the hinge areas.*

INTRODUCTION

Although heart valve implantation is a safe, routine procedure, late valve-related complications such as thromboembolism, tissue overgrowth, hemolysis, endothelial damage, infection, mechanical failure, and paravalvular leakage still hamper complete success.

The majority of these complications are considered related to fluid dynamics [1–4]. Therefore, one way of improving results in heart valve replacement is to optimize the hemodynamic performance of the valves. Design alterations or designing completely new valves must be based on a thorough knowledge of fluid dynamics of the valves used until now. The fluid mechanical characteristics of artificial heart valves have been investigated in more or less advanced steady-state or pulsatile circulation models for description of pressure drops [5], velocity fields [6], energy loss, closing and leakage volume [7], and other fluid mechanical parameters for describing flow disturbances.

Three-dimensional visualizations of velocity fields were first made in vivo by Paulsen et al. [8–10]. Later, Hanle [11] presented similar visualizations, using laser Doppler anemometry in a steady-state and pulsatile flow model.

Extensive comparative hemodynamic studies in the vicinity of artificial heart valves have not gained widespread use in animals [12, 13].

For comparative purposes, linking the information obtained from in vitro studies to in vivo results, we have used an acute swine model for hemodynamic studies of different aortic valve prostheses. This model enabled a dynamic three-dimensional visualization of velocity fields downstream of artificial heart valves implanted in the aortic position.

In this study, velocity fields downstream of an aortic ST. JUDE MEDICAL valve implanted in the model were registered.

MATERIALS AND METHODS

Animal preparation

Mixed Danish Landrace and Yorkshire swine weighing approximately 100 kg were used for implantation of size 25 mm ST. JUDE MEDICAL aortic valves, using cardiopulmonary bypass and cold cardioplegic arrest.

Anesthesia and surgical techniques are described elsewhere [14].

Principle of measurement and analysis

Blood velocity measurements were accomplished in the ascending aorta, two diameters downstream of the aortic valve, immediately before the aortic arch, using an L-shaped 1 mm conical hot-film anemometer needle probe. The probe was inserted into the aortic lumen through a purse string suture in the anterior vessel wall and positioned at 41 predetermined measuring points (figure 12-1).

The hot-film anemometer principle of measurement is that a thin metal film, mounted on the tip of the probe, is heated 5 °C above blood temperature, and the passing blood tends to cool off the film. The effect required to main-

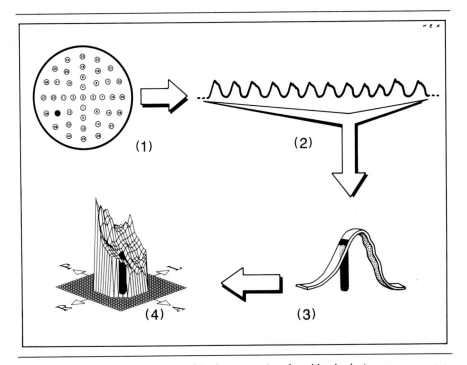

Figure 12-1. Schematic presentation of the data processing, from blood velocity measurements to the three-dimensional visualization of velocity profiles. (1) Velocity is measured at selected points in the cross-sectional area of the vessel. (2) Data was collected at each point for 20 heart cycles. (3) A mean heart cycle was obtained by ensemble averaging for each measuring point. (4) Blood velocity of all measuring points at a specific time in the heart cycle is presented three dimensionally. Velocity is indicated by the height of the profile. Orientations are: A = anterior; P = posterior; R = right vessel wall, and L = left vessel wall.

tain film temperature is an expression of the blood velocity in the measuring point. The hot-film anemometer system was a DANTEC (formerly DISA) system (55 M 01 Main Unit, 55 M 10 Standard Bridge, and 55 M 25 Linearizer), which is described in more detail elsewhere [15].

In each measuring point, 20 heart cycles were registered and recorded on a TEAC XR 510 analog data recorder for later analysis. The recorded data were A/D converted at a sample frequency of 400 Hz, using a seventh order analog 55 Hz low-pass antialiasing filter. The digitized data were stored and processed on an RMX microcomputer, where the heart cycles from each measuring point were subjected to ensemble averaging, giving 41 mean velocity curves as indicated in figure 12-1.

The trigger point in each systole was indicated manually on a graphic screen for visual control.

The ensemble averaged curves were processed by a Cyber CDC computer, enabling a three-dimensional visualization of velocity profiles, as seen in figure

12-1. The software was based on a graphic software package (DISSPLA). By plotting 100 velocity profiles during one mean heart cycle and using animated film techniques, a film that dynamically shows the velocity profile development throughout the heart cycle was made.

RESULTS

Velocity profiles at different times in the heart cycle are seen in figure 12-2.

In the early phases of the systolic acceleration phase, the velocity profiles were generally flat. The valve characteristics were most evidently reflected at top systole, showing high velocity zones downstream of the two major orifices and low velocities in the hinge areas and in the central part of the flow field. In the systolic deceleration phase, the profile was again smoothed and now skewed, revealing higher velocities to the posterior-left than to the anterior-right vessel wall.

DISCUSSION

Although in vitro studies offer very detailed information on velocity fields downstream of artificial heart valves, it is always questionable how comparable the mock circulations are to hemodynamics in humans carrying an artificial heart valve.

As swine have several cardiovascular anatomic and physiologic similarities with humans, we consider this animal a suitable model for hemodynamic studies of artificial aortic valves.

The velocity profiles presented in this study correspond well with those from model studies using a similar technique [6, 16] and with those presented by others using two-dimensional visualization techniques based on laser Doppler anemometry [5, 17].

The velocity profiles reveal large velocity gradients within the flow field, especially in the hinge areas where relative stasis areas were found. These stasis areas correspond with locations for thrombus formation reported clinically [18].

The velocity profile downstream of the ST. JUDE MEDICAL valve is rather uniform and does not present as large velocity gradients in vitro as, for example, tilting or pivoting disc valves [6]. Especially advantageous is the lack of high velocity zones in the area near the wall. This may reduce the risk of endothelial damage due to high turbulent and laminar shear stress levels.

The dynamic three-dimensional visualization, particularly when presented with animated film technique, is very illustrative and imparts a better understanding of the velocity profile development during systole.

The present identification of velocity fields comparable to those obtained from in vitro results, along with a thorough characterization of the swine model [14], encourages more advanced studies of turbulent shear stresses in swine, subjected to different hemodynamic loads after implantation of artificial heart valves.

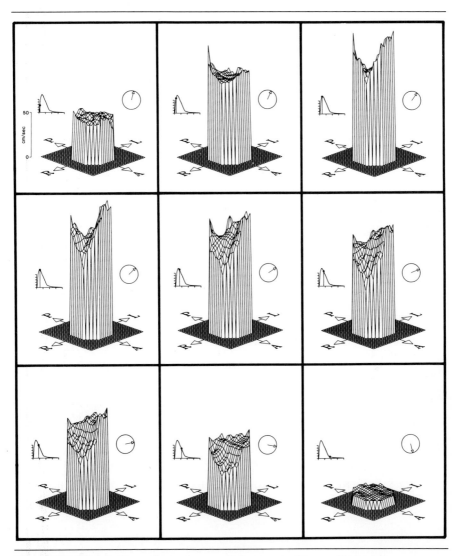

Figure 12-2. The velocity profile development during systole, illustrated by instantaneous profiles shown at time windows 4, 7, 10, 13, 16, 19, 22, 28, and 46 of the 100 comprised in one mean heart cycle. The time in heart cycle is indicated in the small curve in the upper left corner of each profile. The time after start of systole is indicated in the arrowed circle. Orientations are: A = anterior; P = posterior; R = right vessel wall, and L = left vessel wall.

REFERENCES

1. Hung TC, Hochmuth RM, Joist JH, Sutera SP. Shear-induced aggregation and lysis of platelets. Trans Am Soc Artific Internal Organs 1976; XXII:285–291.
2. Yoganathan AP, Corcoran WH, Harrison EC, Carl JR. The Björk-Shiley aortic prosthesis:

Flow characteristics, thrombus formation and tissue overgrowth. Circulation 1978; 58:70–76.

3. Sutera SP, Mehrjardi MH. Deformation and fragmentation of human red blood cells in turbulent shear flow. Biophys J 1975; 15:1–10.

4. Fry DL. Acute vascular endothelial changes associated with increased blood velocity gradients. Circ Res 1968; 22:165–197.

5. Bruss K-H, Reul H, van Gilse J, Knott E. Pressure drops and velocity flow fields at four mechanical heart valve prostheses: Björk-Shiley Standard, Björk-Shiley Concave-Convex, Hall-Kaster and St. Jude Medical. Life Support Syst 1983; 1:3–22.

6. Hasenkam JM, Westphal D, Reul H, Gormsen J, Giersiepen M, Stødkilde-Jørgensen H, Paulsen PK. Three-dimensional visualization of axial velocity profiles downstream of six different mechanical aortic valve prostheses, measured with a hot-film anemometer in a steady state flow model. J Biomech 1987; 20(4):353–364.

7. Knott E, Reul H, Steinseifer U. Pressure drop, energy loss and closure volume of prosthetic heart valves in aortic and mitral position under pulsatile flow conditions. Life Support Syst 1986; Suppl 2(4):139–141.

8. Paulsen PK, Gormsen J. An easy and exact intraluminal positioning of velocity probes in great vessels. Clin Phys Physiol Meas 1981; 2(1):53–56.

9. Paulsen PK, Albrechtsen O. Visualizing velocity profiles in great arteries. A preliminary report. J Biomech 1982; 15:61–63.

10. Paulsen PK, Hasenkam JM. Three-dimensional visualization of velocity profiles in the ascending aorta in dogs, measured with a hot-film anemometer. J Biomech 1983; 16(3): 201–210.

11. Hanle DD. In vitro fluid dynamics of prosthetic aortic valves in steady and pulsatile flow. Ph.D. thesis, California Institute of Technology 1984; Pasadena.

12. Gentle CR, Arundel PA, Hamilton DI, Swales PD. Development of a twin flap, porous ceramic mitral valve prosthesis. J. Biomed Eng 1981; 3:3–8.

13. Arbustini E, Jones M, Moses RD, Eidbo EE, Caroll RJ, Ferrans VJ. Modifications by the Hancock T6 process of calcification of bioprosthetic cardiac valves implanted in sheep. Am J Cardiol 1984; 53:1388–1396.

14. Hasenkam JM, Østergaard JH, Pedersen EM, Paulsen PK, Nygaard H, Schurizek BA, Johannsen G. A model for acute hemodynamic studies in the ascending aorta in pigs. Cardiovas Res, in press.

15. Paulsen PK. The hot-film anemometer—a method for blood velocity determination. I. In vitro comparison with the electromagnetic flowmeter. Eur Surg Res 1980; 12:140–148.

16. Hasenkam JM, Giersiepen M, Reul H. Three-dimensional visualization of velocity fields downstream of six mechanical aortic valves in a pulsatile flow model. J Biomech, in press.

17. Woo Y-R, Yoganathan AP. In vitro pulsatile flow velocity and turbulent shear stress measurements in the vicinity of mechanical aortic valve prostheses. Life Support Syst 1985; 3:283–312.

18. Prabhu S, Friday KJ, Reynolds D, Elkins D, Lazzara R. Thrombosis of aortic St. Jude valve. Ann Thorac Surg 1986; 41:332–333.

13. QUALITY OF LIFE AFTER VALVE REPLACEMENT WITH THE ST. JUDE MEDICAL BIOIMPLANT™ HEART VALVE: A FOUR-YEAR STUDY

S. L. CRONJÉ, C. A. CURCIO

Abstract. *We restricted the use of the St. Jude Medical, Inc. BIOIMPLANT*^{TM} *heart valve to patients in an underdeveloped population group where anticoagulation was not possible and in females anticipating childbearing. Between 1983 and 1986, 158 patients received 180 valves. All patients received at least 1 BIOIMPLANT valve; 17 patients also received ST. JUDE MEDICAL® mechanical valves. Seven MEDTRONIC HALL*^{TM} *valves were implanted in the aortic position. Forty-four patients were male and 114 were female. Mean age was 31 years. The majority of patients were in New York Heart Association (NYHA) Class III or IV. All patients received dipyridamole and aspirin, but not warfarin. The overall perioperative mortality was 5% (8 of 158 patients). Fifteen of the 158 patients could not be contacted, giving a follow-up of 90%. The longest follow-up was 4 years; the minimum was 4 months. One hundred thirty-five patients were followed for a total of 3050 months, with a mean follow-up period of 21 months. Good hemodynamic function and improved quality of life were demonstrated by the low operative mortality (5%), a generally uncomplicated postoperative course, and dramatic improvement in Functional Class. Most patients achieved an improvement of 2 or 3 NYHA Classes. In addition, since these patients did not receive anticoagulants, they were not subject to hemorrhagic complications. There were no late deaths, but 1 mitral valve prosthesis had to be replaced 23 months after insertion, due to diffuse calcification of the valve. The thromboembolic rate was 1.3% per patient-year (3 patients). In summary, although a favorable and encouraging initial experience has been documented, longer term follow-up studies will be required, especially to determine whether the low early failure rate will accelerate.*

INTRODUCTION

When patients require a valve replacement but anticoagulation is contraindicated, they present a difficult problem. On the one hand, there are the thromboembolic complications of mechanical valves and, on the other hand, the expected poor durability of bioprostheses.

We anticipated the risks associated with mechanical valves without anticoagulation to be greater and selected the BIOIMPLANT bioprosthesis for this group of patients.

Apart from low thrombogenicity, the BIOIMPLANT valve had some other attractive qualities: low profile, flexible stent, and low pressure fixation. In the mitral position, the low profile reduces the possibilities of posterior ventricular wall perforation and of aortic outflow tract obstruction. In addition, it makes the valve suitable for patients in which anatomical factors (e.g., a small left ventricle or narrow aortic root) preclude the use of a high profile prosthesis. Our greatest concern was for accelerated valve dysfunction.

PATIENTS AND METHODS

The patients were all from an underdeveloped population group, mostly being referred from rural areas and neighboring African states. The geographic situation, low patient compliance, and unavailability of warfarin were the contraindications for anticoagulation.

From 1983 to 1986, 158 patients received 180 BIOIMPLANT valves. In addition, 24 mechanical valves were implanted in the same group (17 ST. JUDE MEDICAL and 7 MEDTRONIC HALL), a total of 204 valves (table 13-1).

Ninety-seven patients had isolated mitral valve replacement (MVR); 14 patients, isolated aortic valve replacement (AVR); 37 patients, double (aortic and mitral) valve replacement (DVR). One patient had triple valve replacement (aortic, mitral, and tricuspid), 1 patient had mitral and tricuspid valve replacement, and 1 patient had pulmonary valve replacement (table 13-3). The

Table 13-1. Spectrum of valves used in 158 patients

Position	Number of Patients	BioImplant	St. Jude Medical	Medtronic Hall
Mitral	97	97		
Aortic	14	14		
Mitral–aortic	37	50	17	7
Mitral–aortic–tricuspid	1	3		
Mitral–tricuspid	7	14		
Tricuspid	1	1		
Pulmonary	1	1		
Total	158	180	17	7

Table 13-2. Valve sizes and distribution of 180 BioImplant valves

| Position | Sizes of valves (mm) | | | | | | | | | Subtotal |
	19	21	23	24	25	26	28	30	32	
Mitral							71	48	23	142
Aortic			15	6	3	4				28
Tricuspid							3	5	1	9
Pulmonary		1								1
Total										180

Table 13-3. Valve sizes and types of aortic valves

| Position | Sizes of valves (mm) | | | | | Subtotal |
	21	23	24	25	26	
Aortic BioImplant		15	6	3	4	28
Aortic St. Jude Medical (with mitral BioImplant)	5	12				17
Aortic Medtronic Hall (with mitral BioImplant)	1	3		3		7
Total						52

valve sizes, distribution of the valves, and types of aortic valves used are reflected in tables 13-2 and 13-3.

The predominant mitral valve lesions were mixed mitral stenosis and incompetence. The predominant aortic valve lesion was aortic incompetence. The patient who had a pulmonary replacement was in right heart failure due to pulmonary valve incompetence after repair of Tetralogy of Fallot. The isolated tricuspid valve replacement was done for bacterial endocarditis in a 5-year-old child. One patient had an ascending aorta replacement with a 23 mm BIOIMPLANT valve sutured into a 25 mm graft. Sixteen patients (10%) had emergency operations.

The mean age was 31 years for the whole group. The youngest patient was 5-years-old, and all the others were older than 12 years. Eighty-five patients (54%) were younger than 35 years. Forty-four patients were male and 114 female. The majority of patients were in New York Heart Association (NYHA) Class III or IV (table 13-4). A large number of patients had severe pulmonary hypertension (table 13-5).

Valve implantation was performed with standard cardiopulmonary bypass, moderate systemic hypothermia, and cold asanguineous cardioplegic arrest. Mitral prostheses were generally implanted with a continuous suture, except in cases where a previous prosthesis had been implanted or when the anulus was affected by bacterial endocarditis. In the latter, interrupted figure-of-eight

Table 13-4. Preoperative NYHA
Classification of 158 patients

NYHA Class	Number of patients
I	0
II	7
III	105
IV	46

Table 13-5. Preoperative hemodynamic data in 57 patients

Pulmonary artery mean pressure (mm Hg)	Number of patients	
	Isolated mitral valve replacement	Double valve replacement
0–19	—	—
20–29	—	—
30–39	—	—
40–59	3	7
60–79	19	21
80	5	2
Total patients	27	30

or mattress sutures were used. Interrupted figure-of-eight sutures were used for the implantation of aortic prostheses.

RESULTS

Early mortality

Eight of the 158 patients (5%) died within 30 days or during the same hospital admission: 4.1% of the single mitral valve replacement group and 8.9% of the multiple valve replacement group.

An analysis of operative mortality is shown in table 13-6. Four patients were cases of isolated mitral valve replacement, 3 had mitral and tricuspid valve replacement, and 1 had aortic and mitral valve replacement. Four of the operative deaths occurred in patients operated on as emergencies.

Follow-up

Fifteen patients were lost to follow-up (10%). The remaining survivors were followed up for a total period of 3050 months, with a mean follow-up of 21 months.

Thromboembolism

All patients were managed on dipyridamole 50, 100 mg t.d.s. and aspirin 150 mg daily, but no patient was anticoagulated. Thromboembolic events were

Table 13-6. Early mortality involving 8 of 158 patients (5%)

Patient number	Valve position and size	Remarks	Cause of death
1	MVR 28 TVR 30	Severe pulmonary hypertension 115/80 mmHg	Low output; death in operating room
2	MVR 30 AVR 23	advanced endocarditis	Heart failure
3	MVR 30 TVR 28	Two previous MVR	Low output; cause unknown (no PM)
4	MVR 28 TVR 23	Advanced bacterial endocarditis	Pre- and postoperative renal failure
5	MVR 28	—	Low cardiac output
6	MVR 28	Several sudden episodes of ventricular fibrillation	Arrhythmia
7	MVR 32	Clotted mechanical valve	Low cardiac output
8	MVR 28	—	Wound infection, sepsis

Table 13-7. Thromboembolic complications in 3 patients

Patient number	Valve position and size	Time postoperative	Characteristics
1	MVR 30 mm	5 months	Minor
2	MVR 28 mm	10 months	Major, left hemiparesis
3	MVR 30 mm	4 months	Mild, (poor L.V. function, clot in L.V.)

defined as documented episodes resulting in permanent or temporary central nervous system, visceral, or peripheral ischemia.

Three patients had a total of 3 embolic episodes (1.3 per 100 patient-years, table 13-7). Two episodes were mild and 1 serious, leaving the patient with a left hemiparesis. One patient who had a mild embolic episode was found to have a poorly contracting left ventricle with a clot in the left ventricle. The patient is now on permanent warfarin therapy.

After these incidents, all 3 patients were hospitalized and anticoagulated with warfarin sodium (2 patients for 2 months during their hospital stays and the above-mentioned patient, permanently).

Valve failure

One valve failure due to bioprosthetic valve calcification occurred. This 18-year-old male presented with a calcified valve and perforation of a leaflet 23 months after the implantation of a size 28 mitral BIOIMPLANT valve. He also had mild aortic incompetence at the initial operation. Despite the aortic incompetence and the malfunctioning bioprosthesis, the patient deteriorated over a period of a few days and traveled a long distance to be operated on as a semi-emergency.

Late mortality and other complications

There have been no late deaths or late complications, such as endocarditis, paravalvular leaks, thrombotic obstruction, etc. Nevertheless, as the causes for the 10% of patients lost to follow-up are unknown, the number of valve-related deaths and complications may be underestimated.

Pregnancy in 4 patients with BIOIMPLANT valves

Four patients became pregnant and went to term with normal, living new-borns. No thromboembolic or hemorrhagic events occurred. All of them were cases of single mitral valve replacement, were in NYHA Class I, and were in sinus rhythm.

Functional improvement

There was dramatic improvement in clinical status as shown in figure 13-1.

DISCUSSION

We conclude that the quality of life in this group of patients after valve replacement is favorable. We base the conclusion on the gratifying functional improvement, low operative morbidity, low valve failure rate, low thromboembolic rate, absence of other valve-related complications, and uneventful pregnancies. In addition, patients were not subject to the risk of hemorrhagic complications associated with anticoagulants.

Due to the geographic location of patients, long distance traveling at frequent intervals for monitoring of anticoagulation would have been very troublesome and would have influenced the quality of life significantly.

The psychological advantage of the possibility of pregnancy in this group also can not be underestimated.

The problem of durability of tissue valves, in general, is well recognized [1]. Low failure rates initially, which accelerate around the sixth or seventh year after insertion, have been reported [2].

Accelerated calcification of bioprostheses in children is also well recognized [3]. This applies to young adults and has been demonstrated in all age groups under 35 years of age. Reflecting these facts and taking into consideration that 54% of the group of patients discussed here are younger than 35 years, the continuing need for vigilance and further follow-up is emphasized.

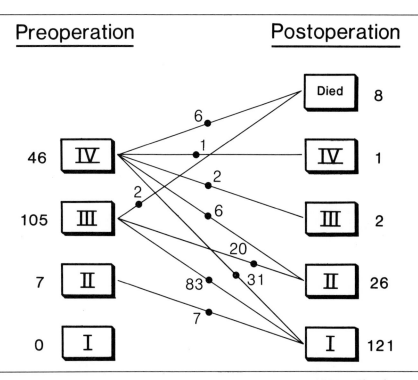

Figure 13-1. Functional improvement in New York Heart Association (NYHA) Classification. The figure shows the number of patients in each category preoperatively and postoperatively, as well as the number of patients transferring between classes.

REFERENCES

1. Magilligan DJ, Lewis JW, Tilley B, Peterson E. The porcine bioprosthetic valve: 12 years later. J Thorac Cardiovasc Surg 1985; 89:499–507.
2. Cowan JC. Valve replacement: Natural history and comparison of prostheses. Current Opinion in Cardiology 1986; 1:228–232.
3. Antunes MJ. Bioprosthetic valve replacement in children: Long-term follow-up of 135 isolated mitral valve implantations. Eur Heart J 1984; 5:913–918.

14. CINEFLUOROSCOPIC FOLLOW UP OF THE ST. JUDE MEDICAL® VALVE IN THE AORTIC POSITION

R. S. HARTZ, S. O'MARA, S. N. MEYERS, D. J. MEHLMAN

Abstract. *Follow-up of patients with prosthetic heart valves is greatly facilitated by noninvasive studies. Since the ST. JUDE MEDICAL® valve is readily visualized radiographically, we performed nonenhanced cinefluoroscopy on 72 occasions in 62 patients after aortic valve replacement with this prothesis. Five patients had serial studies. Both leaflets were adequately visualized in all but 1 patient. The study was grossly normal to objective interpretation in 63 of 72 studies, slightly abnormal (slight stuttering or asymmetry of leaflet motion) in 6, and grossly abnormal in 3. It was possible to measure the opening and closing angles (minimal and maximal interleaflet angles) and to generate leaflet velocities and acceleration. In the 3 patients with grossly abnormal valve motion (leaflet partially or fully immobilized), the fluoroscopic study modified the therapy. The group of patients as a whole modified our approach to postoperative anticoagulation in the ST. JUDE MEDICAL aortic valve patients. In conclusion, the ST. JUDE MEDICAL valve lends itself to easily performed, non-enhanced cinefluoroscopic examination. Our data support routine performance of this test postoperatively and at serial intervals, especially when valve malfunction is suspected.*

INTRODUCTION

Noninvasive visualization of prosthetic heart valves, such as the ST. JUDE MEDICAL valve, can provide valuable information for patient management. A simple technique for cinefluoroscopic visualization has resulted in changes in patient therapy for 3 grossly abnormal cases, as will be discussed.

METHODS

The study group consisted of 62 patients who had aortic valve replacement. The mean patient age was 57 years, in an age range of 22 to 83 years. Patients were initially examined when they returned as outpatients. Subsequently, the study was expanded and visualization was performed postoperatively, prior to patient release. The mean examination time was 19.7 months, in a range of 3 days to 5.5 years -after implantation. Within the group of 62 patients, 72 studies were performed. Five patients underwent serial studies.

The studies were performed in the catheterization laboratory. A patient underwent initial biplane fluoroscopy for 20 to 30 seconds, until both leaflets could be visualized. Nonenhanced cinefluoroscopy followed at 60 frames per second. The frames were adjusted by the angiographer until one of four reference lines, through which neither leaflet passed in diastole, was obtained. A spark pen was used to mark the computer screen at the four reference points representing the two ends of the leaflets. Views both parallel and perpendicular to the leaflets were obtained. Typical examples are shown in figure 14-1. A simple computer program was used to obtain qualitative data on opening and closing angles (minimal and maximal interleaflet angles) and to generate leaflet velocities and accelerations.

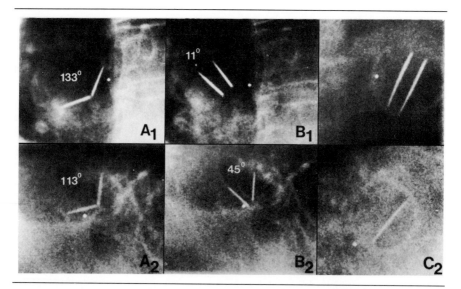

Figure 14-1. Computer-enhanced cinefluoroscopy showing a normally functioning St. Jude Medical aortic valve (upper panel) and a thrombosed St. Jude Medical aortic valve (lower panel). A_1 = closed (left anterior oblique); B_1 = open (left anterior oblique); C_1 = open (craniocaudal); A_2 = closed (left anterior oblique, closing angle diminished); B_2 = open (left anterior oblique, posterior leaflet immobile); C_2 = open (craniocaudal, immobile leaflet not visualized). [Reproduced with permission from Hartz RS, et al. J Thorac Cardiovasc Surg 1986; 92:684–690.]

Parallel views were the basis for the quantitative data. Four angles were measured, those of the first and second leaflets, the interleaflet angle, and the bisected interleaflet angle relative to the horizontal, called the bisector angle, which was used to examine leaflet asymmetrical movement.

It should be stressed that each of these patients made an elective return to the laboratory. None returned urgently with an abnormal valve.

RESULTS

Data from 20 cases were evaluated qualitatively and quantitatively by three different cardiologists: the cardiologist performing the test, a noninvasive cardiologist from the clinical service, and the principal investigator. There was no statistically significant variation among their findings.

In the qualitative analysis phase, one of three interpretations was made. These were: grossly normal; slightly abnormal, in which there was a slight stuttering or asymmetry of leaflet motion; or grossly abnormal, in which case either the opening or the closing angle of the prosthesis was distinctly abnormal or where one leaflet did not move at all.

Both leaflets were well visualized in 61 of 62 patients. Results were grossly normal by objective interpretation in 63 of 72 studies. Slightly abnormal results were found in 6 instances and grossly abnormal results were obtained for 3 patients.

Results of the visualization study prompted changes in therapy for the 3 grossly abnormal patients. The first patient was a 70-year-old man, who related that he had had a myocardial infarction. Visualization showed that one of the valve leaflets was immobile. He had wide-open aortic regurgitation upon physical examination, although he was extremely stable. Immediately after the study he was admitted and subsequently underwent aortic valve replacement with a porcine prosthesis.

The second patient had mild hemolysis. She was being followed by her cardiologist, who presumed that she simply had a small paravalvular leak. When she was examined in the study, marked annular calcification was noted. She related that she had not been taking her COUMADIN®. Given her high risk for reoperation, her anticoagulation therapy was adjusted. She was followed in serial visualizations. Six weeks into COUMADIN therapy, full leaflet motion had returned.

In a third patient who had a small cerebrovascular accident (CVA) while on inadequate COUMADIN therapy, the prothrombin time was adjusted with subsequent return of leaflet motion.

Note that thrombolytic therapy was not used on any of these patients.

DISCUSSION

As a whole, the group of patients modified our approach to postoperative anticoagulation in the ST. JUDE MEDICAL aortic valve patients.

The ST. JUDE MEDICAL prosthesis readily lends itself to simple, nonenhanced cinefluoroscopic examination. Given the useful information that is obtained, we recommend it to all patients with this prosthesis, prior to hospital discharge. Serial examination is encouraged in high-risk patients, especially when leaflet malfunction is suspected or when a patient's anticoagulation therapy must be discontinued.

15. THROMBOEMBOLISM IN ADULTS WITH ST. JUDE MEDICAL® VALVES ON TICLOPIDINE AND ASPIRIN MAINTENANCE

H. M. KIM, K. T. KIM

Abstract. We evaluated the risks of thromboembolism, valve thrombosis, anticoagulant hemorrhage, and sudden cardiac death in two groups of patients. The groups were similar in age, sex, and associated cardiovascular diseases except for the method of prevention of thromboembolism and length of follow-up. The group receiving warfarin consisted of 74 patients with 85 valves. Patients were maintained on long-term warfarin therapy. Eight of the 74 patients in the warfarin group did not survive the operative period, for a mortality of 10.8%. Prevention of thromboembolism was managed solely with warfarin to maintain the prothrombin time of 1.5 times control. The group receiving ticlopidine and aspirin consisted of 88 patients with 93 heart valves. Patients received ticlopidine (500 mg) and aspirin (500 mg) daily for 3 months postoperatively and in half doses thereafter. Three of the 88 patients did not survive the operative period, for an operative mortality of 3.4%. Warfarin was added postoperatively for 3 months for 39 of the 88 ticlopidine and aspirin group patients with high risk factors. Patients were followed-up from 36 to 120 months, with a mean of 33.5 months, in the warfarin group; and 1 to 36 months, with a mean of 8.5 months in the ticlopidine and aspirin group. At the most recent follow-up, 90% of the patients were in New York Heart Association (NYHA) Classes I and II. There were 5 late deaths in the warfarin group, 3 due to thromboembolism and 2 due to anticoagulant-related cerebral hemorrhage. Nonfatal attacks of thromboembolism and anticoagulant-related hemorrhage were noted in 10 other cases during follow-up. There were no late deaths in the ticlopidine and aspirin group during the short period of follow-up, except 1 case 35 days after mitral valve replacement, already included in the operative deaths. There was no case of primary valve failure or anticoagulant-related hemorrhage, except minor epistaxis and hypermenorrhea in the ticlopidine and aspirin group during this follow-up. It is our strong impression that combining ticlopidine and aspirin in low-risk adults has a synergistic effect and had superior results in preventing thromboembolism without anticoagulant-related hemorrhage. Warfarin is also necessary in high-risk adults for preventing early thrombus formation along the valve suture line. We recommend antiplatelet aggregator therapy with ticlopidine and aspirin in low-risk adult patients with ST. JUDE MEDICAL® valves and additional warfarin for 3 months in the high-risk adults with ST. JUDE MEDICAL valves.

INTRODUCTION

Thromboembolism is one of the main complications in the course of prosthetic cardiac valve replacement. Prevention of thromboembolism after valve replacement is mandatory for patients.

Data from Tepley [1] revealed the differences in combined fatal and nonfatal events in two time eras, representing decreased thromboembolism from 6.3% to 4.4% per patient-year with increasing hemorrhage from 1.3% to 4.3% per patient-year. Although the thromboembolism rate falls, we note that the rate of hemorrhage associated with use of anticoagulation is increased. It is not possible to determine if this is a cause and effect relationship, but it tends to suggest that the decrease in the incidence of embolism is associated with an increase in anticoagulation morbidity.

To determine the necessity of long-term prevention of thromboembolism after prosthetic cardiac valve replacement in adults, we evaluated the risks of thromboembolism, valve thrombosis, anticoagulant-related hemorrhage, and sudden cardiac death in two groups of patients.

PATIENTS AND METHODS

Clinical trial profile

The group receiving warfarin consisted of 74 adults with 85 valves, including 60 tissue valves (54 CARPENTIER-EDWARDS® and 6 IONESCU-SHILEY®) and 25 mechanical valves (17 BJÖRK-SHILEY® and 8 STARR-EDWARDS®). The male to female ratio was 34:40 and ages ranged from 18 to 65 years (mean 37.5 years). Patients were maintained on long-term warfarin therapy for 10 years, from October 1976 to September 1986.

The group using ticlopidine and aspirin consisted of 88 patients who received 93 ST. JUDE MEDICAL heart valves (54 mitral, 29 aortic, and 5 double valve replacements) for 3 years, from October 1983 to September 1986. Patients received ticlopidine (500 mg) and aspirin (500 mg) daily for 3 months postoperatively and in half doses thereafter. Patients were 16- to 39-years-old (mean 36.5 years). The male to female ratio was 40:48.

RESULTS

Hospital mortality

Eight of the 74 patients in the warfarin group did not survive the operative period, for a mortality of 10.8% (table 15-1). Five of the 8 deaths occurred because of heart failure (low–output syndrome). Two occurred from cerebral air embolism and 1 from an old cerebral infarction that occurred before operation.

In the ticlopidine and aspirin group, 3 out of the 88 patients did not survive the operative period, for an operative mortality of 3.4% (table 15-2). These deaths were because of pneumonic sepsis on the seventh postoperative day, sudden death with paroxysmal tachycardia on the tenth postoperative day, and a giant left atrial thrombus formation on the 35th day after mitral valve replacement.

Late complications and death

Prevention of thromboembolism in the warfarin group was managed solely with warfarin, to maintain the prothrombin time of 1.5 times control. Anti-

Table 15-1. Hospital mortality (warfarin group)

Operation	No. of patients	Deaths
MVR in MS	13	2 embolism; 2 low-output syndrome
MVR in MR	35	3 low-output syndrome
AVR in ASR	16	
DVR in A + M(T)	9	1 cerebral infarction
TVR in A + M + T	1	
Total	74	8 (10.8%)

MVR = mitral valve replacement; AVR = aortic valve replacement; DVR = double valve replacement; TVR = triple valve replacement; MS = mitral stenosis; MR = mitral regurgitation; ASR = aortic stenoinsufficiency; A = aortic; M = mitral; T = tricuspid; (T) = tricuspid annuloplasty

Table 15-2. Hospital mortality (ticlopidine group)

Operation	No. of patients	Deaths
MVR in MS	18	1 left atrial thrombus
MVR in MR	36	1 sudden death
AVR in ASR	29	
DVR in A + M	5	1 sepsis
Total	88	3 (3.4%)

MVR = mitral valve replacement; AVR = aortic valve replacement; DVR = double valve replacement; MS = mitral stenosis; MR = mitral regurgitation; ASR = aortic stenoinsufficiency; A = aortic; M = mitral

Table 15-3. Patients with high risk factors

	Number of patients	
	Warfarin group 74 patients	Ticlopidine group 88 patients
Atrial fibrillation	28	29
Left atrial thrombus	7	9
Peripheral embolism	3	1
Total	38	39

Table 15-4. Length of follow-up in patient-months

Range
  Warfarin group: 36–120 months
  Ticlopidine group: 1–36 months

Operation	Warfarin group	Ticlopidine group
AVR	324	135
MVR	1,724	225
DVR	396	28
TVR	36	—
Total	2,480	388

AVR = aortic valve replacement; MVR = mitral valve replacement; DVR = double valve replacement; TVR = tricuspid valve replacement

coagulant therapy was extended for 2 years in patients with tissue valves and permanently in patients with mechanical valves. In the ticlopidine and aspirin group, patients received ticlopidine (500 mg) and aspirin (500 mg) daily for 3 months postoperatively and in half doses thereafter. Warfarin was also added postoperatively for 3 months in 39 out of the 88 ticlopidine group patients with high risk factors, such as atrial fibrillation, left atrial thrombus removal during operation, and previous peripheral thromboembolism (table 15-3).

The groups were similar in age, sex, and associated cardiovascular diseases, except for the method of prevention of thromboembolism and length of follow-up. Patients were followed from 36 to 120 months, with a mean of 33.5 months, in the warfarin group; and from 1 to 36 months, with a mean of 8.5 months, in the ticlopidine and aspirin group (table 15-4). The total follow-up on warfarin therapy was 2480 months (AVR 324, MVR 1724, DVR 396, and TVR 36 months).★ The total follow-up on ticlopidine and aspirin therapy

★ AVR = aortic valve replacement; MVR = mitral valve replacement; DVR = double valve replacement (aortic and mitral); TVR = triple valve replacement.

Table 15-5. Late complications and deaths

	Number of complication (deaths)	
Complication	Warfarin group	Ticlopidine group
Thromboembolism	10 (3)	1 (1)*
Hemorrhage	5 (2)	2
Low output syndrome	4	2
Valve failure	5**	
Total	25 (5)	3 (1)

 * Left atrial thrombus 35 days after MVR
** Re-replaced with St. Jude Medical valve

was 388 months (AVR 135, MVR 225, and DVR 28 months). At the most recent follow-up, 90% of the surviving patients were in NYHA Class I to II.

There were 5 late deaths in the warfarin group, 3 due to thromboembolism and 2 due to anticoagulant-related cerebral hemorrhage (table 15-5). Nonfatal attacks of thromboembolism and anticoagulant-related hemorrhage were noted in another 10 cases during follow-up. Out of 5 primary valve failures with tissue valves, we re-replaced 2 valves with ST. JUDE MEDICAL valves. There were no late deaths in the ticlopidine and aspirin group during the short period of follow-up, except 1 case with giant left atrial thrombus formation along the atrial septal suture line, 35 days after mitral valve replacement. The case was already included in the operative death results. There were no cases of primary valve failure or hemorrhage, except minor epistaxis and hyper-menorrhea in the ticlopidine and aspirin group, during this follow-up.

Anticoagulant and/or antiplatelet aggregators

While our clinical experience with the ST. JUDE MEDICAL valve is brief, it is our strong impression that combining ticlopidine and aspirin in low-risk adults has synergistic and superior effects in preventing thromboembolism, without the side effects of anticoagulant-related fatal hemorrhage. Warfarin is also necessary in high-risk adults in the early postoperative 3 months to prevent valve thrombosis and thromboembolism. We recommend antiplatelet aggregator therapy with ticlopidine and aspirin in low-risk adults with ST. JUDE MEDICAL valves and additional warfarin for the early 3 months in high-risk adults with ST. JUDE MEDICAL valves (table 15-6). We suggest a cooperative multicenter trial to help resolve this issue.

DISCUSSION

There is not a great deal of recent data on the morbidity and mortality of patients undergoing long-term anticoagulation. The problem of morbidity following anticoagulaton varies enormously. Still unknown is the actual level

Table 15-6. Regimen of anticoagulant and/or antiplatelet aggregators

Early 3 months with high-risk patients	Warfarin	3–6 mg
	Aspirin	500 mg
	Ticlopidine	500 mg
Early 3 months with low-risk patients	Ticlopidine	500 mg
	Aspirin	500 mg
Late follow-up patients	Ticlopidine	250 mg
	Aspirin	250 mg

of anticoagulation at which a patient is protected from thromboembolism occurring in the presence of a prosthetic valve.

There are five factors that seem to have an effect on the incidence of thromboembolism: valve design, the presence or absence of anticoagulation, cardiac rhythm, and atrial and patient factors. Patient factors include the presence of chronic low cardiac output, predisposing to stasis within the cardiac chambers and thromboembolism.

Edmunds' review of the literature [2] has shown that the incidence of thromboembolism in aortic valve replacement with either a mechanical valve or a bioprosthesis is about 2% per patient-year. In mitral valve replacement, the rate of thromboembolism is about 4% per patient-year for mechanical and bioprosthetic valves.

Cohn's data [3] from analysis of 912 patients over a 12-year period indicated that the percent of embolism and thrombosis per patient-year was about the same for both valve types, bioprosthetic or tilting disc. However, the probability of anticoagulant hemorrhage was much greater in patients with tilting disc valves who required long-term anticoagulation than in the 10% of the patients with bioprostheses who required anticoagulation for chronic atrial fibrillation.

Björk [4] indicated that his 268 patients who received BJÖRK-SHILEY® Monostrut valves, followed for 2 to 3 years, revealed thrombotic complications of 0.6% per patient-year after aortic valve replacement and 2.6% per patient-year after mitral valve replacement in patients given anticoagulation. Bleeding complications occurred at a rate of 1.3% per patient-year.

Kim [5] reported thromboembolic complications of 5.2% per patient-year in aortic valve replacement and 12.4% per patient-year in mitral valve replacement for 4 years with various mechanical and tissue valves.

Arom [6] reviewed 680 patients operated on between 1977 and 1983. Congestive heart failure was the main indication for surgery and accounted for 85% of the patient population. The mean follow-up period was 2 years. There were no cases of mechanical prosthetic failure. Operative mortality was 6.6% for the entire group; overall mortality was 7.7%. The incidence of thromboembolism was 0.7% per patient-year in the aortic valve replacement group and

2.2% per patient-year in the mitral valve replacement group. Bleeding complications occurred in 42 patients, 30 of them in the aortic replacement group.

Recently, we reviewed our personal experience in two serial groups of patients. The group receiving warfarin postoperatively consisted of 74 patients with 85 various valves in various positions over 10 years. Follow-up of 36 to 120 months revealed 3 deaths among 10 cases of thromboembolism and 2 deaths among 5 cases of anticoagulant hemorrhage. Another serial group receiving ticlopidine and aspirin postoperatively consisted of 88 patients with 93 ST. JUDE MEDICAL valves in aortic and/or mitral positions. Analysis revealed only 1 case of giant left atrial thrombus formation along the atrial septal suture line 35 days after mitral valve replacement. There were no cases of primary valve failure or fatal hemorrhage, except minor epistaxis and hypermenorrhea for a 3-year period of observation.

Day's review of the literature [7] has shown that antiplatelet drugs in large, well-controlled clinical trials will show a maximal decrease of 25% to 30% of arterial thromboembolic events. Combinations of drugs known to affect platelet function by inhibiting different pathways of platelet metabolism have added little more than single drugs, such as aspirin, used alone. Of the antiplatelet drugs currently available for clinical investigation, ticlopidine hydrochloride is one of the most potent and has several important advantages over existing agents. Ticlopidine hydrochloride is chemically unrelated to other antiplatelet drugs and appears to have a unique mechanism of action upon the agonist/receptor function of platelets. In contrast to some other drugs, ticlopidine seems to have no effect upon the mechanism that controls calcium mobilization. Poorly active in vivo, the drug must be given systematically to achieve maximal activity. The onset of full activity takes 3 to 5 days of continuous doses, with the onset of action taking at least 7 days.

Kim [8] measured the parameters of platelet function in an aggregation curve of platelets with a platelet aggregator (Chronolog Aggregometer, model no. 430). The mean maximum platelet aggregability induced by 10 μmol/L epinephrine in the patient group saturated with ticlopidine was 15.6%. In the normal control group without ticlopidine, the maximum platelet aggregation induced by 10 μmol/L epinephrine was 69%. Ticlopidine produced a significant inhibition of platelet aggregation in the presence of ADP and epinephrine in this study.

Cardiac rhythm appears to be critical in determining thromboembolism in the mitral valve area because of the large number of patients with chronic atrial fibrillation drawing a worse long-term survival rate than control patients who did not have atrial fibrillation. In the long-term study by Gajewski and Singer [9], 3500 patients with atrial fibrillation from many different conditions, including mitral stenosis, were evaluated against a standard expected curve of survival in patients who did not have atrial fibrillation. If the patients are in chronic atrial fibrillation and need a mitral valve replacement, they probably will require long-term anticoagulation regardless of the valve substitute chosen. Other intraoperative atrial factors, such as the presence of intra-atrial clot, previous embolism, or a large, dilated left atrium are indicative of the need for anticoagulation. The presence of one or more of these atrial factors places patients at a very high risk for embolism, regardless of the type of valve used, and anticoagulation must be prescribed.

We maintained 39 high-risk patients with warfarin, in addition to the ticlopidine and aspirin menu, for at least 2 years after prosthetic valve replacement.

CONCLUSIONS

There was no primary valve failure in adults receiving ST. JUDE MEDICAL valves in 88 consecutive cases for 388 patient-months. Maintenance on ticlopidine and aspirin in adults with ST. JUDE MEDICAL valves was very effective for prevention of thromboembolism without fatal hemorrhage. Warfarin addition is necessary for the early 3 months in high-risk patients with ST. JUDE MEDICAL valves.

REFERENCES

1. Tepley JF, Grunkemeier GL, Sutherland HD, et al. The ultimate prognosis after valve replacement: An assessment of twenty years. Ann Thorac Surg 1981; 32:111–119.
2. Edmunds LH Jr. Thromboembolic complications of current cardiac valve prostheses. Ann Thorac Surg 1982; 34:96.
3. Cohn LH. Thromboembolism after cardiac valve replacement. In Matloff JM (ed): *Cardiac Valve Replacement*. Martinus Nijhoff Publishing, Boston 1984; pp 9–16.
4. Björk VO, Lindblom D. The monostrut Björk-Shiley heart valve. Scand J Thorac Cardiovasc Surg 1985; 19(1):13–19.
5. Kim JH. Cardiac valve replacement and anticoagulant therapy. J Korea Thorac Cardiovasc Surg 1978; 11:303–312.
6. Arom KV, Nicoloff DM, Kersten TE, et al. Six years of experience with the St. Jude Medical valvular prosthesis. Circulation 1985 Sep; 72(3pt 2):II 153–158.
7. Day HJ. Overview: Clinical experiences with ticlopidine. In Gordon JI (ed): *Ticlopidine: Quo Vadis?* AAS 15, Birkhauser Verlag, Basel 1984; p 287.
8. Kim KT, Kim HM. A clinical and experimental study on prevention of thromboembolism with antiplatelet drug after cardiac valve replacement. Korea Univ Med J 1987; 24:1–12.
9. Gajewski J, Singer RB. Mortality in an insured population with atrial fibrillation. JAMA 1981; 245:1540–1544.

16. MIDTERM FOLLOW-UP OF THE ST. JUDE MEDICAL® HEART VALVE

A. PAVIE, C. CABROL, A. TABLEY, V. BORS, M. FONTANEL, I. GANDJBAKHCH

Abstract. *From November 1978 to September 1984, 200 ST. JUDE MEDI-CAL® valves were implanted in 177 patients (102 AVR, 55 MVR, 20 MuVR).* * *The use of this low profile prosthesis is particularly appropriate in special anatomical conditions, e.g., when the aortic anulus is larger than the ascending aorta or in a small ventricular cavity. The hospital mortality was 9.8%. The 153 operative survivors were followed over a period of 3 months to 6 years (408.8 patient-years). Actuarial analysis of late results indicates an expected survival rate at 6 years of 83.1% for the whole group (AVR 81.6%, MVR 97.5%, MuVR 71.5%). Freedom from thromboembolism was 94.5% (AVR 97.3%, MVR 91.4%, MuVR 85.7%). Two patients underwent reoperation (1 endocarditis, 1 paravalvular leak). The actuarial rate of freedom from all complications was 90.1%. Postoperatively, 94% of patients were in New York Heart Association (NYHA) Class I or II. In conclusion, this midterm follow-up at 6 years shows very satisfactory results in terms of thrombo-embolism and survival.*

INTRODUCTION

Between November 1978 and September 1984, 200 ST. JUDE MEDICAL® valves were implanted in 177 patients; 102 patients had isolated aortic valve

---

* AVR = aortic valve replacement; MVR = mitral valve replacement; MuVR = multiple valve replacement.

replacement, 55 isolated mitral valve replacement, and 20 multiple valve replacement.

PATIENTS AND METHODS

The patients who had aortic valve replacement were mainly men, age 20- to 78-years-old (mean age 52 years); 62% of them were in New York Heart Association (NYHA) Class III or IV. The main cause for valvular replacement was calcified aortic stenosis. Aortic insufficiency also prompted valve replacement. Nine cases involved endocarditis, and there were 7 reoperations for failure of another prosthesis.

The patients who had mitral valve replacement were mainly women, with a mean age of 48 years. A greater proportion of these patients, 89%, were in NYHA Class III or IV. Valvular replacement was undertaken for primary mitral stenosis or insufficiency, but in a significant number of cases reoperation was necessary, especially if a previous mitral commissurotomy had been performed.

Patients receiving multiple valve replacement were mainly women, younger (mean age 38 years) than in the preceding groups. Again, a significant proportion of them, 84%, were in NYHA Class III or IV. Seventeen had a double (mitral-aortic) valve replacement and 3 had a triple (aortic-mitral-tricuspid) replacement.

Associated lesions requiring concomitant procedures were: tricuspid repair using annuloplasty in 21 patients, mitral repair in 7 patients, aorto-coronary bypass in 4 patients, a left ventriculomyotomy in 2 patients, a total replacement of the ascending aorta (according to our technique) in 2 patients, and the use of a supracoronary valvular conduit in 1 case of endocarditis.

There was preferential use of the ST. JUDE MEDICAL valve in small aortic orifices because of the excellent hemodynamic performance of the small valve sizes. In aortic valve replacement, sizes varied from 19 mm to 27 mm tissue anulus diameter. For the mitral and tricuspid valve replacements, most valves were 27, 29, and 31 mm.

RESULTS

Early overall mortality at 1 month was 9.6%, most being cases of mitral valve replacement (12%). Fewer early deaths were observed in patients with multiple valve replacement (5%). Due to its excellent hemodynamic performance, we used the ST. JUDE MEDICAL valve in our early experience for the most difficult cases, such as emergency cases, thrombosis of another prosthesis, infection, reoperation, and poor ventricular function. Most of these patients died of low cardiac output, recurrent infection, or thrombosis.

We followed 96% of the survivors from 1 to 6 years after surgery, for a total of more than 400 patient-years (280 years for aortic, 91 years for mitral, and 36 years for multiple valve replacement). Late mortality was 8.5%, mainly due to congestive heart failure, but also to sudden death, anticoagulation accident, and noncardiac causes.

The actuarial survival rate at 6 years was best for mitral replacement at 97%, less for aortic replacement at 81%, and for multiple valve replacement only 71%. The overall survival rate was 83% for all patients (figure 16-1). Actuarial survival rates were established according to the Kaplan-Meier method [1]; early mortality was excluded from this analysis. Standard deviation for each data was calculated using the Greenwood formula [2].

All patients were treated with anticoagulants. Three cases of thrombo-

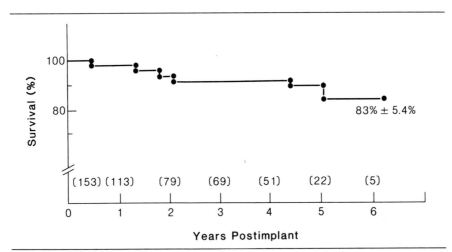

Figure 16-1. Actuarial survival curve.

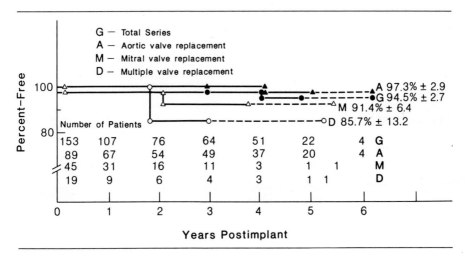

Figure 16-2. Patients free of thromboembolism.

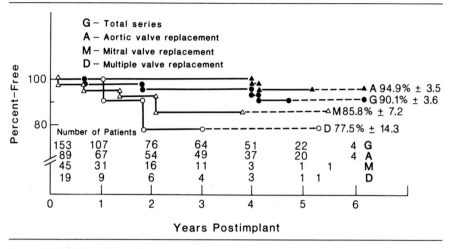

Figure 16-3. Patients free of all complications.

embolism have been observed at 10, 24, and 54 months after surgery. This equals 1.36% per patient-year. Actuarial analysis shows that 94% of patients are free of any thromboembolism at 6 years; 97% for aortic, 91% for mitral, and 85% for multiple valve replacements (figure 16-2). Two patients were reoperated on, one at 1 year for mitral paravalvular leak and another at 4 years for aortic endocarditis. No deterioration of the prosthesis was observed. Overall, more than 90% of the patients were free of any complication at 6 years, almost 95% for aortic, 85% for mitral, and 77% for multiple valve replacement (figure 16-3).

As usual, functional improvement after valvular replacement was important. Before operation, 75% of the patients were in NYHA Class III or IV; after operation more than 93% were in NYHA Class I or II.

In our experience the ST. JUDE MEDICAL valve is one of the best mechanical valve prostheses we have ever used and the only low profile valve we use now in mitral valve replacement.

REFERENCES

1. Kaplan EL, Meier P. Nonparametric estimation from incomplete observations. Am Stat Assoc J 1958; 53:457–481.
2. Dixon WJ (ed). *BMDP Statistical Software*. University of California Press, Berkeley, 1983; p 557–577.

PART II. DISCUSSION

DENNIS F. PUPELLO, MODERATOR

ORIENTATION

GEORGE REUL, JR.: Dr. Hartz, in your patient with the subaortic myocardial proliferation, could this have been prevented by orienting the valve in a different direction? Also, have you noticed any difference in leaflet movement according to the orientation of the valve?

RENEE HARTZ: The first patient with an immobilized leaflet was a patient with severe left ventricular hypertrophy. He was operated on before recommendations concerning orientation of the ST. JUDE MEDICAL® valve in the aortic position were published. There is no question that in his case the prosthesis was improperly oriented for his anatomy. It was placed with the long apis parallel to the septum rather than perpendicular. At reoperation there was a very small amount of thrombus at the right pivot guard, which, it seemed, had originated at the posterior leaflet and had immobilized the leaflet. Since the recommendations for orienting the prosthesis were made, we have been very careful about orientation with respect to both positions. We try to orient aortic valves by placing one pivot guard at the center of the right coronary cusp as recommended by Professor Eugene Baudet and the mitral valves in the anti-anatomical orientation.

PH. MIKAELOFF: Based on your experience with disc valves, can you say that a bileaflet valve is superior to a disc valve in terms of follow-up with your nonenhanced cinefluoroscopic technique?

RENEE HARTZ: We have a very limited experience with disc valves. We prefer the ST. JUDE MEDICAL valve for most mechanical valve reoperations where we previously used a caged-ball prosthesis. We have an extremely limited experience with the BJÖRK-SHILEY® valve. Recently we began to use the MEDTRONIC HALL™ valve, which visualizes as nicely as the ST. JUDE MEDICAL valve fluoroscopically. We also have limited follow-up with this valve, so I can't really say too much yet. One interesting observation we've made is that the ST. JUDE MEDICAL valve seems to open more fully and close more completely in isolated aortic valve replacement than it does in double valve replacement in the aortic position, with a porcine valve in the mitral position. This has been true for 5 or 6 of our patients receiving this combination. When there are two ST. JUDE MEDICAL prostheses in place, the aortic valve seems to open and close more completely. I think that perhaps the bigger sewing ring on the porcine mitral valve might interfere a little with the opening and closing of the other prosthesis.

GEORGE REUL, JR.: I think it is important to record the orientation of the valve when we are giving valve thrombosis rates, so we can see if there is any difference in these rates according to the orientation. There is very little data on this and it's a very important technical point.

MVR WITH NATURAL VALVE PRESERVATION

ANTONIO PUCCI: Dr. Cabrol, I know that you almost routinely leave a posterior leaflet of the mitral valve in place when performing a mitral valve replacement. Did you have any problem using the ST. JUDE MEDICAL prosthesis in mitral valve replacement with this technique?

CHRISTIAN CABROL: I learned from my master, Dr. Walt Lillehei, to leave the posterior leaflet *and* the chordae tendineae in place, and if it is not possible to leave all of the leaflet, to leave the mural chordae tendineae. If you do not, you risk stretching the left ventricular wall and having rupture on that side. A week ago during a valve replacement, to avoid cutting all the chordae tendineae, I left the posterior leaflet in place and I had no problem. The ST. JUDE MEDICAL valve is one of the best designed valves for this purpose, because the leaflets move inside the orifice ring. The EDWARDS-DUROMEDICS™ leaflets open into the ventricle. But the design of the ST. JUDE MEDICAL valve is, in fact, an atrial valve, because the struts are in the atrial side in the mitral position, and the leaflets open and close within the orifice ring.

ANTONIO PUCCI: Do you use it in the anti-anatomical position or the anatomical position?

CHRISTIAN CABROL: I will try all the valve positions. The important thing is to have a good output channel for each large orifice. Sometimes, if you position the valve anatomically, the mural channel is very small and one valve leaflet is facing the mural wall of the left ventricle. I think an antianatomical position would be the best.

ANTICOAGULATION

ANDRE WESSELS: Dr. Hartz, concerning that patient with the clotted ST. JUDE MEDICAL valve in the aortic position, was the opening click of that valve audible on auscultation?

RENEE HARTZ: No. The valve was not normal on auscultation. The surgical service follows all of our patients once a year, specifically to listen to their prostheses. This patient had experienced a myocardial infarction, so even before I listened to him I suspected that something would be wrong. The click was gone and there was aortic insufficiency. The same thing occurred with the second woman; there was no click. She had a history of hemolysis, but, immediately upon listening to her, it was clear to me she had aortic insufficiency and the hemolysis was due to the stuck leaflet rather than any paravalvular leak. The click returned in the second patient and, subsequently, in a third patient, when the leaflet was freed by anticoagulation therapy.

J. CLELAND: If you have a patient with a malfunctioning valve, or a clotted valve that is not causing hemodynamic distress, would you give that patient any anticoagulants first, rather than operating immediately?

RENEE HARTZ: Absolutely. We've only operated on 1 of the 3 patients we have seen with this condition. This patient was the first one I discussed. He was 74 at the time, and we did not feel that we should use thrombolytic therapy; because of his age we thought it was a high risk. We kept him on heparin over the weekend and operated on Monday morning. The second woman, with the marked annular calcification, simply would not come into the hospital, so she was put on COUMADIN® therapy. As you saw, within 6 weeks, her valve functioned normally. The real question in my mind is, where did the clot go? If indeed this was a clot, which we presume it was, I wonder if thrombolytic therapy may be more dangerous than is gradual anticoagulation, because it releases fragments of the thrombus. We have been lucky because only one leaflet has been stuck in our patients' valves.

NORBERTO GONZALEZ DE VEGA: I was excited about Dr. Acinapura's results but note that procedures were done only with sizes 25 and 31 mm aortic and mitral valves. There is also a sharp contrast between Dr. Acinapura's results of 1.6% per patient-year for thromboembolic complications in the mitral position without anticoagulation therapy and those of Dr. Cleland with a 4.6% per patient-year thromboembolic complication rate in the mitral position with 80% of patients anticoagulated. I would ask for an explanation for these very different results.

ANTHONY ACINAPURA: We do not use anything less than a 25 mm porcine aortic valve because we found higher gradients (in excess of 25 to 30 mm Hg) when we used a size 23 porcine valve, especially in adults weighing more than 75 kg. However, that's not to say that the 23 mm valve should not be utilized. As far as the porcine valve in the mitral position is concerned, I found it relatively uncommon not to be able to insert a size 31 porcine valve in that position. The heart is very relaxed, especially with myocardial protection with cardioplegia, and we have not had any problems with a strut rupturing the ventricle or atrioventricular (A-V) groove rupture.

Regarding anticoagulation and thromboembolic problems with the mitral prosthesis, we have not reported many major thromboembolic complications. There may be many that we do not record because they are considered minor. It is very hard to give an accurate report on the amount of thrombotic complications, but I feel that it is important to ligate the left atrial appendage or oversew it from within, because that is where most of the thrombus formation occurs.

PULMONARY VALVE REPLACEMENT

S. K. GANDHI: This question is for the whole panel. I have been faced with an interesting patient recently: a 52-year-old lady who came in with a recent onset of cyanosis on exertion. She has a ventricular septal defect, a right ventricular hypertrophic outflow tract obstruction, and a pulmonary valve obstruction. Right ventricular hypertropy is present. I cannot tell whether her pulmonary valve is normal. At surgery would you replace the pulmonary valve? And if so, with what type?

RENEE HARTZ: I wouldn't replace a normal pulmonary valve. If she has organic pulmonary valvular stenosis, it's an easy decision. If she needs a pulmonary outflow enlarging procedure, it's also a relatively easy decision. If she has simple, straight-forward infundibular stenosis, I think it's a little more complicated.

S. K. GANDHI: The valve is stenotic.

J. CLELAND: In the situation with a pulmonary valve or an infundibular stenosis, it is rarely necessary to replace the pulmonary valve. Frequently, a pulmonary valvotomy and resection of the infundibular obstruction is all that's necessary. If the stenosis is very severe, then an outflow patch is the next option. If you have to go to a valve replacement, which is, again, extremely rare, a homograft is probably the best solution.

TISSUE VALVE FIBROSIS

KENNETH ROSS: We've had 2 patients in the last 2 years, both in their 60s, who had CARPENTIER-EDWARDS® valves inserted, and within 3 and 4 months after insertion, each had aortic stenosis with gradients of 80 mm Hg to 100 mm Hg. Both valves were replaced with ST. JUDE MEDICAL valves. The CARPENTIER-EDWARDS valves were leatherized—they were not calcified, but they were just very thick, leathery valves. Some people have said that if you do not use calcium in the postoperative period, maybe this will not occur. Both patients have been anticoagulated with COUMADIN and are doing very well. Dr. Acinapura, have you seen this?

ANTHONY ACINAPURA: We have not seen tissue fibrosis to that degree, that early. We have observed cases of accelerated stenosis in young patients, who were in their 20s and, in those situations, we stopped using the valves. But certainly, we have seen no one in their 60s and 70s. I really don't have any explanation for it.

All the patients we presented, by the way, had no other associated procedures, and we excluded all of the young patients with accelerated stenosis who had valve replacement. None were given any kind of calcium channel blockers.

III. VALVE REPLACEMENT IN THE ELDERLY (AGE 66 AND OLDER)

17. COMBINED VALVE AND CORONARY ARTERY BYPASS PROCEDURES IN SEPTUAGENARIANS AND OCTOGENARIANS: RESULTS IN 119 PATIENTS

R. J. GRAY, T.-P. TSAI, C. M. CONKLIN, J. M. MATLOFF

Abstract. *A consecutive series of 96 septuagenarians (Group I, mean age 74) and 23 octogenarians (Group II, mean age 83) underwent coronary artery bypass (CAB, mean 2.6 grafts per patient) and valve operations using hypothermia and hyperkalemic cardioplegia in a 45-month period. Most patients (57% of Group I and 91% of Group II) were in New York Heart Association (NYHA) Class IV preoperatively. The early deaths were 19% for Group I and 39% for Group II; late deaths were 13% and 30%, respectively (mean 25 months). Of 91 survivors, 86% of Group I and 71% of Group II improved by one or more NYHA Classes postoperatively. Overall, of 56 patients with combined CAB and aortic valve replacement, 19 (33%) died; of 38 with combined CAB and mitral valve replacement, 23 (61%) died; 3 of 13 (23%) with combined CAB and double valve replacement died; and 3 of 12 (25%) with CAB and mitral valve repair died. In comparison, among patients less than 70 years of age having isolated valve replacement in the same period, 2 of 30 (7%) in the AVR group died, 5 of 17 (29%) in the MVR group died, and 2 of 7 (33%) in the DVR group died. The risk of combined valve procedures and bypass surgery was significantly increased in the elderly and may warrant a less aggressive procedure, especially in the mitral position.*

INTRODUCTION

At the present time, 72% of cardiovascular deaths occur in people over age 65, and in the United States, patients in this age category use the majority of our health care resource dollars. The aging of our population is the inevitable result of success due, among other things, to public health measures and, of course, high quality medical care. A recent patient contemplating cardiac surgery put this issue into personal perspective, saying, "I don't want to be younger, doctor, please make me older." That important realization is being heard more and more from patients who are 65, 70, and even 80 years of age.

At our institution in Los Angeles fully one-third of patients undergoing cardiac surgery are now over age 70. Thus, we are now compelled to treat patients who are increasingly more aged and more complex. Therefore, the purpose of this chapter is to describe a group of patients who are older and to define more clearly the results and complications of surgery.

This analysis addresses the results of combined bypass and valve replacement during 3.5 years ending in 1984. These include 96 people, 70 to 79 years of age, who will be referred to as Group I, and 23 individuals in the 80- to 89-year old category, who will be referred to as Group II. The average ages are 74 and 83 years, respectively. In Group II, fewer patients were male (35% compared to 66% in Group I), indicating the greater preponderance of females surviving to older age.

SURGICAL PROCEDURES

We have divided the type of valves implanted into the ST. JUDE MEDICAL® and porcine valve categories. Of the 27 patients receiving porcine valves, 26% were CARPENTIER-EDWARDS® and 74% were HANCOCK® (standard orifice).

Thirty-one patients over 70 years of age (Group I) and 7 patients over 80 years of age (Group II) had mitral valve replacement and coronary bypass. Mitral valve repair and coronary bypass was performed in 9 patients in Group I and in 3 patients in Group II. Forty-three patients in Group I and 12 patients in Group II underwent aortic valve replacement and coronary bypass surgery. Twelve in Group I and one in Group II had coronary bypass combined with double valve replacement utilizing either 2 ST. JUDE MEDICAL valves or a ST. JUDE MEDICAL aortic valve with mitral repair. Unfortunately, the number of double valve recipients is too small to accurately define this population, and they will not be further analyzed.

PATIENT DESCRIPTION

In general, these patients are highly symptomatic, as depicted in table 17-1. Unstable angina, defined as progressive angina requiring hospitalization, was present in 74% of Group I and 87% of Group II. Dyspnea, indicating the severity of valve disease, was present in 70% of Group I and 91% of Group II; previous myocardial infarction was present in 39% of Group I and 65% of Group II. The NYHA Functional Class of all patients (table 17-2) indicates that the majority of patients in both groups are NYHA Class IV. Only 7 of the 96 patients in Group I were in Class I or II, and none of the patients in Group II were in Class I or II.

Table 17-1. Preoperative symptoms

	Group I	Group II
Unstable angina	74%	87%
Dyspnea	70%	91%
Prior myocardial infarction	39%	65%

Table 17-2. Preoperative NYHA Classification

NYHA Class	Group I (n = 96)	Group II (n = 23)	Total (%) (n = 119)
I–II	7	0	7 (6%)
III	34	2	36 (30%)
IV	55	21	76 (64%)

Table 17-3. Follow-up duration

	Group I	Group II
Range (months)	2–54	2–51
Mean (months)	26	21

Group I patients as a whole have a high proportion of associated cardio-vascular risk factors: 43% have hypertension; 38% have been, or presently are, cigarette smokers; 19% are under treatment for diabetes mellitus; history of hyperlipidemia is present in 9%; and 40% have a family history of premature coronary atherosclerosis.

Follow-up ranges from 2 months to approximately 4.5 years for both of these two cohorts, with an average of approximately 2 years (table 17-3).

OUTCOME

Even by conservative standards, these patients had lengthy hospital stays, with an average of 22 days for Group I and 24 days for Group II (table 17-4).

Postoperative complications are shown in table 17-5. Supraventricular arrhythmias, most commonly atrial fibrillation, occur very frequently (43% of Group I; 30% of Group II). Heart block requiring prolonged early postoperative pacing occurred in 29% overall; ventricular arrhythmias requiring

Table 17-4. Results

	Group I	Group II
Hospital stay (days)	9–102 (22 average)	10–46 (24 average)

Table 17-5. Postoperative complications

Complication	Number of patients		
	Group I	Group II	Total
Supraventricular arrhythmia	41	7	48
Transient heart block	28	7	35
Ventricular arrhythmia	21	4	25
Myocardial infarction	23	5	28
Psychoses	2	3	5
Sternal dehiscence	2	1	3
Renal failure	4	2	6
Bleeding	6	5	11
Pericarditis	2	2	4
Pulmonary insufficiency	3	2	5
Wound infections	8	4	12
CVA or thromboembolism	2	2	4
Sepsis	2	2	4
Cardiac rupture	1	0	1

treatment occurred in 21% of patients; perioperative myocardial infarction occurred in 24% overall; and postoperative psychosis occurred in 5 individuals. Eleven patients (9%) had postoperative bleeding requiring return to the operating room, and 12 patients (10%) had serious postoperative wound infection.

Preoperative and postoperative Functional Class for Group I is shown in figure 17-1. Overall, 54 of 63 patients, or 86%, have improved by at least

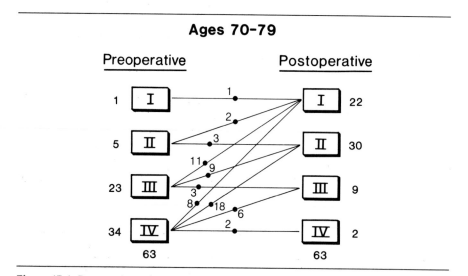

Figure 17-1. Preoperative and postoperative NYHA Classification in Group I.

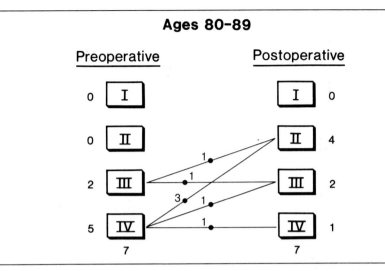

Figure 17-2. Preoperative and Postoperative NYHA Classification in Group II.

one NYHA Classification. Data for Group II is shown in figure 17-2. All are in Class III or IV preoperatively; unfortunately, none became asymptomatic (Class I). Thus, in this small cohort of 80-year-old patients, few experience dramatic symptomatic improvement.

Mortality, divided into early (hospital) and late events, is shown in table 17-6. The overall mortality for mitral valve replacement is 61%, of which a large part is in the early period (15 of 23 deaths occurred early). Unfortunately, all 7 of the 80-year-olds having mitral valve replacement and coronary bypass died

Table 17-6. Mortality

	MVR and CABG					
	Group I			Group II		
	Early	Late	Total	Early	Late	Total
St. Jude Medical	9/20	0/11	45%	1/3	2/2	100%
Porcine	2/11	5/9	64%	3/4	1/1	100%

	AVR and CABG					
	Group I			Group II		
	Early	Late	Total	Early	Late	Total
St. Jude Medical	3/33	7/30	30%	2/9	2/7	44%
Porcine	2/10	0/8	20%	1/3	1/2	67%

Table 17-7. Causes of death in patients undergoing mitral valve replacement or repair

	Group I			Group II		
	Cardiac	Valve	Noncardiac	Cardiac	Valve	Noncardiac
St. Jude Medical	7	0	2	1	0	2
Porcine	2	4	1	2	0	2
Repair	1			1	0	1

(4 early, 3 late). Mitral valve repair and coronary bypass is much better tolerated. Of 9 patients having these procedures in Group I, the mortality is 11%, occurring predominantly in the early postoperative period, and of the 3 in Group II having mitral repair and coronary bypass, 1 died early and 1 died late for a total mortality of 67%. Because of the small number of patients in Group II, additional patients will obviously be needed to confirm these results.

The results from aortic valve replacement and bypass are more encouraging. There is a 33% overall mortality with ST. JUDE MEDICAL replacement and bypass, and a 31% overall mortality for porcine valve replacement. The overall mortality is 30% for ST. JUDE MEDICAL aortic valve replacement in Group I and 20% for porcine aortic valve recipients. In Group II, overall mortality is 44% for ST. JUDE MEDICAL and 67% for porcine valves.

Analysis of the causes of death, for mitral valve replacement or repair, and for coronary bypass, reveals no valve-related causes in the ST. JUDE

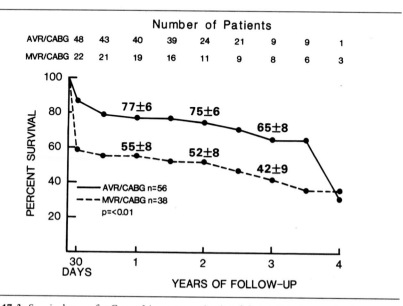

Figure 17-3. Survival curve for Group I (septuagenarians) and Group II (octogenarians).

MEDICAL cohort of either group (table 17-7). Four patients in Group I having mitral valve replacement with CARPENTIER-EDWARDS prostheses died of valve-related causes. These were due either to stroke resulting from thromboembolism (2 patients) or serious hemorrhagic complications (2 patients). None in Group II had valve-related causes of death.

The causes of death in patients having aortic valve replacement and coronary artery bypass were cardiac non-valve-related or noncardiac in both the ST. JUDE MEDICAL and porcine recipients.

The actuarial data is shown in figure 17-3. Both groups have not been separated because the numbers of patients are small. The top line represents the survival curve for all patients having aortic valve replacement and bypass; the dashed line represents all those with mitral valve replacement and bypass. Included here are those having mitral valve repair and bypass. Survival is better with aortic valve replacement (p < .01). The principal difference is seen in the early or surgical-related mortality, but after that the two survival curves are parallel. Beyond 3.5 years the number of patients does not warrant any additional analysis.

SUMMARY

Based upon these results, we conclude that combined valve procedures and coronary bypass is associated with high early mortality, especially in Group II individuals having mitral replacement and bypass. The preoperative NYHA Classification is advanced, especially in Group II individuals, suggesting refractoriness to medical therapy and the requirement for convincing surgical indications. While these factors reflect current decision-making policy in the elderly, an important question remaining is whether the observed higher surgical risk is due to more advanced disease or to age itself.

Because the results are not always as gratifying as similar procedures in younger patients, perhaps one may choose not to offer surgery to patients over 80-years-old. A better choice is to accept the challenge to determine the surgical risk of age alone and to define precisely which elderly patients may benefit from surgery and have a more meaningful extension of life.

18. THE IONESCU-SHILEY® XENOBIOPROSTHESIS AS AN AORTIC VALVE SUBSTITUTE IN PATIENTS 66 YEARS OF AGE AND OLDER

L. GONZALEZ-LAVIN, L. B. McGRATH, S. AMINI, B. LEWIS,
J. GONZALEZ-LAVIN, S. CHI

Abstract. A cohort of 107 patients, aged 66 years and over, from a series of 240 patients receiving an IONESCU-SHILEY® bioprosthesis (ISBPV) in the aortic position, were studied in isolation. The procedures were performed from 1977 to 1983. The mean age of this group was 72.7 ± 5.2 years (range: 66 to 88 years; median: 71 years). The average preoperative New York Heart Association (NYHA) Functional Class was III. Concomitant procedures were performed in 54 patients (50.5%). Hospital mortality was 8.4% (n = 9). Univariate analysis revealed that risk factors for hospital mortality were older age (p = 0.04), higher preoperative NYHA Class (p = 0.06), and earlier year of operation (p = 0.05). Patients dismissed from the hospital were followed for a total of 4652.35 months (mean 43.5 ± 2.5). Follow-up was 100% complete. Late mortality occurred at a rate of 7.7% per patient-year. Significant univariate risk factors for late mortality were earlier year of operation (p = 0.03) and concomitant procedures (p = 0.06). Late mortality due to valve-related complications was 0.8% per patient-year. Where numbers permitted, univariate and multivariate risk factors were assessed for each valve-related complication. Pertinent findings were abstracted. The univariate risk factor for intrinsic valve failure was elective operation (p = 0.04); an indicator was younger age, for example, 69 vs. 72.9 years (p = 0.08). The only multivariate risk factor for intrinsic valve failure was previous operation (p = 0.04). Multivariate risk factors for any valve-related complication were younger age (p = 0.04 for 68.9 years vs. 73.2 years), previous operation (p = 0.04), and concomitant procedures (p = 0.01). Our conclusion is that results of aortic valve replacement with ISBPV in older patients are good. Older age increases the risk of hospital death. Actuarial survival and freedom from valve-related events are good.

INTRODUCTION

The design of the standard IONESCU-SHILEY® bovine pericardial valve (ISBPV) provides superior hydraulic function with simultaneous and symmetrical opening of the three pericardial cusps [1–3]. This particular feature has provided excellent hemodynamic performance even in small-sized valves. In the clinical setting, these fluid dynamic characteristics concede minimal gradients [4] and low thrombogenicity [5]. These advantages make the choice of this xenobioprosthesis particularly appealing for use in elderly patients, who are recently being referred with increasing frequency for aortic valve replacement (AVR). Avoidance of aortic root enlargement and postoperative anticoagulant therapy after isolated AVR are distinct advantages that should decrease operative and postoperative morbidity and mortality. To corroborate these presumptions, 107 patients, aged 66 years and over, were isolated from a series of 240 patients receiving an ISBPV in the aortic position and studied retrospectively. The analysis of this cohort of patients is the basis of this report.

DEMOGRAPHY

Between February 1977 and December 1983, 240 patients underwent AVR with an ISBPV at Ingham Medical Center and Palo Alto Medical Center [6]. Of these, 107 patients were 66 years of age or older. The cohort consisted of 55 males and 52 females (p = 0.40). Ages ranged from 66 to 88 years of age, mean ± standard error 72.7 ± 5.2 years, median 71 years. Eight patients (7.5%) had previous cardiac procedure(s). According to the criteria set forth by the New York Heart Association (NYHA), 81 patients (76%) were in Class III or IV at the time of operation, the average being Class III. Valve sizes implanted were: 17 mm, 5 patients; 19 mm, 28; 21 mm, 41; 23 mm, 23; 25 mm, 3; 27 mm, 5; 29 mm, 2. Fifty-four patients (50.5%) underwent a concomitant procedure.

FOLLOW-UP AND STATISTICAL ANALYSIS

This cohort of 107 patients have been followed for 4652.35 months (mean 43.5 ± 2.5 months); follow-up was 100%. Sixty-four percent have been followed for at least 3 years (70% confidence limits [CL]: 59.7%–69.3%).

Occurrence of valve-related events are expressed as a linearized rate (percent per patient-year) and as actuarial freedom. Probability of surviving and freedom from the events were calculated using the method of Kaplan-Meier [7]. Censoring of data was by date of analysis. Follow-up was 100%, with the status of all patients ascertained. Actuarial comparison of events and survival functions was performed according to the method of log rank, Mantel-

Haenszel, and Cox's proportional hazards model [8, 9]. A p valve of < 0.05 was considered statistically significant. Univariate (UVA) and multivariate (MVA) analyses such as Fisher's exact test [10], two sample t-tests, and Cox linear logistic regression analysis [11] were performed to assess the influence of risk factors on hospital and late mortalities, as well as other valve-related and non-valve-related events [12]. The factors considered were: age, gender, previous cardiac procedures, predominant lesion, preoperative NYHA Classification, concomitant procedure, year of operation, institution, surgeon, status at operation (elective, urgent, or emergency intervention), cardiopulmonary bypass and cross–clamp time, xenobioprosthetic size, and follow–up time.

RESULTS

Hospital mortality

Nine patients died within 30 days of operation (8.4%). Of the 53 patients undergoing isolated AVR, 3 hospital deaths occurred (5.7%), compared to 11.1% for those having a concomitant procedure (p = 0.25). Univariate analyses revealed that incremental risk factors (IRF) for hospital death were older age (p = 0.04), higher preoperative NYHA Class (p = 0.06), and earlier year of operation (p = 0.05). Both earlier year of operation (p = 0.05) and older age (p = 0.07) were also found to be IRF by MVA.

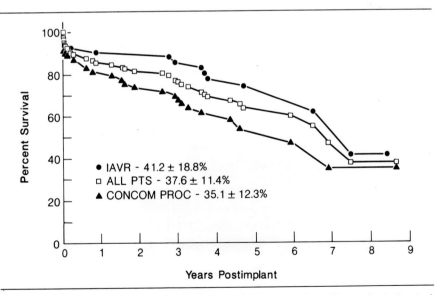

Figure 18-1. Comparative actuarial patient survival with the original xenobioprosthesis. Survival of patients who had undergone isolated aortic valve replacement (IAVR) was significantly better than those who had had a concomitant procedure (p = 0.03).

Late mortality

Late death occurred in 30 patients (30.6%, 70% CL: 25.5%–36.2%), a linearized rate of 7.7% per patient-year. Seventeen were cardiac-related (17.3%, 70% CL: 13.3%–22.2%, 4.4% per patient-year. One of these was due to a complication of intrinsic valve failure (1.02%, 70% CL: 0.13%–3.4%), 0.3% per patient-year. Significant IRF identified by UVA for late mortality were: earlier year of operation (p = 0.03) and concomitant procedure (p = 0.06). The only IRF by MVA was earlier year of operation (p = 0.028).

Patient survival with original prosthesis

Actuarial patient survival with the original prosthesis is 81.7%, 63.4%, and 37.6% at 2, 5, and 8.7 years, respectively (figure 18-1). Survival of patients with the original xenobioprosthesis, who had undergone isolated AVR, was significantly better than those who had undergone a concomitant procedure (p = 0.03). There is an indication that patients with larger-sized xenobio-prostheses (> 21 mm) have a higher chance of survival (p = 0.09). Of the survivors, 95.2% (70% CL: 90.5%–97.7%) are in NYHA Class I or II (figure 18-2).

Valve-related events (table 18-1)

INTRINSIC VALVE FAILURE (IVF). Following the definition of IVF as outlined by Borkon et al. [13], 6 valves failed (6.1%, 70% CL: 3.6%–9.7%), for a rate of 1.5% per patient-year. These occurred in patients aged 66 to 77 years of age (mean 69 ± 1.7 years) at time of implantation, 32 to 91 months (mean 51.5 ± 9.1 months) after operation. Two were males and 4 were females. Five of the valves were calcified, 1 of which also had a tear. One patient experienced a myocardial infarction and expired because of a calcific embolus to the circumflex coronary artery from the xenobioprosthesis [14]. The other valve

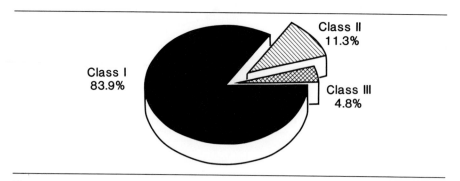

Figure 18-2. Clinical status of the surviving patients, as assessed by New York Heart Association (NYHA) Functional Classification.

Table 18-1. Incidence of valve-related events, expressed as actuarial freedom from complications and linearized rate

Event	N	2 years	5 years	8.7 years	% per pt-yr
Intrinsic valve failure	6	96.6 ± 1.9%	90.2 ± 4.6%	67.7 ± 19.8%	1.5
Thromboembolism	5	98.8 ± 1.2%	92.6 ± 4.0%	84.9 ± 8.3%	1.3
Infective endocarditis with valve failure	3	96.9 ± 1.8%	96.9 ± 1.8%	96.9 ± 1.8%	0.8
Total valve-related events	14	95.7 ± 2.1%	84.0 ± 4.9%	49.2 ± 20.8%	3.6
Late mortality due to valve-related events	3	97.9 ± 2.1%	96.3 ± 2.2%	96.3 ± 2.2%	0.8
Mortality and reoperation	9	96.9 ± 1.8%	90.6 ± 3.5%	65.3 ± 19.2%	2.3

had a perforation of the right coronary cusp at 91 months; there was no calcification or infective endocarditis. The typical pathological changes have been studied [15, 16].

Actuarial freedom from IVF was 96.6 ± 1.9%, 90.2 ± 4.6%, and 67.7 ± 19.8% at 2, 5, and 8.7 years after implantation, respectively (figure 18-3). Reoperation for IVF did not significantly affect patient survival (p = 0.21).

The early phase risk of instantaneous IVF, as assessed by life table estimate of hazard function, started 30 to 40 months after implantation and increased during 40 to 50 months postimplantation.

The only significant IRF identified by UVA for IVF was elective operation (p = 0.04). An indicator was younger age (p = 0.08); the mean patient age for those experiencing IVF was 69 years, compared to 72.9 years for those who did not. Having had a previous operation was identified as an IRF by MVA (p = 0.04).

THROMBOEMBOLISM (TE). Thromboembolism was defined as all new focal neurological deficits, either transient or permanent, as well as any clinically detectable noncerebral emboli [5]. Patients who had undergone isolated AVR did not receive anticoagulant therapy; patients with multivalve replacements received long-term sodium dicumarol therapy.

Thromboembolism occurred in 5 hospital-discharged patients (5.1%, 70%

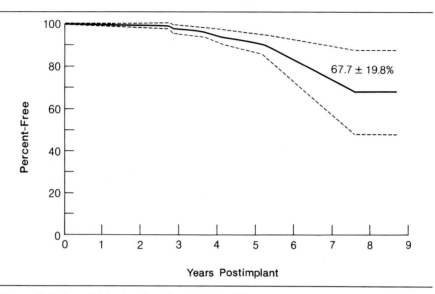

Figure 18-3. Actuarial freedom from intrinsic valve failure.

CL: 2.8%–8.5%), a linearized rate of 1.3% per patient-year. All were nonfatal; only 1 episode was considered a major event. Actuarial freedom from TE was 98.81 ± 1.2%, 92.6 ± 4.0%, and 84.9 ± 8.3% at 2, 5, and 8.7 years, respectively (figure 18-4). The instantaneous risk of TE plotted

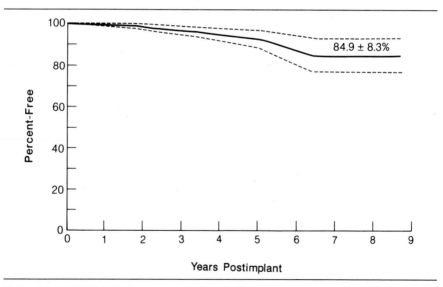

Figure 18-4. Actuarial freedom from thromboembolism.

by hazard function disclosed that the incidence of TE started at about 20 months after operation and linearly increased to about 1% at 70 to 80 months postoperatively.

Longer survival time with the original prosthesis was found to be an IRF by UVA (p = 0.057).

No known anticoagulant hemorrhages (ARH) occurred.

INFECTIVE ENDOCARDITIS (IE). Nine patients experienced infective endo-carditis 6 weeks to 50 months after operation (9.2%, 70% CL: 6.2%–13.2%), a linearized rate of 2.3% per patient-year. Six patients survived (66.6%). Infective endocarditis compromised the performance of the bio-prosthesis in 3 instances, 0.8% per patient-year. Actuarial freedom from IE affecting the valve substitute (IEVF) was 96.9 ± 1.8% at all intervals (2, 5, and 8.7 years after operation) as shown in figure 18-5. Incremental risk factors by UVA for IE not affecting the valve were: earlier year of operation (p = 0.01), concomitant procedure (p = 0.099), and longer survival time (p = 0.08). The only IRF by MVA for IE not affecting the valve was year of operation (p = 0.01). No IRF could be identified by UVA or MVA for IE affecting the valve.

The hazard function for prosthetic valve endocarditis peaked just after operation. Infective endocarditis not affecting the valve occurred in a constant but lower rate for up to 60 months after operation.

CUMULATIVE VALVE-RELATED EVENTS (VRE). The accumulation of all valve-related events (IVF, TE, ARH, IEVF) totaled 14 events (14.3%, 70% CL:

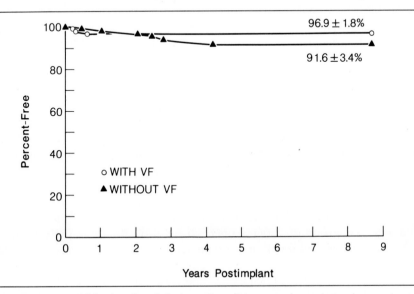

Figure 18-5. Actuarial freedom from infective endocarditis, comparing patients who experienced valve failure with those who did not.

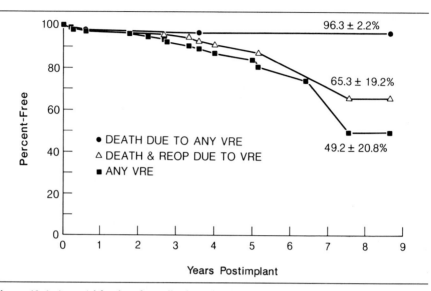

Figure 18-6. Actuarial freedom from all valve-related events (VRE) plotted along with freedom from death due to VRE and death or reoperation due to VRE.

10.6%–18.9%) or 3.6% per patient-year. The linearized rate for mortality resulting from all VRE was 0.8% per patient-year. The respective actuarial freedoms are plotted in figure 18-6. Hazard function for VRE revealed a constant, but low, chance of VRE occurrence. The peak incidence was 70 to 90 months after operation. Incremental risk factors for any VRE identified by MVA were younger age (p = 0.02, 69.8 vs. 73.2 years), previous operation (p = 0.04), and concomitant procedure (p = 0.01).

DISCUSSION

Several requisites are imperative for a thorough assessment of the performance and behavior of a given valve substitute, as well as the clinical results of a particular group of patients receiving a given device. Time frame, preferably longer than 8 years, is mandatory to allow sufficient time lapse for the occurrence of all possible events. Complete follow-up (> 98%) assures accurate documentation of the frequency of a given event. Stringent investigation of all valve-related events should provide complete data to execute sophisticated statistical analyses. If feasible, such analyses should be performed within a homogenous group of patients operated upon during the same time frame. The present study fulfills all the aforementioned requisites in a group of elderly patients (median age 71 years) undergoing AVR with one type of xenobioprosthesis, the IONESCU-SHILEY bioprosthesis valve (ISBPV).

With changing demography, older patients are being referred for operation with increasing frequency; the outcome deserves in-depth study. From this analysis several conclusions can be drawn: Older age, per se, was found to be an incremental risk factor for hospital death by univariate analysis (p = 0.04), as was higher NYHA Functional Class (p = 0.06). Incremental risk factors for late mortality were concomitant procedures and earlier year of operation. When operating upon this cohort of patients it is reasonable to expect a higher operative mortality, as shown in this experience. Regarding the valve substitute itself, the ISBPV performs well, with a low incidence of valve-related events. It appears to be a safe valve substitute in this age group, given that the linearized rate of mortality due to valve-related events is less than 1 occurrence per hundred patient-years (0.8% per patient-year). The ISBPV permits AVR, avoiding aortic annular enlargement and concomitant prolonged aortic cross-clamp time.

Eighty-five percent of the patients were free from thromboembolism at 10 years; 4 of the 5 events were considered minor and none were fatal. Patients with isolated AVR did not receive anticoagulant therapy. This emphasizes the safety of the ISBPV in the elderly, in whom anticoagulant-related events can reach significant incidence. In an analysis of mechanical prostheses undertaken at our institution, the incidence of anticoagulant-related events outnumbered the incidence of emboli [17].

When hazard functions compared the instantaneous risk for valve-related events with that of a contemporaneous group of 133 patients less than 66 years of age, the hazard function peaked at 55 to 65 months after operation for the younger group and at 70 to 90 months for those 66 years of age and older.

CONCLUSIONS

The IONESCU-SHILEY bovine pericardial valve is a reliable valve substitute in the aortic position in patients 66 years of age and older. Older age increases the risk of hospital death. Actuarial survival and freedom from valve-related events is good.

This xenobioprosthesis allows for isolated AVR without the need for anticoagulant therapy and consequent threat of anticoagulant hemorrhage. In addition, there is no need for aortic root enlargement.

REFERENCES

1. Walker DK, Scotten LN, Modi VJ, et al. In vitro assessment of mitral valve prostheses. J Thorac Cardiovasc Surg 1980; 79:680.
2. Wright JTM. Hydrodynamic evaluation of tissue valves. In Ionescu MI (ed): *Tissue Heart Valves*. Butterworth, London 1979; pp 29–88.
3. Rainer WG, Christopher RA, Sadler TR Jr, et al. Dynamic behavior of prosthetic aortic tissue valves as viewed by high-speed cinematography. Ann Thorac Surg 1979; 28:274.
4. Tandon AP, Smith DR, Mary DAS, et al. Sequential hemodynamic studies in patients having aortic valve replacement with the Ionescu-Shiley pericardial valve. Ann Thorac Surg 1977; 24:149.
5. Gonzalez-Lavin L, Tandon AP, Chi S, Blair TC, McFadden PM, Lewis B, Daughters G, Ionescu MI. Risk of thromboembolism and hemorrhage following mitral valve replacement. A comparative analysis between porcine xenograft and Ionescu-Shiley bovine pericardial valves. J Thorac Cardiovasc Surg 1984; 87:340.

6. Gonzalez-Lavin L, Chi S, Lewis B, et al. An 8-year experience with the standard Ionescu-Shiley pericardial valve in the aortic position. In Bodnar E and Yacoub M (eds): *Biologic Bioprosthetic Valves: Proceedings of the Third International Symposium.* Yorke Medical Books, New York 1986; pp 199–213.
7. Kaplan EL, Meier P. Nonparametric estimation from incomplete observations. Am Stat Assoc J 1958; 53:457–481.
8. Cox, DR. Regression models and life tables (with discussion). J Roy Stat Soc B 1972; 34:187–220.
9. Mantel N, Haenszel W. Statistical aspects of the analyses of the data from retrospective studies of disease. J Nat Canc Inst 1959; 22:719–748.
10. Fleiss JL. *Statistical Methods for Rates and Proportions.* John Wiley and Sons, New York 1973.
11. Cox DR. *Analysis of Binary Data.* Methuen and Co., London 1970.
12. Lee ET. *Statistical Methods for Survival Data Analysis.* Lifetime Learning Publications, Belmont 1980.
13. Borkon, AM, McIntosh CL, Von Reuden TJ, et al. Mitral valve replacement with the Hancock bioprosthesis: Five- to ten-year follow-up. Ann Thorac Surg 1981; 32:127.
14. Johnson D, Gonzalez-Lavin L. Myocardial infarction secondary to calcific embolization. An unusual complication of xenobioprosthetic degeneration. Ann Thorac Surg 1986; 42:102.
15. Johnson DE, Billingham ME, Gonzalez-Lavin L. Pathologic changes in dysfunctional Ionescu-Shiley bovine pericardial heterograft valves. In *Cardiac Prostheses Symposium III.* Shiley, Inc., Irvine, 1987; p 135–45.
16. Schoen FJ, Fernandez J, Gonzalez-Lavin L, Cernaianu A. Causes of failure and pathologic findings in surgically removed bovine Ionescu-Shiley standard pericardial heart valve bioprostheses: emphasis on progressive structural deterioration. Circulation 1987; 76-III-618.
17. Gonzalez-Lavin L, McGrath LB, Fernandez J, Quinlan WC. Strut fracture and other related valve-related events following valve replaceemnt with the 60° Convexo-Concave Björk-Shiley prosthesis. Circulation 1986; 74:II-337.

19. VALVE REPLACEMENT IN THE ELDERLY: OPERATIVE RISK AND EARLY POSTOPERATIVE RESULTS

R. KÖRFER, U. POTT, K. MINAMI, U. GLEICHMANN

Abstract. *From the opening of our institution in November 1984 to December 1986, 2770 open heart procedures for congenital and acquired heart disease have been performed. There were 680 patients who had valve replacement; isolated or in combination with other operations, i.e., myocardial revascularization, thromboendarterectomy of carotid artery [TEA]. Of these, 182 patients (69 male and 113 female) were between 66 and 82 years of age (mean age 71.3 years). Early mortality (within 30 days postoperation) was 3.1% (2 patients). Eight patients have required reoperation. It is our policy to use bioprostheses in patients of more than 65 years of age, except in those who are on anticoagulation for special reasons. Nevertheless, all patients have anticoagulant therapy for at least 3 months postoperatively. Operative risk and rate of perioperative complications in this age group are similar to those in younger patients. Thus, older patients with good motivation, a desire for an improved lifestyle, in good mental status, and with no other major disease are good candidates for valve replacement and additional procedures if necessary.*

INTRODUCTION

The purpose of this study is to present the operative results of cardiac valve replacement obtained in patients more than 66 years of age. Patients of this group, especially septuagenarians and octogenarians, are often considered poor candidates for valvular surgery and subsequently are not accepted for operation.

147

PATIENTS AND METHODS

Since the opening of our institution in November 1984 up to December 1986, nearly 3000 open heart procedures for congenital and acquired heart disease have been performed (table 19-1). There were 680 patients who had 685 valvular operations, either isolated or in combination with other operations (i.e., myocardial revascularization or thromboendarterectomy of carotid artery). Of these, 182 patients with 185 valve replacements (69 male and 113 female) were between 66 and 82 years of age (mean age 71.3 years). More detailed analysis of age distribution of elderly patients showed that 87 patients were between 66 and 70 years of age, 69 patients were between 71 and 75 years of age, and 26 patients were beyond 76 years of age. Additional procedures were performed in nearly 40% of the operations (table 19-2).

The majority of patients suffered from aortic valve disease, a smaller number had mitral valve disease, and only a few patients had double (aortic and mitral) valve disease. One patient had a reoperation for prosthetic tricuspid valve dysfunction. One hundred eleven patients were in New York Heart Association (NYHA) Functional Class III, 40 patients were in Class III to IV, and 29 patients were in Functional Class IV. Only 5 patients were in Functional Class II to III. All had aortic valve disease together with coronary heart disease and had simultaneous operations (table 19-3). One hundred twenty valve replacements without concomitant procedures were performed. The most frequent operation was aortic valve replacement for aortic stenosis. Five patients did not survive, resulting in a mortality rate of 4.2% (table 19-4).

Sixty-five concomitant procedures, mostly myocardial revascularization, were performed. In the subgroup with mitral valve replacement, there were 6

Table 19-1. Quota of valve replacement on patient population

2973	operations with ECC
685	operations for valvular heart disease (valve reconstructions excluded)
185	valve replacements in the elderly (> 66 years of age)

Table 19-2. Age distribution and percentage of additional procedures

Age range (years)	No. of patients	Additional procedures No. of patients (90%)
66–70	87	34 (39.1%)
71–75	69	26 (37.7%)
> 76	26	11 (42.3%)

Table 19-3. Valve disease and preoperative NYHA Functional Class

Valve disease	New York Heart Association Functional Class			
	II–III	III	III–IV	IV
Aortic	5	85	24	22
Mitral		22	12	4
Tricuspid			1	
Aortic + mitral		4	3	3
Total	5	111	40	29

Table 19-4. Results of isolated valve replacement in the elderly

Operation	No. of patients	Mortality No. of patients (%)
AVR	86	2 (2.3%)
MVR★	26	1 (3.8%)
TVR	1	
AVR + MVR	7	2
Total	120	5 (4.2%)

AVR = aortic valve replacement; MVR = mitral valve replacement; TVR = tricuspid valve replacement
★ Ten patients with additional tricuspid valve annuloplasty

patients who suffered from ischemic mitral valve regurgitation. Again, most of the valve replacements were performed in the aortic position. Three patients had a thromboendarterectomy of the carotid artery in addition to their myocardial revascularization (table 19-5). The number of peripheral anastomoses ranged from 1 to 5, with a mean of 2.3. Mortality rate was 3.1% (2 patients).

RESULTS

The causes of death are summarized in table 19-6. Four patients died due to their cardiac disease; 3 patients developed multi-organ failure. The 82-year-old woman described was the former head nurse of a hospital in the neighborhood. She came into the hospital with pulmonary edema and cardiogenic shock. To give her at least a chance, a double valve replacement was performed as an emergency operation without any invasive examination, but she died *in tabula*.

Neurological disorders were the most frequent nonfatal complications. Most of these patients had some signs of disorientation for a maximum of 3 days. Twelve patients had transient hemiplegia for a maximum of 7 days, and only 1 patient had a tetraplegia, which improved remarkably during the

Table 19-5. Results of valve replacement with concomitant procedures in the elderly

Operation	No. of patients	No. of peripheral anastomoses (mean range)	Mortality
AVR + CABG	47	2.3 (1–5)	2 (4.3%)
MVR* + CABG	11	2.7 (1–5)	
MVR + CABG + VAR	1	3.0	
AVR + MVR + CABG	3	2.0 (1–3)	
AVR + CABG + TEA (carotid artery)	3	1.3 (1–2)	
Total	65	2.3 (1–5)	2 (3.1%)

AVR = aortic valve replacement; MVR = mitral valve replacement; CABG = coronary artery bypass graft; VAR = ventricular aneurysm resection; TEA = thromboendarterectomy of carotid artery
* Three patients with additional tricuspid valve annuloplasty

Table 19-6. Cause of death in elderly patients with valve replacement

Patient	Sex	Age (years)	Operation	Cause of death
1	Male	73	AVR	Cardiac failure, 2 days postop
2	Male	72	AVR + CABG × 3	Respiratory and renal failure, 10 days postop
3	Male	72	AVR + CABG × 3	Cardiac failure, 4 days postop
4	Female	66	MVR	Cardiac failure, 6 hours postop
5	Female	76	AVR	Cerebral death, 3 days postop
6	Male	67	AVR + MVR	Respiratory and renal failure, 30 days postop
7	Female	82	AVR + MVR	Cardiac failure (in tabula)

hospital stay. Patients with renal failure were successfully treated by hemodialysis or hemofiltration. Postoperative bleeding required rethoracotomy in 9 cases. All other complications disappeared after adequate treatment (table 19-7).

Table 19-7. Nonfatal complications in elderly patients after valve replacement

Type of complication	No. of patients
Neurological disorders	49
Postoperative bleeding	9
Arrhythmias	7
Gastrointestinal bleeding	3
Renal failure	3
Respiratory insufficiency	3

Eight patients out of 182 had a reoperation. Five primary operations were done elsewhere and 3 primary operations were performed in our clinic. The types of primary operation and indications for reoperation are summarized in tables 19-8 and 19-9.

Within the group of patients who had their previous operation elsewhere, 1 patient is rather interesting. The woman had a double valve (mitral and tricuspid) replacement with ST. JUDE MEDICAL® (SJM) prostheses. Five years postoperatively a thrombosis of the tricuspid prosthesis occurred and she was operated upon urgently. The mechanical valve was replaced by a xenograft (St. Jude Medical, Inc. BIOIMPLANT™).

In our own series, we had to reoperate on 2 patients with thrombosis of their xenograft valves in the aortic position, at 17 months and 22 months postoperatively. One of these valves was replaced by a mechanical valve along with another triple aortocoronary bypass. In the other case, a porcine valve was replaced by a pericardial valve. One patient with an excessively calcified mitral valve apparatus developed a small paravalvular leak with severe hemolysis. This was the reason for re-replacement of the valve 8 months later.

For various reasons, biological as well as mechanical valves were used for valvular replacement (table 19-10). Basically, a bioprosthesis was the valve of choice in patients more than 65 years of age. If there was a need for anticoagulaton therapy, mechanical valves were implanted. An overview of the results of valve replacements in our clinic is given in table 19-11. Note that there is no significant difference in mortality between the age groups. Interesting, but not unexpected, is the high amount of female patients among the older age group.

CONCLUSION

Valve replacement can be performed in elderly patients with acceptable results. The risk of operation is comparable to the risk of operation in younger patients. Additional procedures, i.e., myocardial revascularization, do not increase the risk of the procedure. The postoperative morbidity is characterized by an increased number of mostly transient neurological disorders. With respect to life expectancy of these patients, the question for the surgeon remains which type of prosthesis should be use.

Table 19-8. Reoperation for valvular heart disease in the elderly done elsewhere

Patient	Sex	Age (years)	Primary operation	Indication for reoperation	Type of reoperation
8	Male	67	CABG	Aortic stenosis, graft closure, 17 months postop	AVR – SJM CABG x 1
9	Female	67	MVR, TVR – SJM	Thrombosis of tricuspid prosthesis, 5 years postop	TV re-replacement – BioImplant
10	Male	71	MVR – Hancock	Xenograft dysfunction, TV regurgitation, 8 years postop	MV re-replacement – SJM; TV reconstruction
11	Female	66	MV Commissurotomy	MV restenosis, 18 years postop	MVR – SJM
12	Female	69	MV Commissurotomy	MV restenosis, TV regurgitation 18 years postop	MVR – Mitroflow, TV reconstruction

CABG = coronary artery bypass graft; MV = mitral valve; TV = tricuspid valve; MV = mitral valve; MVR = mitral valve replacement; TVR = tricuspid valve replacement; SJM = St. Jude Medical

Table 19-9. Reoperation for valvular heart disease in the elderly performed in our clinic

Patient	Sex	Age (years)	Primary operation	Indication for reoperation	Type of reoperation
13	Male	70	AVR – BioImplant CABG x 1	Xenograft thrombosis, 17 months postop	AV re-replacement – SJM, CABG x 3
14	Male	71	AVR – BioImplant	Xenograft thrombosis, 22 months postop	MV re-replacement – Mitroflow
15	Female	72	MVR – SJM	Paravalvular leak hemolysis, 8 months postop	MV re-replacement – SJM

Table 19-10. Type of valve prostheses★

	Type of valve	Number implanted
Mechanical valves n = 52	St. Jude Medical Bjork-Shiley Duromedics	36 15 1
Biological valves n = 143	Mitroflow Hancock BioImplant	93 28 22

★ Ten double valve replacements

Table 19-11. Patient population and mortality within 30 days postoperatively: a summary of all patients with valve replacements including isolated, multiple, with concomitant procedures and re-replacements

Age range (mean)	No. of patients	No. of operations	Male/Female No. of patients	Mortality No. of patients (%)
6–65 (56.4)	498	500	296/202	16 (3.2%)
66–82	182	185	69/113	7 (3.8%)
6–82 (60.6)	680	685	365/315	23 (3.4%)

It is absolutely unclear whether the solution of using bioprostheses in all patients more than 65 years of age is a good one. Keeping in mind the limited durability of bioprostheses, many of these patients will survive their xenograft and subsequently have to be reoperated.

20. AORTIC VALVE REPLACEMENT IN PATIENTS 75 YEARS AND OVER

B. BLAKEMAN, A. MONTOYA, H. SULLIVAN, M. BAKHOS, J. GRIECO, B. FOY, R. PIFARRE

Abstract. *A select group of 65 patients in the eighth decade of life who had aortic valvular replacement (AVR) from 1975 through 1984 were retrospectively studied. Preoperatively, 58 of the 65 patients were in New York Heart Association (NYHA) Class III or IV. This group included isolated AVR cases (26 patients) and AVR with concomitant procedures (39 patients). Perioperative mortality (30 days) was 1.5% and perioperative morbidity (62%) involved 54 complications in 40 patients. Long-term follow-up was available for 55 patients, including 40 survivors. Thirty-eight of 40 medium-term survivors (72%) are now in NYHA Class I or II. Perioperative mortality and improved quality of life support aortic valve replacement in this older population.*

INTRODUCTION

Because of advancements in cardiovascular surgery, we have become more aggressive in extending various procedures to the older population. This decision is continuously scrutinized by society, government, third-party payers, hospital administrators, and other medical personnel as costs continue to escalate. In order to justify our therapy, it becomes necessary to re-evaluate our results with these patients.

With this background, we reviewed a select group of patients in their eighth decade of life with aortic valvular disease. Sixty-five patients over the age of 75 had aortic valve replacement with or without concomitant procedures in the

10-year period from 1975 through 1984. The prescribed intent was to evaluate perioperative morbidity and mortality as well as long-term survival.

MATERIALS AND METHODS

The records of 65 patients, 75 years of age and older, with aortic valve replacement were reviewed. This included concomitant procedures and spanned a 10-year period.

Patient ages ranged from 75 to 89 years, with a mean of 77.6 years. Seven of the patients were over 80-years-old. Fifty-eight of 65 patients were categorized in Class III or IV of the New York Heart Association (NYHA) Functional Classification for cardiac symptoms.

The 65 aortic valve replacements represented 9.2% of the total aortic valves replaced for this 10-year period at our institution (706 total aortic valve replacements). This group of 65 patients comprised 23% of the total cardiac surgery performed in this age group (285 total cases).

Symptoms for this group of patients included: heart failure in 43 patients, syncope in 17 cases, and angina in 25 cases. The distribution of cases by year can be seen in figure 20-1; 1984 is the leading year, with 20 cases.

Thirty-two patients had aortic stenosis only, 4 had insufficiency only, and 29 had a fixed-valve orifice with both stenosis and insufficiency.

Mean catheterization data for the group revealed a cardiac index of 2.2 L/M/M², a peak-to-peak gradient across the valve of 65 mm, a valve index of 0.3 cm²/M², pulmonary artery pressure of 42/19 mm Hg and left ventricular end-diastolic pressure of 19 mm Hg.

Procedures performed were: aortic valve replacement only in 26 patients; valve replacement, with an average of 2.06 bypasses, in 32 patients; AVR,

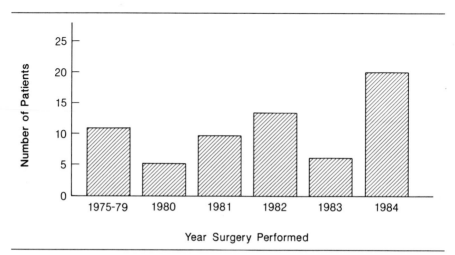

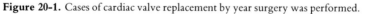

Figure 20-1. Cases of cardiac valve replacement by year surgery was performed.

MVR, and one bypass in 2 patients; AVR with permanent pacemaker in 4 patients; and a valve conduit in 1 patient. Fifty-one patients were given a mechanical valve (47 BJÖRK-SHILEY® tilting disc and 4 ST. JUDE MEDICAL®) and 14 received a bioprosthesis.

RESULTS

Sixty-four of the 65 patients survived the surgery in the perioperative period. The 1 operative death was a 77-year-old female with a peak-to-peak gradient across the valve of 120 mm Hg, a valve index of 0.2 cm^2/M^2, and a cardiac index of 1.95 $L/M/M^2$ by the Fick method. The procedure performed was an aortic valve replacement done on an emergency basis with a #21 BJÖRK-SHILEY disc, a single bypass to the left anterior descending vessel, and exploration of the mitral valve for possible stenosis. Because of poor ventricular function, the patient was not able to be weaned from cardiopulmonary bypass, despite maximum drug support and an intra-aortic balloon pump.

There were 54 complications in the 40 patients, a complication rate of 62%. Fifteen of these postoperative complications required surgical intervention: 6 patients returned for bleeding, 4 required permanent pacemakers, 3 needed pericardial effusions drained, and 2 required surgery for gastrointestinal bleeding.

Thirty-nine complications were nonsurgical. The most common were arrhythmias in 17 patients, which were controlled with medication, and 5 complications were due to urinary tract problems (table 20-1).

The length of postoperative confinement ranged from 9 to 48 days, with an average of 15.8 days per patient.

Because of age and the fact that several patients left our region, we have long-term follow-up on only 55 of the 64 patients (86%). Forty of the 55

Table 20-1. Nonsurgical perioperative complications among 40 surviving patients

Complication	No. of patients
Arrhythmias	17
Urinary	6
Gastrointestinal bleeding	4
Postpericardiectomy syndrome	3
Leg hematoma	3
Drug rash	1
Renal failure	1
Cardiac arrest	1
Pneumothorax	1
Pneumonia	1
Pseudoaneurysm	1
Right groin	1

patients were alive at the time that this follow-up was performed. The postoperative time span for 40 long-term survivors ranges from 5 to 81 months, with a mean of 27.5 months. Thirty-eight of 40 patients are now in NYHA Classes I or II. In this group of 40, there have been 11 complications. Three complications were directly related to the heart: 2 valvular and 1 arrhythmia. The 2 valvular complications were endocarditis in 1 patient, which was treated surgically, and a paravalvular leak in another patient, which required reoperation. Both patients survived surgery without significant problems. The arrhythmia problem was resolved with medical treatment.

There were 8 noncardiac complications in the surviving patients; 5 bleeding problems (2 cerebral, 2 extremity, and 1 ocular), 2 other neurological problems (1 syncope and 1 embolic stroke), and 1 patient who was re-admitted with hepatitis. All patients with bleeding problems were on COUMADIN® at the time.

Fifteen patients were known dead at the time of this follow-up. The postoperative time ranged from 1.5 to 62 months, with a mean of 24.7 months. The causes of death were cardiac-related in 5 patients: 2 with myocardial infarct, 2 with prosthetic valve endocarditis, and 1 of cardiac failure. There were 10 patients with noncardiac deaths: 2 cancer, 2 stroke, 1 trauma, 1 sepsis, and 4 unknown.

DISCUSSION

The many advancements in cardiovascular surgery, in particular the ability to provide better protection of the heart with cardioplegia, have allowed cardiac procedures to be extended to an ever-increasing group of patients. We were particularly interested in the group of patients over the age of 75, who were operated on for aortic valvular disease. The last few years have seen a literal explosion of papers on this topic [1–19]. Our own data indicates that the average age of patients for aortic valve replacement continues to increase. In 1970, the mean age for an aortic valve replacement was 50 years; in 1975, 56 years; in 1980, 62 years; and by 1984 (the last year of our study), 63.5 years. The literature reflects a similar change in the definition of elderly. Spencer et al., in 1964, published a report of 4 patients with aortic valve replacement in which the elderly patients ranged in age from 54 to 62 years [7]. Ahmad and Starr published a report in 1969 of 91 patients over the age of 60 [14]. By 1980, the same group reported a series of "elderly" patients over the age of 75 [2]. So the definition of elderly has changed as the techniques of surgery have improved.

When making a decision to replace the aortic valve or do any procedure in this older age group, one must justify the decision by considering several aspects. First, one must get the patient through surgery with minimal problems. Second, the postoperative quality of life has to be significantly improved. Finally, the morbidity of the procedure must not significantly affect the patient's life.

Considering the disease and symptoms of our patients, mortality of 1.5% and morbidity of 62% are consistent with the results of others. The 30-day perioperative mortality reported in the literature ranges from a low of 4.8% by Arom, 4.8% by Bessone, and 5.3% by Craver to a high of 23% by Teply [1–3, 12]. In all fairness, it should be noted that the series of Teply dates back to 1964, when the ability to protect the myocardium was not as advanced. These figures include isolated AVR and concomitant procedures. Commerford, in 1981, did have a perioperative mortality of only 3.3% in a group of patients for isolated AVR. The causes of death cited include low cardiac output (cause in our case), amyloidosis, pancreatitis, pancytopenia, pulmonary embolus, multiple systemic failure, sepsis, cerebral infarct, myocardial infarction, renal failure, and arrhythmia [1–17, 19].

The most frequent causes of death were low cardiac output with or without myocardial infarction and sepsis, usually resulting in multiple organ failure. Likewise, with the perioperative deaths in the literature, it is very difficult to pinpoint those patients who are in the high-risk category or should not be operated on based on hemodynamic data. However, an operative mortality of 1.5% would seem to be very acceptable and should be a standard to try to achieve.

Second, the morbidity must be minimal. A complication rate of 62% was not too different from the 40% by Bhattacharya, 45% by Kanepa-Anson, and 57.4% by Bessone [8, 9, 12]. The problem of bleeding (9.4%) is higher than our routine result for all hearts (3.5%), but not significantly different than that found by Bessone at 9.3% [12]. None of these patients had further bleeding problems or infection problems. The other very common problem of arrythmias, in 17 patients (25%), is not much different from the complication rate in our entire postoperative cardiac population. The fact that our mean postoperative stay was only 15.8 days indicates that these problems were handled easily and expeditiously. The postoperative stay compares favorably with other figures in the literature: Arom 14 days, Teply and Starr 19 days, and Bergdahl and Björk 18 days [1, 2, 16].

Next, the quality of life was markedly improved in the group of patients who were operated on, with 38 of 40 medium-term survivors in New York Heart Association (NYHA) Class I or II. This is a marked improvement over the 89% which were in Class III or IV preoperatively.

However, this group of survivors had 11 significant complications, 9 of which were directly related to their treatment. These included 2 valvular complications, 5 bleeding problems, 1 stroke, and 1 case of hepatitis presumed secondary to transfusion. With bleeding the most common problem and COUMADIN® being used in all patients, consideration has to be given to the use of a bioprosthetic valve and lack of COUMADIN, when thought feasible by the surgeon or cardiologist.

Finally, at an average follow-up of 2 years, 72% of our medium-term follow-up patients were alive. This is significantly better than the natural history of this disease. Ross and Braunwald, in 1968, estimated that in all age groups, the average length of survival after symptoms was 3 years and only 1.5 to 2 years after congestive heart failure [20]. Sixty-six percent of our patients presented with heart failure. Similarly, Rothman et al. estimated the average life span to be 4 years when symptoms began [21], while Frank and Ross observed an 83% mortality within 5 years of symptoms [22]. Certainly, measuring survival by the natural history of the disease justifies aortic valve replacement.

REFERENCES

1. Arom KV, Nicoloff DM, Lindsay WG, Northrup WF, Kersten TE. Should valve replacement and related procedures be performed in elderly patients? Ann Thor Surg 1984; 38:466.
2. Teply JF, Grunkemeier GL, Starr A. Cardiac valve replacement in patients over 75 years of age. Thor CV Surgeon 1981; 29:47.
3. Craver JM, Goldstein J, Jones EL, Knapp WA, hatcher CR. Clinical, hemodynamic, and operative descriptors affecting outcome of aortic valve replacement in elderly versus young patients. Ann Surg 1984; 199:733.
4. Glock Y, Pecoul R, Cerene A, Laquerre J, Puel P. Aortic valve replacement in elderly patients. J Cardiovasc Surg 1984; 25:205.
5. Santinga JT, Flora J, Kirsh M, Baublis J. Aortic valve replacement in the elderly. J Am Geriat Soc 1983; 31:211.
6. Carlson RG, Shafer RB, Eliot RS, Sellers RD, Lillehei CW. Results of cardiac surgery in 273 older patients. Geriatrics 1967; 22:173.
7. Spencer FC, Trinkle JK, Eiseman B, Reeves JT, Surawicz B. Aortic valve replacement in elderly patients with cardiac failure. JAMA 1964; 189:103.
8. Bhattacharya SK, Teskey JM, Cohen M, Kim SW, Barwinsky J. Risks and benefits of open-heart surgery in patients 70 years of age and older. Can J of Surg 1984; 27:150.
9. Canepa-Anson R, Emanuel RW. Elective aortic and mitral valve surgery in patients over 70 years of age. Br Heart J 1979; 41:493.
10. Austen WG, DeSanctis RW, Buckley MJ, Mundth ED, Scamell JG. Surgical management of aortic valve disease in the elderly. JAMA 1970; 211:624.
11. DeBono AH, English TA, Milstein BB. Heart valve replacement in the elderly. Br Med J 1978; 2:917.
12. Bessone LN, Pupello DF, Blank RH, Harrison EE, Sbar S. Valve replacement in patients over 70 years. Ann Thorac Surg 1977; 24:417.
13. Hildner FJ, Linhart JW, Samet P, Piccinini J, et al. Clinical and hemodynamic comparisons of valve replacement in patients over and under age 60. Ann Thorac Surg 1969; 7:438.
14. Ahmad A, Starr A. Valve replacement in geriatric patients. Br Heart J 1969; 31:322.
15. Commerford PJ, Curcio A, Albanese M, Beck W. Aortic valve replacement in the elderly. SA Med J 1981; 27:975.
16. Bergdahl L, Björk VO, Jonasson R. Aortic valve replacement in patients over 70 years. Scand J Thorac Cardiovasc Surg 1981; 15:123.
17. Oh W, Hickman R, Emmanuel R, McDonald L, et al. Heart valve surgery in 114 patients over age of 60. Br Heart J 1973; 35:174.
18. Gann D, Colin C, Hildner FJ, Samet P, et al. Coronary artery bypass surgery in patients seventy years of age and older. Thorac Cardiovasc Surg 1977; 73:237.
19. Copeland JG, Griepp RB, Stinson EB, Shumway NE. Isolated aortic valve replacement in patients older than 65 years. JAMA 1977; 237:1578.
20. Ross J, Braunwald E. Aortic stenosis. Circulation 1968; 38(Suppl 5):61.
21. Rothman M, Morris JJ, Behar VS, et al. Aortic valvular disease: Comparison of types and their medical and surgical management. Am J Med 1968; 51:241.
22. Frank S, Ross J. Natural history of severe acquired valvular aortic stenosis. Am J Cardiol 1967; 19:128.

21. DURABILTY AND LONG-TERM RESULTS OF AORTIC VALVE REPLACEMENT IN THE ELDERLY

Y. LOGEAIS, A. LEGUERRIER, C. RIOUX, J. F. DELAMBRE, T. LANGANAY

Abstract. *Isolated aortic valve replacement for aortic stenosis was performed on 355 elderly patients (53.5% female), age 70–85 years, between January 1971 and December 1985. One-third of the patients (112) received mechanical valves; 243 patients received bioprostheses. Since April 1981, biological prostheses have been used as the substitute of choice in this group of patients. There was 100% follow-up of the 319 operative survivors for nearly 12 years, for a total of 1107 patient-years and a mean of 3.2 years. The overall survival rate at 5 years is 70.8% (operative deaths included) and the functional result is excellent. Late deaths and complications are reviewed and comparison is made between the two types of prostheses.*

INTRODUCTION

The incidence of valve replacement in elderly patients is increasing. Results of aortic valve replacement for aortic stenosis, in patients aged 70 years and older, are presented.

METHODS

Between January 1971 and December 1985, 355 patients underwent isolated aortic valve replacement (AVR) but had no other valve or coronary surgery. The majority of patients (53.5%) were female. Most were less than 76 years old; 12 patients were between 80 and 85 years of age. The mean age was 73.7 years, as shown in figure 21-1.

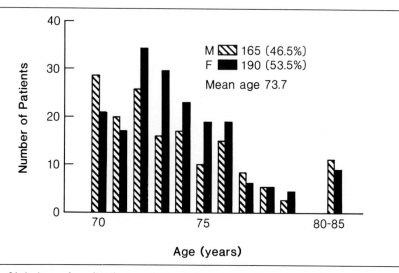

Figure 21-1. Age and sex distribution of 355 elderly patients with aortic stenosis.

As table 21-1 indicates, the majority of patients had advanced stenosis. Some had an associated aortic insufficiency (AI) of mild degree. Thirty-five patients had an associated lesion of the ascending aorta, and 19 of them had associated surgery for that reason. The aortic valve was found to be heavily calcified in 85% of the cases. Most patients had fused commissures, as well as massively calcified and stenosed bicuspid valves. The Monckeberg type has been uncommon [1].

Table 21-2 shows the distribution of Functional Status according to the New York Heart Association (NYHA) Classification and related ECG data. Length of symptoms averaged 4.2 years.

Surgical techniques are described in table 21-3. Mean ECC time was 86 minutes. Aortic cross-clamp time was 55 minutes. Since December 1976, cardioplegia was utilized on 340 patients or nearly 96% of the patients.

Table 21-1. Aortic stenosis and pathology in 355 elderly patients

	No. of patients	Percent
Pure aortic stenosis	279	78.6
Mild associated aortic insufficiency	73	20.6
Etiology		
Calcified	300	84.5
Rheumatic	32	9.0
Bicuspid	36	10.1
Associated lesions of the ascending aorta	35	9.9

Table 21-2. Functional status and related data for 355 patients age 70–85 years with aortic stenosis

| Sex | 165 males (46.5%) |
| | 190 females (53.5%) |

| Age | 70–85 years (mean 73.7 years) |

Preoperative New York Heart Association Classification

Class	No. of patients	Percent
I	3	0.8
II	129	36.3
III	187	52.6
IV	38	10.6

| Average length of symptoms | 4.2 years | |

	No. of patients	Percent
ECG rhythm: S	315	88.7
AF	23	6.5
AV or B. B. Block	158	44.5

Table 21-3. Surgical methods in aortic valve replacement

Extracorporeal circulation (average time)	86 minutes
Aortic cross-clamping (average)	55 minutes
Myocardial protection	
1971–1976: Blood coronary perfusion	15 (4.2%)
Dec. 1976: Crystalloid cold cardioplegia	
± topical cooling	340 (95.8%)
Emergency	12 (3.4%)

Mechanical valves were used almost exclusively from 1972 to April 1981. During that time, 112 patients (32%) received BJÖRK-SHILEY® or ST. JUDE MEDICAL® valves (figure 21-2 and table 21-4). From April 1981 to the present, bioprostheses were used almost exclusively. CARPENTIER-EDWARDS® and some IONESCU-SHILEY® valves were implanted in 243 (68%) of the 355 patients.

RESULTS

Thirty-six patients (10.1%) died in the postoperative period. Causes are listed in table 21-5. Note that 13 (36%) of these deaths were due to myocardial-related causes.

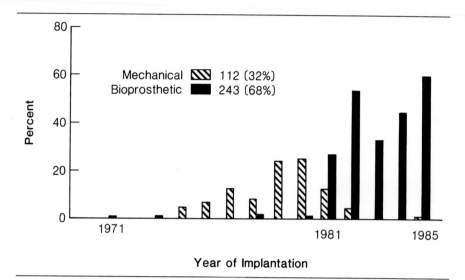

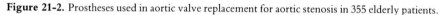

Figure 21-2. Prostheses used in aortic valve replacement for aortic stenosis in 355 elderly patients.

Table 21-4. Prostheses used in isolated aortic valve replacement

1971–1982: Mechanical valves in 112 patients (32%)

Björk-Shiley	
Standard	95 patients
Convexo-Concave	14 patients
St. Jude Medical	3 patients

April 1981–December 1985: Bioprostheses in 243 patients (68%)

Carpentier-Edwards	
Model 2625	81 patients
Model 2650	111 patients
Ionescu-Shiley	51 patients

In addition, there were 3 cases of early thrombosis. We found this higher incidence of postoperative thrombosis following isolated AVR with IONESCU-SHILEY valves not only in this series, but also in our total experience. This complication arose in 4 of 54 patients (7.4%) with IONESCU-SHILEY valves as compared to 1 of 1458 patients (0.07%) with other valves.

All 319 survivors have been accessible, allowing a follow-up of 100% for nearly 12 years. This is a total of 1107 patient-years and an average of 3.2 years. Cases are almost equally distributed between mechanical valves and bioprostheses (474 and 453, respectively).

Table 21-5. Cause of hospital mortality following isolated aortic valve replacement in 355 elderly patients

Deaths 36/355 patients (10.1%)		
Cause	No. of patients	Percent
Myocardial	13	36
Cerebral	5	14
Ionescu-Shiley thrombosis	3	8
Infection	3	8
Technical	6	17
Miscellaneous	6	17

Table 21-6. Causes of late deaths among 60 of 355 elderly patients following isolated AVR

Type of valve	Mechanical		Bioprosthesis	
Number of patients	100		219	
Cause	No. of patients	Percent	No. of patients	Percent
Cardiac	6	20.6	10	32.2
Cerebral	6	20.6	6	19.4
Cancer	1	3.5	6	19.4
Miscellaneous	5	17.3	5	16.1
Unknown	11	37.9	4	12.9
Total (patients)	29		31	
No. of patient-years	474		543	
Percent per patient-year	6.12		5.71	
	(Difference is not significant)			

Late deaths occurred in 60 patients, 29 in patients with mechanical prostheses and 31 among bioprosthesis recipients (table 21-6). This gives similar linearized rates of 6.12% and 5.71% per patient-year, respectively. The difference is not significant. Cardiac, cerebral, and unknown causes of death were the most common.

It is interesting to focus on valve-related (VR) complications leading to death; that is, thromboembolism, anticoagulant hemorrhage, central nervous system complications, prosthetic valve endocarditis, and alteration of the prosthesis (figure 21-3). Incidence was 1.5% per patient-year among mechanical valve patients and 1.3% per patient-year in the bioprostheses group. There was no significant difference between the 2 groups. In actuarial terms, at 5 years, 94.1% of the mechanical group patients were free of VR deaths com-

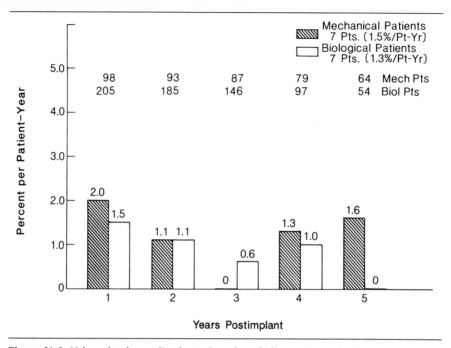

Figure 21-3. Valve-related mortality due to thromboembolism, anticoagulant hemorrhage, central nervous system complications, prosthetic valve endocarditis, and alteration of the prosthesis following AVR.

pared to 96% for the bioprostheses group. This difference was not significant.

Valve-related nonfatal complications were examined. In the mechanical group, 1 valve thrombosis was cured with fibrinolytic treatment. In the bioprostheses group, 1 patient developed alteration of the valve at 4 years and died of cancer. Two patients with prosthetic valve endocarditis (PVE) were managed by heavy antibiotic treatment. One patient in each group developed strokes attributed to systemic emboli and, curiously, patients in both groups had hemorrhagic accidents, more or less related to anticoagulant Tt (5 mechanical and 3 bioprosthesis patients). None of the patients in either group had to be reoperated upon for any type of complication. A few of them had small periprosthetic leaks that were well tolerated.

Morbidity for the two groups was 1.5% per patient-year for the mechanical group and 1.3% per patient-year for the bioprostheses group, as shown in figure 21-4. In actuarial terms, at 5 years, 94.5% of the mechanical patients were free of valve-related morbidity and 93% for the bioprostheses group, a difference that was not significant.

The addition of valve-related morbidity and mortality shows no significant difference between the two groups of prostheses, as shown in figure 21-5. Results were 2.95% per patient-year for mechanical valves, with actuarial

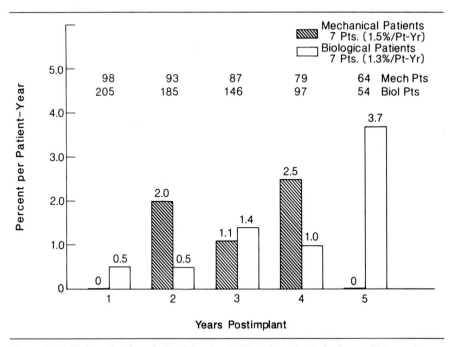

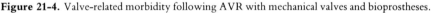

Figure 21-4. Valve-related morbidity following AVR with mechanical valves and bioprostheses.

freedom from valve-related complications (VRC) at 5 years of 88.9%, and 2.6% per patient-year for bioprostheses, with actuarial freedom from VRC at 5 years of 89%.

Figure 21-6 shows the overall actuarial survival curve for the whole group, irrespective of the type of prosthesis. At 5 years, 70.8% of the patients survived (operative deaths included).

Actuarial survival for the two subgroups is shown in figure 21-7. Among patients with mechanical valves, the survival rate was 69.2% at 5 years and 57% at 8 years, while for bioprostheses the survival rate was 72% at 5 years. The end of the curve has been interrupted because the number of patients exposed to risk was too small. At 5 years, the difference between the two subsets is not significant.

The functional results could be evaluated in all the long-term survivors, as shown in table 21-7. NYHA Classification shows drastic improvement: 99.6% of the patients were in Class I or II postoperatively.

Of 130 known ECG tracings, 112 (86%) were in sinus rhythm (table 21-8). The overall result was considered excellent or good in 253 of the 259 survivors (97.7%). It is important to note that they remained stable over time, which parallels the curve of a normal population.

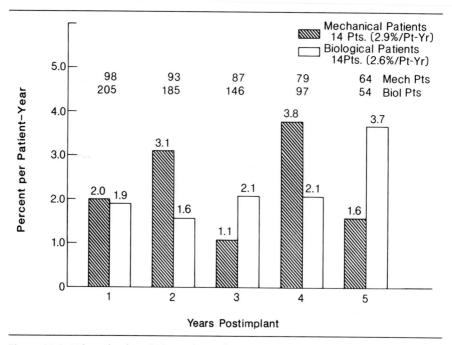

Figure 21-5. Valve-related morbidity and mortality.

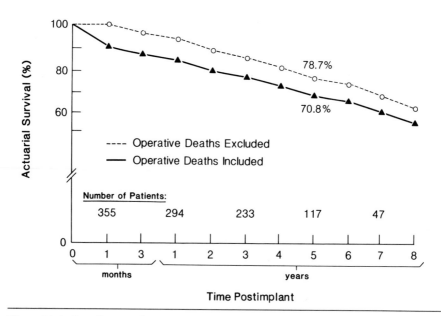

Figure 21-6. Overall actuarial survival following AVR.

Table 21-7. Functional results in 259 survivors following isolated AVR

NYHA Classification	Preoperative		Postoperative	
	No. of patients	Percent	No. of patients	Percent
I	2	0.8	199	76.8
II	106	40.9	59	22.8
III	135	52.1	1	0.4
IV	16	6.2	0	

Mechanical = 71 patients; Bioprostheses = 188 patients

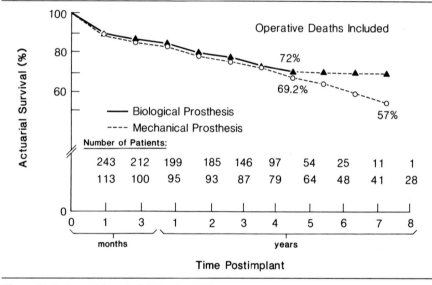

Figure 21-7. Actuarial survival following AVR.

Table 21-8. Long-term results in 259 survivors following isolated AVR

ECG Rhythm in 130 patients

Sinus rhythm in 112 patients (86.0%)
Atrial fibrillation in 14 patients (10.8%)

General result	No. of patients	Percent
Excellent	222	85.7
Good	31	12.0
Unchanged	5	1.9
Deteriorated	1	0.4

DISCUSSION

The incidence of valve replacement in elderly patients is progressively increasing, as shown in absolute numbers (figure 21-8) or in percentages (figure 21-9). This correlates with extensive use of bioprostheses in recent years.

Age has an increasing role in surgical risk. Mortality in AVR is shown

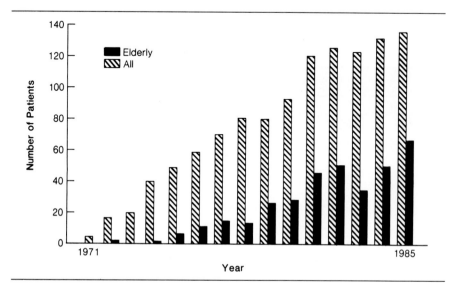

Figure 21-8. Incidence of AVR in elderly patients among 1130 cases of AVR.

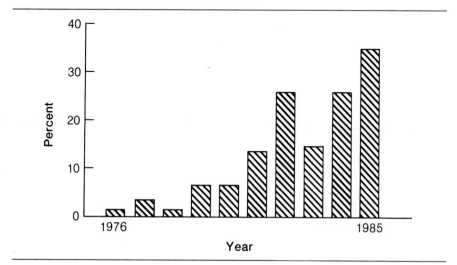

Figure 21-9. Incidence of AVR shown as percent-per-year in patients age 75 years and older.

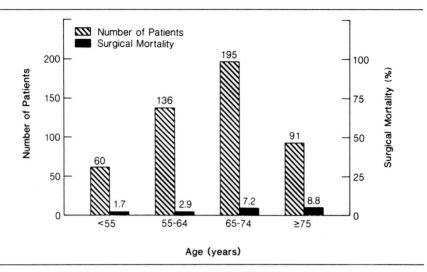

Figure 21-10. Surgical mortality and age in 482 cases of AVR for aortic stenosis.

in figure 21-10 for 482 isolated aortic valve replacements performed between 1982 and 1985. Surgical mortality steadily increased, from 1.7% in patients below age 55 years to 8.8% after 75 years of age.

Long-term results of surgery appear very good and show excellent durability in spite of old age. Surgery is an effective treatment (vs. valvuloplasty).

In 1981, to avoid anticoagulation hemorrhage, we made the choice of using bioprostheses for patients more than 65 years of age. Analysis of this series, with a significant 5-year follow-up, does not confirm the hope for better results at this time. Furthermore, bioprostheses include an increased risk for other complications such as alteration, infection, and reoperations.

Surgery remains an excellent treatment in elderly patients with aortic stenosis. The number of these patients will increase in the future. The economic expense is justified considering the life expectancy. In France, at age 70, it is 10.5 years for males and 13.6 years for females.

REFERENCES

1. Edwards JE. Pathology of acquired valvular disease of the heart. Semin Roentgenol 1979; 14:96.

PART III. DISCUSSION

EUGENE M. BAUDET, MODERATOR

VALVULOPLASTY

CARLOS E. RUIZ: I agree with you, Dr. Logeais, that if the patient is younger than 70 years of age, valve replacement will definitely offer a much better solution than valvuloplasty. But for patients over 70-years-old I think the data reported in the literature do not support your statement that valvuloplasty may not offer the same long-term results that valve replacement does, even though valvuloplasty is repeated in the event of severe stenosis. The costs of both procedures are markedly different, and the complication rate for valvuloplasty seems to be much lower than that for aortic valve replacement. Discharge at 24 to 48 hours after valvuloplasty vs. at least 10 days hospitalization for valve replacement, plus relative comfort compared to the pain a valve replacement patient experiences, support valvuloplasty in the over-70 age group.

YVES LOGEAIS: I agree that my conclusion was deliberately provocative. In our series, indications for valvuloplasty were rather uncommon because the type of lesion has to be considered. The Mönckeberg lesion with intact commissures may be an indication for valvuloplasty. But this type of lesion was not often encountered in our experience. We had to deal with heavily calcified, and almost always, bicuspid aortic valves with fused commissures and friable calcium. While valvuloplasty may help the patient, I am not sure that it would be beneficial long-term.

CARLOS E. RUIZ: In our experience on valvuloplasties, when we have fusion of the commissures, we get the best results. The problem is that most patients do not have commissure fusion and have very stiff cusps. Those are the ones in whom the results are the poorest, so far. Preoperatively, just on the basis of ventriculography or echocardiography, it is very difficult to make that differentiation when they are so heavily calcified.

TISSUE VALVE FAILURE

GEORGES STALPAERT: I would like to ask Dr. Gonzalez-Lavin a question and add some more data about the IONESCU-SHILEY® valve. In an experience of 473 patients with an average age of 60 years, we have compared the standard model with the low profile model. In the standard model, we have seen 3 calcifications in the aortic replacement and 2 cusp ruptures in aortic and mitral replacement. With the low profile valve, we have observed 1 calcification in aortic replacement and 2 in aortic and mitral. We have no tears and no cusp ruptures in aortic IONESCU-SHILEY low profile valves in a follow-up of 6 years. We also have had no cusp ruptures in 137 mitral valve replacements. The only ruptures we have seen are in aortic and mitral valve replacement, and these occurred in 4 of 82 cases. This is statistically significant with a p value of 0.01. In other words, freedom from tissue failure in 6 years was 93% for the standard valve and 98% for the low profile valve. My question is, have you seen the same thing, and what is the reason we see ruptures more frequently in double value replacement with the IONESCU-SHILEY valve?

LORENZO GONZALEZ-LAVIN: Our data parallel your results. I presented a series of patients with aortic valve replacement using the IONESCU-SHILEY standard model, and there were no cusp tears and there was only 1 perforation in the 6 failures. We are in the process of analyzing our mitral and double valve implants. I do not have that information at the present time.

GEORGE REUL, JR.: The valve failure rate among our double valves replacement patients was very low, in fact, lower than either group as a subgroup. The problem with analyzing the IONESCU-SHILEY valve was that we had excellent data at a mean follow-up of about 5 years (60 months), but at a mean of about 58 months the aortic calcifications and ruptures of the leaflets occurred. So you have to extend your data, but you have a precipitous drop at the mean follow-up of 6 years, if you have enough patients who are statistically significant. The main problems with the aortic valve occurred on an average of about 58 months, and these were tears, not degeneration, at the sewing area of the upper portion of the cusp. In the mitral position, the occurrence of the tears was at a mean time of about 44 months, but some occurred a few months after surgery. In the aortic position in the elderly, we found that these tears were occurring without calcification or any other condition, at the sewing area. That supposedly has been corrected in the low profile valve.

GEORGES STALPAERT: Yes, but even with the low profile valve, we have seen the same results as with standard valves. I'd like to add another comment. We have checked patients with the IONESCU-SHILEY valve in sinus rhythm with anticoagulants. In sinus rhythm with anticoagulants, the incidence of thromboemboli was 7.3% per patient-year, while without anticoagulants in sinus rhythm, the incidence was only 1.2%. This is statistically significant, with a p value of 0.01. However, if you give anticoagulants to patients who are not in sinus rhythm, the incidence is 8%, and in patients not anticoagulated and not in sinus rhythm, the incidence is even lower, at

5.7%, but that's not statistically significant. So, for this biological valve, I think it is more important not to give anticoagulants than to use them.

LORENZO GONZALEZ-LAVIN: I would thoroughly agree with that last statement. We have to come up with very solid evidence. We are currently conducting a prospective randomized study of patients undergoing mitral valve replacement with pericardial valves and have established two groups: patients who received warfarin anticoagulants and patients without anticoagulants. We will be able to tell you the results in a couple of years.

YVES GOFFIN: Dr. Gonzalez-Lavin, in your series of aortic valve replacements, you have no case of rupture, at the strut or the hinge line, which is remarkable, but you had a perforation. That perforation, for me as a pathologist, is very exceptional. Could you give more information about it?

LORENZO GONZALEZ-LAVIN: The perforation occurred 91 months after implantation and the valve was not calcified. This valve has been sent to Dr. Schoen, a pathologist at Harvard, and he will be presenting several views on it. On gross examination the valve appeared perfectly normal, other than having a punched-out hole in one of the leaflets. Histological examination revealed no evidence of infection. The patient had no murmurs until 91 months.

MORBIDITY AND MORTALITY AMONG OCTOGENARIANS

GEORGE KOBINIA: Dr. Gray, has age alone accounted for the higher morbidity and mortality in your octogenarian group or did these patients have worse hemodynamics than the other group? Have you compared hemodynamic data like ejection fraction and cardiac index in the octogenarian age group with those in the middle age group?

RICHARD GRAY: That's perhaps the most important question to address and we've begun to look at it. Comparing those patients that have a normal ejection fraction with those who have an abnormal ejection fraction, we found that the early postoperative mortality in this cohort of 119 elderly patients is the same, irrespective of a cutoff point in ejection fraction. In our experience, age, itself, is a factor. As one gets older, the mortality is higher. As clinicians, we are forced or obligated to take care of such patients, and we have to decide whether or not to operate on them. How do we predict, prior to surgery, which of these older patients will have a good outcome? So far, I would say that ejection fraction is not the determinant. New York Heart Association Classification is an important factor with the cohort we presented. Being in Class IV vs. Class III did make a difference, in terms of early postoperative survival. Examining averages in groups of 30 to 50 patients is not the way to find the answer. I think you have to review very small subsets of patients to find the answers to these questions.

IV. CONSIDERATIONS IN HEART VALVE REPLACEMENT

22. MECHANICAL OR TISSUE VALVES: FACTORS INFLUENCING DIFFERENTIAL THERAPY

D. HORSTKOTTE, H. D. SCHULTE, W. BIRCKS

Abstract. *The late outcome of heart valve replacement can be determined by subjective improvement, improvement of functional capacity and central hemodynamics, normalization of impaired ventricular function by the frequency of complications related to or induced by the prosthesis, and by postoperative survival. According to these advantages and disadvantages of bioprostheses and mechanical valves, a differential therapy and an individualized approach should be preferred. Considering the durability of bioprostheses currently available, mechanical valves are favorable in patients younger than 35-years-old and particularly in children, in whom rapid calcification must be expected. Regarding valve implantation in older patients, recent improvement in life expectancy has to be considered, indicating a high probability of reoperation even in patients with bioprosthetic valve replacement at the age of 65 years. Weighing the risks and benefits, anticoagulation has to be recommended in a substantial number of patients with mitral bioprostheses, which means that these patients would not receive enough benefit from bioprosthetic valve implantation. In atrioventricular valve replacement and in aortic valve implants, in which only small-sized prostheses can be used, the hemodynamic disadvantage of bioprostheses may limit the overall operative success. In these patients, for hemodynamic reasons, a modern mechanical valve should be preferred. Moreover, an expected high risk of reoperation would discourage tissue valve implantation.*

179

INTRODUCTION

Comparison between mechanical and tissue valves should assess the late outcome of heart valve replacement by determining the subjective improvement of the patients, the improvement of functional capacity and central hemodynamics, and a normalization of impaired left and/or right ventricular function, as well as the frequency of those complications that are likely to be valve-related.

Subjective improvement

The subjective postoperative improvement of individual symptoms is obviously dependent on the degree of postoperative normalization of hemodynamics, especially of pressures in the pulmonary circulation [1–5].

After mitral valve replacement, patients report dyspnea, and pressures in the pulmonary circulation do not correlate in all individual cases; however, on the average, a good correlation can be found [5, 6]. In the group of patients showing no or only little clinical improvement, preoperative and postoperative mean pulmonary artery pressures (PAP) are not different. On the other hand, PAP at rest are normalized in patients whose conditions are improved by one New York Heart Association (NYHA) Functional Class. PAP in these patients decreased from 38 ± 12 mm Hg to 20 ± 8 mm Hg. The reduction of PAP is more significant in patients who reported an improvement of two NYHA classes. In this group, PAP decreased from 42 ± 8 mm Hg to 20 ± 6 mm Hg.

The hydraulic performance of the artificial valve is more important for postoperative clinical improvement in mitral valve replacements than in aortic valve replacements [6–10]. On the average, one can expect a clinical improvement of one NYHA Class [11] after mitral valve implantation. A more significant decrease in symptoms and increase in functional capacity can be expected only in a small group of patients. Absence of symptoms after valve replacement for chronic mitral lesions, which would allow patients to be placed in NYHA Class I, is rarely observed. Many patients have symptoms, for example, of atrial fibrillation or dyspnea during strain imposed by ordinary day-to-day activities, which is consistent with NYHA Class II or III.

During a 6-year follow-up of consecutive patients with mechanical mitral valve prostheses, the percentage of patients in NYHA Class III or IV was not significantly altered and was 36.5% after 6 years. At that time 11.1% of patients were classified as NYHA Class I and 52.4% as Class II (figure 22-1).

Our limited experience with tissue valves has shown that some of these patients deteriorate clinically between the fourth and sixth years postoperatively. Up to the fourth year after tissue valve implantation, the percentage of patients in NYHA Class I or Class II is very similar to that in the group with mechanical valves. At 6 years postoperatively, there is an increasing number of patients who again show a deterioration of clinical symptoms, so that the percentage of patients in NYHA Classes I and II decreases from 72% after 4

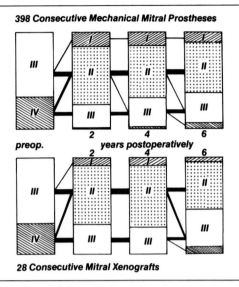

398 Consecutive Mechanical Mitral Prostheses

28 Consecutive Mitral Xenografts

Figure 22-1. NYHA classification of consecutive patients receiving mitral valve prostheses.

years to 54% after 6 years (figure 22-1). The mean age of these patients at the time of surgery was 53.7 ± 12.9 years, so increased calcium metabolism with unusual rapid calcification of tissue valves, as seen frequently after 6 years in young patients [12–14], can be excluded. These findings are in accordance with echocardiographic studies, which have shown a progressive thickening and rigidity of the tissue valve cusps, resulting in a decrease of valve orifice areas even a few years after valve implantation [15]. The risk of reoperation and the psychological problems imposed on the patients are thus not the only disadvantages to be taken into account when implanting bioprostheses.

It has often been stressed that a patient's active lifestyle is confined after mechanical valve implantation because of the inconvenience and dangers associated with anticoagulant therapy. For obvious reasons, there are only a few patients who have experience with both a bioprosthesis and a mechanical device. In 29 of our patients there was such a change in valve type at reoperation performed for prosthetic valve endocarditis, primary valve failure, or valve thrombosis. Within this group, the percentage of patients who did better, respectively, with a bioprosthesis or a mechanical valve, or who reported no differences in their quality of life were more or less the same. However, if anticoagulation was necessary with either valve type (mostly mitral valve lesions with atrial fibrillation persisting postoperatively), two-thirds of the patients did better with a mechanical substitute, while 50% of the patients in whom anticoagulation was not indicated with a bioprosthesis implanted were in favor of their tissue valve (table 22-1). From these findings we can conclude that anticoagulation is one of the main factors that reduces

Table 22-1. Quality of life with bioprostheses (BP) and mechanical valves (MV) (29 patients* having experience with both valve types)

	Anticoagulation indicated				
	With either valve type	With mechanical prostheses only	Mitral	Aortic	Total
Better with BP	n = 1 (11%)	n = 10 (50%)	n = 3 (23%)	n = 8 (50%)	n = 11 (38%)
Better with MV	n = 6 (67%)	n = 4 (20%)	n = 8 (62%)	n = 2 (12.5%)	n = 10 (34%)
No difference	n = 2 (22%)	n = 6 (30%)	n = 2 (15%)	n = 6 (37.5%)	n = 8 (28%)

* Patients with irreversible impaired left ventricular function excluded

quality of life after valve replacement. On the other hand, patients who need anticoagulation because of factors that cause thromboembolism derive greater benefit from mechanical valve implantation.

Improvement of functional capacity

Evaluation of the improvement of patients who have undergone heart valve replacement can be made objectively by comparing functional capacities before and after surgery [16].

After mitral valve replacement, we found significant differences in the increase of functional capacity depending on the implanted valve type (figure 22-2). With the ST. JUDE MEDICAL® (SJM) prosthesis and identical tissue anulus diameters, functional improvement was more favorable than with the IONESCU-SHILEY® (IS) valve. Selection of either a tissue or mechanical valve had been made only on the basis of the thromboembolic and hemorrhagic risks. Although valve implantation was not performed on a randomized basis, these 60 consecutive patients had identical preoperative clinical and hemodynamic findings. Functional capacity was evaluated by having patients climb stairs until the appearance of dyspnea. The increase of this capacity was 74% in the group with bioprostheses but 181% in the group with mechanical

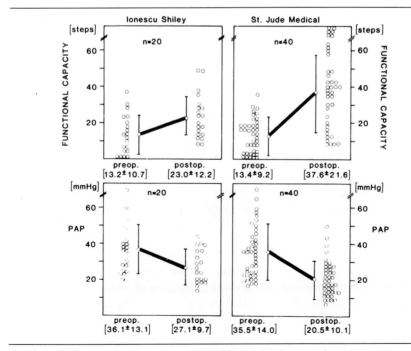

Figure 22-2. Functional capacity (appearance of dyspnea) and mean pulmonary artery pressure after mitral valve replacement.

valves. This greater increase correlates closely to the significantly greater decrease of the PAP at rest from 35.5 ± 14.0 mm Hg preoperatively to 20.5 ± 10.1 mm Hg postoperatively in patients with ST. JUDE MEDICAL prostheses. After IONESCU-SHILEY implantation, PAP dropped from 36.1 ± 13.1 mm Hg to only 27.1 ± 9.7 mm Hg (figure 22-2). Left ventricular dysfunction was not found in any of these patients by angiocardiography and/or echocardiography.

Although the conclusions drawn from these findings may be restricted due to the fact that this is not a randomized comparison, increase of functional capacity and the correlation between functional capacity and PAP are obvious.

In another study we compared the PAP at rest and during bicycle exercise (supine position) of patients with IS and SJM mitral prostheses [6, 17]. Both of these study groups also consisted of consecutively operated patients without specific selection, with identical preoperative clinical and hemodynamic status and without left ventricular impairment postoperatively. Tissue valves had been implanted in patients with a high thromboembolic and/or hemorrhagic risk and in those who wanted to receive a bioprosthesis.

In the SJM group, PAP increased from 19.7 ± 9.1 mm Hg at rest to 26.1 ± 9.9 mm Hg at 30 watts bicycle exercise and 37.4 ± 13.9 mm Hg at 150 watts. Twelve percent of patients with SJM prostheses had stopped exercising at the 30-watt level, while 51% could experience 150 watts or more.

In contrast, in the IS group, PAP increased from 24.7 ± 5.9 mmHg at rest to 37.3 ± 7.5 mm Hg at 30 watts bicycle exercise and to 58.1 ± 14.0 mmHg at 150 watts. Twenty-five percent of these patients had to stop at the 30-watt level, while only 22% experienced 90 watts and none reached the 150-watt level.

These differences must be due to different left atrial pressures caused by obstruction from the mitral prosthesis [18–23].

Improvement of central hemodynamics

The success of heart valve replacement depends, in part, on the degree to which normal central hemodynamics can be restored. Generally, physiological hemodynamic conditions are not restored. It must be expected that differences in postoperative subjective and functional improvement, with respect to the implanted valve type, are due to the different hemodynamics of the prosthesis concerned.

In native mitral valves, clinical signs and symptoms of mild stenosis are present if the mitral valve opening is reduced to less than 2.5 cm² in adults [14]. Most of the commonly used mitral valve prostheses of 29 mm outer diameter studied in vivo have an effective valve orifice area (EOA) between 2 cm² and 3 cm². That is why slight changes in the design, and consequently in the valve's hemodynamics, may determine whether a prosthesis will produce signs and symptoms of mitral stenosis.

Taking reported effective valve orifice areas of different mechanical tissue

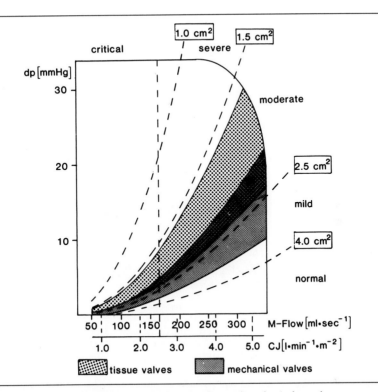

Figure 22-3. Effective valve opening areas of tissue valves and mechanical prostheses measured in vivo by different investigators.

valves into account, it can be demonstrated that all prostheses are mild to moderately obstructive (figure 22-3). For mitral prostheses with an outer diameter of 29 mm, effective valve orifice areas (EOA) have been reported to be 2.2 to 2.5 cm² for BJÖRK-SHILEY®; 1.9 to 3.2 cm² for MEDTRONIC HALL™; and 2.8 to 3.4 cm² for ST. JUDE MEDICAL prostheses. For 29 mm bioprostheses, the effective orifice areas for the IONESCU-SHILEY valve have been reported from 1.9 to 2.0 cm²; for the HANCOCK® prosthesis from 1.3 to 2.7 cm²; and for the CARPENTIER-EDWARDS® from 2.2 to 3.0 cm² [20, 23–30].

To compare the flow-pressure relationship of different mitral valve prostheses under identical condition, at rest and during exercise, we compared 5 mechanical valves and the IS pericardial valve with a tissue anulus diameter of 29 mm (or a corresponding size, when 29 mm sized prostheses were not available). The flow-pressure relationship at rest and under bicycle exercise for these equally sized mitral prostheses are given in figures 22-4 and 22–5. The survey demonstrates that, with regard to flow-pressure relationship, modern mechanical valves have some advantages over bioprostheses.

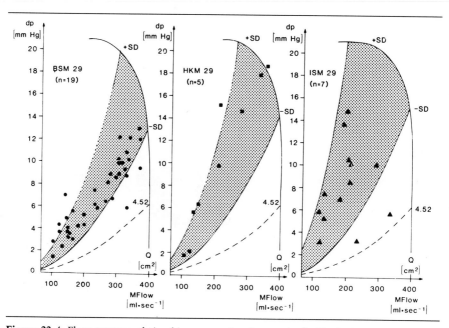

Figure 22-4. Flow-pressure relationship at rest and under exercise for Björk-Shiley (BSM), Medtronic-Hall (HKM), and Ionescu-Shiley (ISM) mitral valves. Mean flow (ml/sec) is plotted against transprosthetic gradient dp (mm Hg).

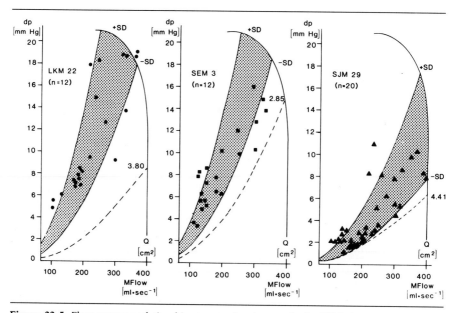

Figure 22-5. Flow-pressure relationship at rest and under exercise for Lillehei-Kaster (LKM), Starr-Edwards (SEM), and St. Jude Medical (SJM) mitral valves.

The flow-pressure relationship after aortic valve replacement is similar to that of mitral valve prostheses. However, residual transaortic gradients are only of minor significance with the usual valve sizes and normal prosthetic function [31]. However, in the small aortic anulus, which allows the implantation of a valve less than 21 mm in outer diameter, high residual transaortic gradients may endanger postoperative results [32–34]. To ensure an adequate EOA, additional surgical procedures are recommended [35–38]. However, according to the less favorable flow-pressure relationship, tissue valves should only be used if a 23 mm prosthesis fits well into the aortic anulus [39].

For the 25 mm SJM aortic prosthesis, we did not find a significant difference between effective and geometric orifice areas (figure 22-6). In comparison with the equally sized IONESCU-SHILEY pericardial valve, the systolic pressure gradient was significantly lower (figure 22-7).

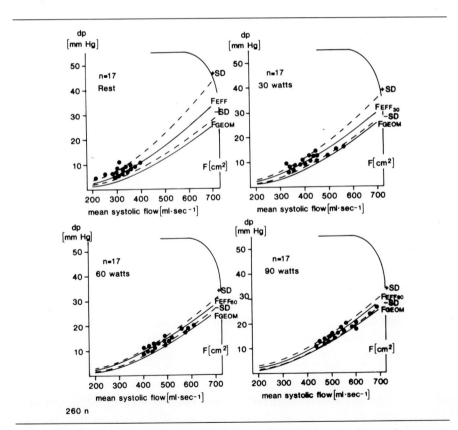

Figure 22-6. Flow-pressure relationship in 25 mm St. Jude Medical aortic valve prostheses at rest and during bicycle exercise with 30, 60, and 90 watts. Mean systolic flow (ml/sec) is plotted against the transprosthetic gradient dp (mm Hg) calculated from simultaneous records after retrograde and transseptal catheterization. The geometric orifice area (F_{Geom}) and the calculated mean effective valve orifice areas (F_{EFF}) ± SD are given.

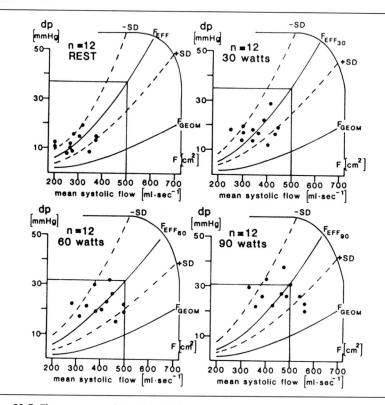

Figure 22-7. Flow-pressure relationship in 25 mm Ionescu-Shiley valve prostheses at rest and during bicycle exercise. For further explanations and abbreviations see figure 22-6.

In the IONESCU-SHILEY valve with an anulus diameter of 25 mm, orifice diameter is 2.14 mm and geometric orifice area is 3.60 cm^2 [40]. It is emphasized that, due to the design and the thinness of the pericardium, the effective/geometric valve orifice ratio of this pericardial bioprosthesis is superior to all other tissue valves commercially available in recent years [40].

Nevertheless, in our in vivo hemodynamic measurements this geometric orifice area of 3.6 cm^2 is far from being reached. At rest, the mean EOA was calculated to be only 1.9 ± 0.4 cm^2. Moreover, in contrast to most mechanical valves (except the OMNISCIENCE® and OMNICARBON® valves [41–43]), a variety of EOA measurements were found, not only at rest, but also with increasing exercise. This points toward a considerable different in design from valve to valve. In some of the prostheses studied hemodynamically, effective orifice areas are only slightly smaller than the geometric valve orifice area, while in others there is a significant discrepancy (figure 22-7).

Improvement of left ventricular function

The postoperative clinical and functional result is determined not only by the restoration of valve function, but also by the degree to which impaired left ventricular pump function can be restored. Left ventricular impairment postoperatively is probably related to the compromised left ventricular inotropic state prior to surgery or to intraoperative myocardial damage. Thus, the optimal time for surgical intervention prior to irreversible myocardial damage has to be chosen. In some studies, however, a residual obstruction to forward blood flow caused by the prosthetic valve itself has been found to also be responsible [4].

Primary prosthetic valve dysfunction

Prosthetic valve dysfunction is rare with mechanical valves used today. In our own patients operated on between 1972 and 1983, the cumulative rate of primary mechanical dysfunction is 0.096 after 11 years. The major disadvantage of tissue valves is their limited durability due to calcification and degeneration of the biological material [44].

For mitral bioprostheses, freedom from primary tissue failure after 5 years was reported to be 98% [45] and after 8 years between 98% and 63% [45–50]. At 10 years published rates of freedom from tissue failure vary from 77% to 68% [46, 48, 51]. Ionescu reported a 15% rate of tissue failure in hospital-made pericardial valves after 12 years [47].

In biological aortic valve implants, a wide range of cumulative rates for freedom from tissue failure is reported, with cumulative rates after 5 years of 95% to 68% [45, 52], after 8 years of 99% to 66% [45–50, 52], and after 10 years of 86% to 42% [48, 52, 53]. Figure 22–8 gathers the reported incidences and illustrates that durability can differ widely, depending on individual determinants of the patients, preservation techniques, and designs of the bioprostheses. Some of these reported failure rates, however, may be imprecise due to the small samples of patients and insufficient follow-up periods [54].

Most of the long-term results that have been published after tissue valve replacement allow no definite conclusion on durability of the bioprosthesis in the individual patient. Furthermore, due to the inconstant hazard rate of this complication, an adequate follow-up period can be estimated only for bioprostheses of the first and second generations. Finally, an extrapolation of the rate of dysfunctions, so far observed, appears to be difficult, because reoperation due to valve failure is not a linear function of time and obviously increases exponentially when more than 10 years have elapsed since implantation [54–57].

An indication for the use of bioprostheses that is accepted from most centers is a patient-age of 60 to 65 years. However, according to recent life expectancy statistics, 60-year-old females have an average life expectancy of an additional 22 years and males of an additional 19 years. Thus, in a substantial number of these patients a reoperation will be necessary at older ages (figure 22-9).

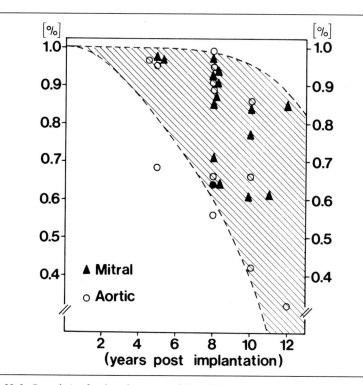

Figure 22-8. Cumulative freedom from tissue failure following aortic or mitral valve replacement, as reported in literature.

Complications likely to be valve-related

Despite the hemodynamic improvement with heart valve substitutes developed in recent years, late complications, which are likely to be valve-related, are still limiting factors to the overall success of valve replacement. However, it is more than difficult to distinguish between complications that are valve-related and those that are related to the underlying heart disease. This holds especially true for thromboembolic complications after mitral valve replacement [58].

Complications directly caused by artificial valves may be a consequence of hemodynamic disturbances persisting after surgery, such as is the case with intravascular hemolysis. They may also be a consequence of the artificial material implanted (primary valve dysfunction) or of both factors, such as is the case with prosthetic valve endocarditis or thromboembolic events. Complications indirectly associated with prosthestic implantations are most often attributed to the side effects of anticoagulation therapy [59].

Although these complications occur without malfunction of the prosthesis, their incidence or extent is more or less increased in the case of malfunctioning prostheses [60, 61].

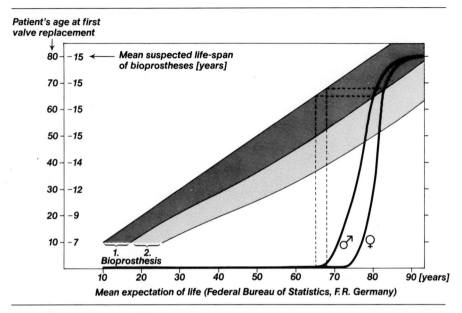

Patient's age at first
valve replacement

80 – 15 ← **Mean suspected life-span
of bioprostheses [years]**

70 – 15

60 – 15

50 – 15

40 – 14

30 – 12

20 – 9

10 – 7

1.   2.
Bioprosthesis

10   20   30   40   50   60   70   80   90 [years]

Mean expectation of life (Federal Bureau of Statistics, F. R. Germany)

Figure 22-9. Expectation of life (Federal Republic of Germany, 1985) and suspected durability of bioprostheses.

Chronic intravascular hemolysis

Without valve malfunction, hemolysis is a reliable parameter of the valve's functional integrity [62, 63]. The degree of hemolysis does not play a role in the indication for reoperation. Even with high rates of hemolysis persisting for years, consecutive pathological effects have not been seen. The only criterion for reoperation is a clinically noncompensated anemia.

Prosthetic valve endocarditis

Prosthetic valve endocarditis (PVE) continues to constitute a severe complication with poor prognosis. In our patients, the frequency of early PVE has decreased, the frequency of late PVE has increased since the mid 1970s. Among other reasons, this is due to a consequent perioperative prophylaxis. The rates of prosthetic valve endocarditis in patients operated on between 1965 and 1975, and 1976 to 1986, are given in figure 22-10.

While PVE affects the sewing cuff and the adjacent endocardium in mechanical valves, pathogenesis of prosthetic infection is more complex [67]. It has been suggested that an infection of tissue valves can be confined to the cusps, with only a slight tendency to involve the sewing cuff and to form abscesses, as is frequently observed with endocarditis of mechanical valves [68, 69]. Furthermore, differences in morphological features of infection in porcine and pericardial bioprostheses have been found [67]. In porcine bioprostheses, vegetations are more prominent on the inflow surfaces; in pericardial bio-

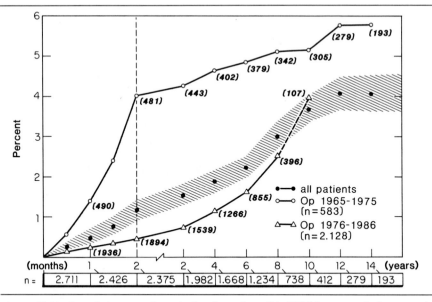

Figure 22-10. Cumulative rates of prosthetic valve endocarditis (PVE) in consecutively operated patients (1965–1986). The shadowed area gives the PVE rate and its confidence limits for all 2711 patients. ○ = patients operated on between 1965 and 1975; △ = patients operated on between 1976 and 1986.

prostheses, they are more prominent on the outflow surfaces of the cusps. Moreover, invasion of deeper layers of the cusps is more common in porcine valves [67].

These differences in the pathogenesis of prosthetic valve endocarditis between mechanical and biological valves may explain the higher incidence of PVE reported in bioprostheses, but the poorer prognosis of PVE in mechanical prostheses.

Thromboembolic complications

Reduction of thrombocyte survival time and the generation of thrombus formation are supported by effects of turbulent flows on formed blood elements [70, 71]. As the flow pattern remains more significantly disturbed after bioprosthetic valve implantation, the basic risk of thromboembolism is present.

The incidence depends on the type of prosthesis implanted (table 22-2). A mean incidence of 4.79 events per 100 patient-years can be calculated for mechanical mitral prostheses. In bioprostheses, 0.9% to 3.5% per patient-year is reported, which results in a calculated incidence of 2.41% per patient-year (table 22-3).

In aortic valve replacements with mechanical valves, on the average, a thromboembolic rate of 2.45% per patient-year must be expected (table 22-4).

Table 22-2. Incidence of thromboembolic events in patients with mechanical mitral prostheses

Author	Reference	Valve Type	Follow-up (patient-years)	Incidence of valve thrombosis (% per pt-yr)	Incidence of TE events (% per pt-yr)	Percent free from TE events (actuarial)
Starr	72	SE	684	1.2	4.6	88 after 5 years
Oxman	73	SC	1085	0.3	8.0	71 after 5 years
Horstkotte	2	SE★	169	—	4.6	83 after 5 years
Björk	74	BS	912	1.3	5.5	81 after 5 years
Horstkotte	75	BS	725	0.4	2.8	91 after 5 years
Horstkotte	2	BS★	165	0.6	2.9	85 after 5 years
Marvasti	76	LK	278	—	2.9	
Horstkotte	2	LK★	171	0.6	3.8	89 after 5 years
Nicoloff	77	SJM	112	—	3.6	96 after 3 years
LeClerc	78	SJM	420	—	3.9	93 after 3 years
Horstkotte	75	SJM	273	—	0.9	98 after 4 years
				0.57	4.79	

SE = Starr-Edwards; SC = Smeloff-Cutter; BS = Björk-Shiley; LK = Lillehei-Kaster; SJM = St. Jude Medical
★ Randomized comparison

Table 22-3. Incidence of thromboembolic events in patients with biological mitral prostheses

Author	Reference	Valve type	Follow-up (patient-years)	Incidence of valve thrombosis (% per pt-yr)	Incidence of TE events (% per pt-yr)	Percent free from TE events (actuarial)
Ionescu	30	IS	515	—	0.9	97 after 5 years
Janusz	79	CE	422	—	1.9	96 after 3 years
Oyer	80	"p"	1302	0.2	2.9	92 after 5 years
Hetzer	81	H	546	—	3.5	
				0.01	2.41	

IS = Ionescu-Shiley; CE = Carpentier-Edwards; "p" = porcine; H = Hancock

Table 22-4. Incidence of thromboembolic events in patients with mechanical aortic prostheses

Author	Reference	Valve type	Follow-up (patient-years)	Incidence of valve thrombosis (% per pt-yr)	Incidence of TE events (% per pt-yr)	Percent free from TE events (actuarial)
Lee	82	SC	650	—	3.7	
Starr	72	SE	855	—	5.4	78 after 5 years
Zwart	83	LK	153	0.7	2.8	
Björk	74	BS	555	0.3	1.0	97 after 5 years
Cheung	84	BS	1925	0.2	1.8	
Horstkotte	75	BS	734	0.4	1.9	95 after 5 years
Nicoloff	77	SJM	145	—	0.7	98 after 5 years
LeClerc	78	SJM	454	—	0.6	99 after 3 years
Horstkotte	75	SJM	271	—	0.7	98 after 4 years
				0.17	2.54	

SC = Smeloff-Cutter; SE = Starr-Edwards; LK = Lillehei-Kaster; BS = Björk-Shiley; SJM = St. Jude Medical

With aortic bioprostheses, the average risk of 1.2% per patient-year is significantly lower (table 22-5).

In our own experience, we found no significant difference between the cumulative thromboembolic rates following tissue or mechanical mitral valve replacement, although the incidence of atrial fibrillation was 49% in patients with tissue valves and 78% in patients with mechanical prostheses. The incidence reported by Gallucci et al. [48] for a much larger number of mitral bioprostheses than we have followed-up is given in figure 22-11.

The thromboembolic rates reported for aortic valve replacement differ widely. For mechanical valves we found a cumulative thromboembolic rate after 8 years of 8%, while it was less than 3% in the 73 patients after aortic valve replacement using bioprostheses. This is in accordance with the results published by Ionescu [85] for a larger number of patients with bovine pericardial xenografts (figure 22-12).

Significant differences in published complication rates indicate the difficulties in determining exact hazard rates for these events, especially for thromboembolic complications. Many published studies emphasize the use of strict definitions but pretend an accuracy of their follow-up, which is not given because of insufficient follow-up techniques. Table 22-6 is intended to show differences in the thromboembolic hazard in an identical patient group followed for the same period. The differences were due to the follow-up technique (clinical examination vs. questionnaires).

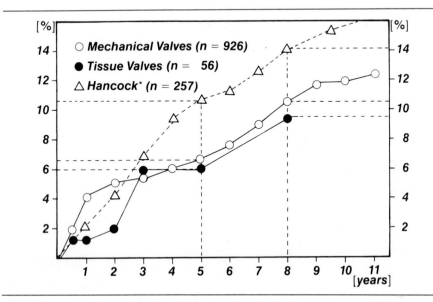

Figure 22-11. Cumulative thromboembolic rates after mitral valve replacement with 926 mechanical and 56 biological valves (mostly Ionescu-Shiley), performed in Düsseldorf. *The data are compared to the results after Hancock mitral valve replacement published by Gallucci in 1982.

Table 22-5. Incidence of thromboembolic events in patients with biological aortic prostheses

Author	Reference	Valve type	Follow-up (patient-years)	Incidence of valve thrombosis (% per pt-yr)	Incidence of TE events (% per pt-yr)	Percent free from TE events (actuarial)
Ionescu	30	IS	735	—	0.4	99 after 5 years
Janusz	79	CE	530	—	0.9	98 after 3 years
Oyer	80	"P"	1121	0.1	1.9	94 after 5 years
				0.05	1.22	

IS = Ionescu-Shiley; CE = Carpentier-Edwards; "P" = porcine

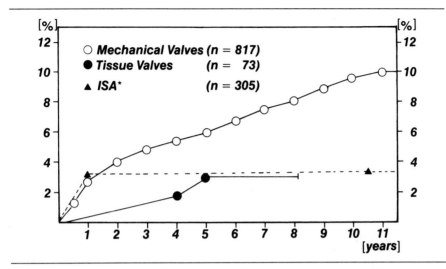

Figure 22-12. Cumulative thromboembolic rates after aortic valve replacement with 817 mechanical and 73 biological valves (mostly Ionescu-Shiley) performed in Düsseldorf. The data are compared to the results published by Ionescu in 1983 for 305 Ionescu-Shiley aortic prostheses (ISA).

Bleeding complications

The rate of thromboembolic events has to be compared with the risk of bleeding complications due to anticoagulant treatment. Thromboembolic complications mostly occur if the effectiveness of anticoagulation is not guaranteed. In 82% of our patients with valve thromboses or thromboembolic

Table 22-6. Documentation of TE events with either clinical examinations or questionnaires during three years of follow-up (1982–1985) after randomized mitral valve replacement in the same group of patients. Rates are % per patient-year

	Outpatient examinations every 6 months	Question-naires every year	Question-naires every 2 years
Follow-up months	4436	4497	4581
Transient TE	1.62 (n = 6)	0.80 (n = 3)	0.52 (n = 2)
Reversible TE (disturbance < 8 weeks)	1.62 (n = 6)	0.80 (n = 3)	0.52 (n = 2)
Reversible TE (disturbance > 8 weeks)	0.81 (n = 3)	0.53 (n = 2)	0.52 (n = 2)
TE, irreversible impairment	0.81 (n = 3)	0.53 (n = 2)	0.52 (n = 2)
Prosthetic valve thrombosis	0.54 (n = 2)	0.53 (n = 2)	0.52 (n = 2)
Fatal TE	0.54 (n = 2)	0.53 (n = 2)	0.52 (n = 2)
	5.95 (n = 22)	3.74 (n = 14)	3.14 (n = 12)

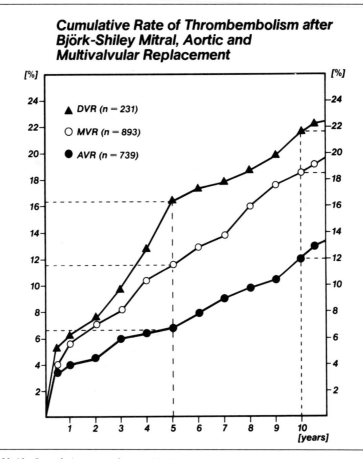

Cumulative Rate of Thrombembolism after Björk-Shiley Mitral, Aortic and Multivalvular Replacement

▲ DVR (n = 231)

○ MVR (n = 893)

● AVR (n = 739)

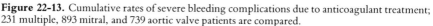

Figure 22-13. Cumulative rates of severe bleeding complications due to anticoagulant treatment; 231 multiple, 893 mitral, and 739 aortic valve patients are compared.

events, where information about the coagulation conditions at the time of the event was available, there was ineffective anticoagulation [75]. In the majority of these cases, anticoagulation was interrupted because of minor interventions or minor bleeding complications.

Figure 22-13 illustrates the incidence of severe hemorrhagic events in patients with mechanical valves under anticoagulant therapy. After 10 years, the incidence was 17.7 ± 4.2% in patients with aortic valve replacements, 23.8 ± 6.7% in patients with mitral and aortic valve replacements, and 25.2 ± 7.9% in patients with isolated mitral valve replacement.

Rate and risk of reoperation

Frequency of reoperation per patient-year due to paravalvular leakage was 0.35% for mechanical valves and 0.58% for tissue valves. Due to infective endocarditis, the reoperation rates in our patients were 0.41% for mechanical valves and 0.39% for bioprostheses. Valve dysfunction was responsible for reoperations at a rate of 0.05% per patient-year in mechanical valves but 1.15% in bioprostheses. These incidences cause an overall reoperation rate in mechanical valves of 1.06% per patient-year; in tissue valves it was 2.02% per patient-year.

The perioperative mortality did not differ in our patients with reoperation of mechanical or bioprostheses. This contrasts with the general opinion that tissue valve failure progresses slowly so that reoperation can be done electively with low risk. It is likely that progressive tissue valve degeneration either is not recognized in due time and reoperation has to be performed as an emergency or that valve incompetence occurs suddenly by perforation or leaflet tearing, which immediately causes ventricular dilatation [44, 86].

The reoperation incidences in our series of patients operated on between 1973 and 1983 did not change distinctly when compared to the section of patients operated on between 1978 and 1983, including all consecutively operated BJÖRK-SHILEY, ST. JUDE MEDICAL, and IONESCU-SHILEY prostheses. The actuarial curves for patients free from reoperation indicate for the mitral (figure 22-14) and the aortic positions (figure 22-15) that there are only very small differences between both mechanical valves within a follow-up time of up to 6 years. In aortic as well as mitral replacements, the cumulative reoperation rate due to prosthetic valve endocarditis, mechanical dysfunction, and valve thrombosis was below 2%.

Other influencing factors

Although the indication for long-term anticoagulation in patients with mitral bioprostheses and chronic atrial fibrillation is not as strict as it is in mechanical prostheses, it has to be kept in mind that atrial fibrillation is accepted, by itself, as a cause of thromboembolism, especially if atrial fibrillation is associated with mitral valve stenosis. In mitral tissue valve replacement, several observers found a significantly higher incidence of thromboembolic complications in patients with atrial fibrillation than with sinus rhythm [87–89]. Thus, after weighing the risks and benefits, anticoagulation has to be recommended in a substantial number of patients with mitral bioprostheses, which means that these patients do not receive enough benefit from a tissue valve implantation.

In atrioventricular valve replacement and in aortic valve implants in which only small-sized prostheses can be used, the hemodynamic disadvantage of bioprostheses may limit the overall success of the operative intervention. In these patients, too, for hemodynamic reasons, a modern mechanical valve with a favorable performance index should be preferred. An expected high risk of reoperation should also discourage tissue valve implantation (figure 22-16).

With valve replacement necessary in active infective endocarditis, a lower reoperation rate has been documented for mechanical valves, so some authors

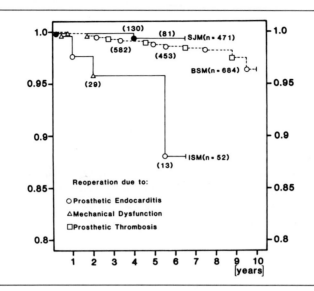

Figure 22-14. Cumulative reoperation rate due to prosthetic valve endocarditis, mechanical dysfunction, or prosthetic valve thrombosis in 52 patients with Ionescu-Shiley (ISM), 684 patients with Björk-Shiley (BSM), and 471 patients with St. Jude Medical (SJM) mitral valve prostheses.

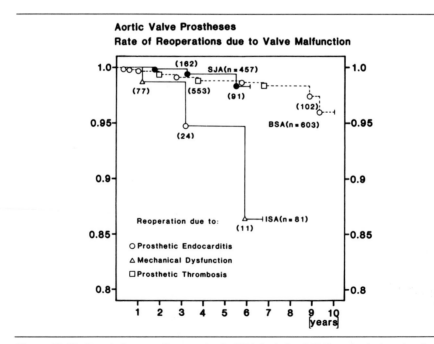

Figure 22-15. Cumulative rate of reoperation in 81 biological and 1060 mechanical aortic valve prostheses.

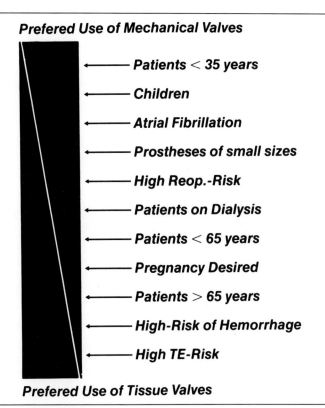

Prefered Use of Mechanical Valves

←————— *Patients < 35 years*

←————— *Children*

←————— *Atrial Fibrillation*

←————— *Prostheses of small sizes*

←————— *High Reop.-Risk*

←————— *Patients on Dialysis*

←————— *Patients < 65 years*

←————— *Pregnancy Desired*

←————— *Patients > 65 years*

←————— *High-Risk of Hemorrhage*

←————— *High TE-Risk*

Prefered Use of Tissue Valves

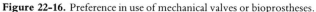

Figure 22-16. Preference in use of mechanical valves or bioprostheses.

recommend the use of mechanical valves in these circumstances. In our institution, indication for use of either bioprostheses or mechanical valves in active infective endocarditis followed the same principles as for patients without endocarditis.

The use of bioprostheses can be advantageous in patients endangered by stroke, bleeding, or thromboembolic complications (figure 22-16).

REFERENCES

1. Haerten K, Horstkotte D. The influence of operative procedures on the long-term follow-up and the prognosis of mitral valve disease. Herz/Kreisl 1982; 7:475.
2. Horstkotte D, Haerten K, Herzer JA, Loogen F, Scheibling R, Schulte HD. Five-year results after randomized mitral valve replacement with Björk-Shiley, Lillehei-Kaster and Starr-Edwards prostheses. Thorac Cardiovasc Surg 1983; 31:206.
3. Horstkotte D, Haerten K, Seipel L. Central hemodynamics at rest and during exercise after mitral valve replacement with different prostheses. Circulation 1983; 68(II):161.
4. Horstkotte D, Delaye J. The limits of central hemodynamic improvement by heart valve replacement. In Horstkotte D and Loogen F (eds.): *Update in Heart Valve Replacement.* Steinkopff, Darmstadt 1986; p 43.
5. Horstkotte D, Loogen F, Bircks W. Is the late outcome of heart valve replacement influenced

by the hemodynamics of the heart valve substitute? In Horstkotte D and Loogen F (eds): *Update in Heart Valve Replacement*. Steinkopff, Darmstadt 1986; p 55.

6. Horstkotte D, Loogen F. *Erworbene Herzklappenfehler*. Urban & Schwarzenberg, München, Berlin, Baltimore 1987.

7. Horstkotte D, Nitter-Hauge S. Patient management in valvular heart disease: What has changed in the last decade? Proceedings, International Workshop on "Patient management decisions in valvular heart disease." Bari 1987.

8. Horstkotte D. Prosthetic valves or tissue valves—a vote for mechanical prostheses. Z Kardiol 1985; 74(6):19.

9. Huhmann W, Köhler J. Klappenöffnungsflächen bei künstlichen Herzklappen. Z Kardiol 1978; 67:672.

10. Rothlin ME, Krayenbühl HP, Messmer BJ, Senning A. Langzeitverlauf nach Aorten- und Mitralklappenersatz. Herz 1977; 2:268.

11. New York Heart Association. The criteria committee of the New York Heart Association "Diseases of the heart and blood vessels" (nomenclature and criteria for diagnosis) (6th ed.). Little, Brown & Co., Boston 1964.

12. Thandroyen FT, Whitton IN, Pirie D, Rogers MA, Mitha AS. Severe calcification of glutaraldehyde-preserved porcine xenografts in children. Am J Cardiol 1980; 45:690.

13. Geha AS, Laks H, Stansel HC, Cornhill JF, Kielman JW, Buckley MJ, Roberts WC. Late failure of porcine valve heterografts in children. J Thorac Cardiovasc Surg 1979; 78:351.

14. Silver MM, Pollock J. Silver MD, Williams WG, Trusler GA. Calcification in porcine xenograft valves in children. Am J Cardiol 1980; 45:685.

15. Alam M, Goldstein S, Lakier JB. Echocardiographic changes in the thickness of porcine valves with time. Chest 1981; 79:663.

16. Horstkotte D, Loogen F. Erfolgsbeurteilung mit invasiven und nichtinvasiven Methoden nach Herzklappenoperationen. Z Kardiol 1983; 72(II):16.

17. Horstkotte D. Belastbarkeit von Patienten mit erworbenen Herzklappenfehlern präoperativ und nach prothetischem Klappenersatz. In Rost R and Webering F (eds.): *Kardiologie im Sport*. Deutscher Ärzte-Verlag, Köln 1987; p 78.

18. Carstens V, Behrenbeck DW, Hilger HA. Exercise capacity before and after cardiac surgery. Cardiology 1983; 70:41.

19. Horstkotte D, Schulte HD, Körfer R, Bircks W, Loogen F. Mitral valve replacement using different prosthetic valves. Int J Artif Organs 1982; 5:177.

20. Horstkotte D, Haerten K, Schulte HD, Seipel L, Krian A, Loogen F. Hemodynamic findings at rest and during exercise after implantation of different mitral valve prostheses with equal tissue annulus diameter. Z Kardiol 1983; 72:385.

21. Horstkotte D. Improvement of prognosis and quality of life by mitral and aortic valve replacement. Comparative long-term follow-up study after implantation of different prostheses. In D'Alessandro LC (ed.): *Heart Surgery 1987*; Casa Editrice Scientifica Internazionale, Rome 1987; p 11.

22. Horstkotte D, Pippert H, Bircks W, Loogen F. Erworbene Herzklappenfehler: Konservative Therapie, Indikation zur chirurgischen Intervention, postoperative Ergebnisse. In Loskot F (Hrsg.): *Herzerkrankungen*. Steinkopff, Darmstadt 1986; p 419.

23. Rashtian MY, Stevenson DM, Allen DT, Yoganathan AP, Harrison EC, Edmiston WA, Faughan P, Rahimtoola SH. Flow characteristics of four commonly used heart valves. Am J Cardiol 1986; 58:743.

24. Bruss KH, Reul H, Van Gilse J, Knott E. Pressure drop and velocity fields at four mechanical heart valve prostheses: Björk-Shiley standard, Björk-Shiley convex-concave, Hall-Kaster and St. Jude Medical. Life Supp Syst 1983; 1:3.

25. Heiliger R, Richter HA, Mittermayer C. Hydrodynamic test of bioprostheses in the mitral position. Life Supp Syst 1985; 3:327.

26. Horstkotte D, Schulte HD, Bircks W, Loogen F, Budde Th. Rest and exercise hemodynamics after mitral valve replacement using allo- and xenografts. Life Supp Syst, Proceedings IX Annual Meeting ESYO. Saunders, London 1982; p 128.

27. Horstkotte D, Haerten K, Seipel L, Körfer R, Budde Th, Bircks W, Loogen F. Central hemodynamics at rest and during exercise after mitral valve replacement with different prostheses. Circulation 1982; 68(II):161.

28. Gabbay S, Yellin L, Frishman WH, Frater WM. In vitro hydrodynamic comparison of St.

Jude, Björk-Shiley and Hall-Kaster valves. Transact ASAIO 1980; 26:231.

29. Björk VO, Henze A. Prosthetic heart valve replacement. Nine years' experience with the Björk-Shiley tilting disc valve. In Ionescu MI (ed); *Tissue Heart Valves*. Butterworth, London 1979; p 3.

30. Ionescu MI, Tandon AP. Long-term clinical and hemodynamic evaluation of the Ionescu-Shiley pericardial xenograft heart valve. In Sebening F, Klövekorn WP, Meisner H, Struck E (eds): *Bioprostheses Cardiac Valves*. Deutsches Herzzentrum, Munich 1979; p 109.

31. Horstkotte D, Haerten K, Körfer R, Spiller P, Budde Th, Bircks W, Loogen F. Hemodynamic findings at rest and during exercise after implantation of different aortic valve prostheses. Z Kardiol 1983; 72:429.

32. Björk VO, Henze A, Holgren A, Szamosi A. Evaluation of the 21 mm Björk-Shiley tilting disc valve in patients with narrow aortic roots. Scand J Thorac Cardiovasc Surg 1973; 7:203.

33. Wortham DC, Tri TB, Bowen TE. Hemodynamic evaluation of the St. Jude Medical valve prosthesis in the small aortic anulus. J Thorac Cardiovasc Surg 1981; 81:615.

34. Teoh KH, Fullop JC, Weisel RD, Ivanov J, Tong CP, Slattery SA, Rakowski H. Aortic valve replacement with a small prosthesis. Circulation 1987; 76(III):111.

35. Schulte HD, Bircks W, Frenzel H, Horstkotte D, Jungblut RM, Oubari M. Patch-graft enlargement of the aortic root using autologous pericardium (long-term results). Thorac Cardiovasc Surg 1983; 31:219.

36. Konno S, Imai Y, Iida Y, Nakajima M, Tasuno K. A new method for prosthetic valve replacemnt in congenital aortic stenosis associated with hypoplasia of the aortic valve ring. J Thorac Cardiovasc Surg 1975; 70:909.

37. Stenseth JH, Danielson GK, McGoon DC. Pericardial patch enlargement of the aortic outflow tract. J Thorac Cardiovasc Surg 1971; 62:442.

38. Bigelow WG, Trimble AS, Auger P, Marquis J, Wigle ED. The ventriculomyotomy operation for muscular subaortic stenosis. J Thorac Cardiovasc Surg 1966; 52:514.

39. Schaff HV, Borkon AM, Hughes C. Clinical and hemodynamic evaluation of the 19 mm Björk-Shiley aortic valve prosthesis. Ann Thorac Surg 1981; 32:50–57.

40. Ionescu MI, Tandon AP. The Ionescu-Shiley pericardial xenograft heart valve. In Ionescu MI (ed): *Tissue Heart Valves*. Butterworth, London 1979; p 201.

41. Ohlmeier H, Mannebach H, Greitemeier A. Postoperative klinische Verlaufsbeobachtung nach Omniscience-Klappenersatz: Ist diese Prothese empfehlenswert? Z Kardiol 1982; 71:350.

42. Rabago G, Fraile J, Martinell J. Mitral Valve Replacement. Comparative clinical results with the Omniscience, Medtronic-Hall and Björk-Shiley (c-c 70°) prostheses. Eur Heart J 1985; 6(1):74.

43. Scotten LN, Racca RG, Nugent AH. New tilting disc cardiac valve prostheses. J Thorac Cardiovasc Surg 1981; 82:136.

44. Milano A. Bortolotti U, Talenti E, Valfre C, Arbustini E, Valente M, Mazzucco A, Gallucci V, Thiene G. Calcific degeneration as the main cause of porcine bioprosthetic valve failure. Am J Cardiol 1984; 53:1066.

45. Bloch G, Vouhe PR, Menu P. Poulain H, Cachera JP, Aubry Ph, Heurtematte Y, Loisance DY, Vernant P, Galey JJ. Long-term evaluation of bioprosthetic valves: 615 consecutive cases. Eur Heart J 1984; 5(Suppl D):73.

46. Oyer PE, Stinson EB, Miller CD, Jamieson SW, Mitchell RS, Shumway NE. Thromboembolic risk and durability of the Hancock bioprosthetic cardiac valve. Eur Heart J 1984; 5(Suppl D):81.

47. Ionescu MI, Tandon AP, Chidambaram M, Yakirevich VS, Silverton NP. Durability of the pericardial valve. Eur Heart J 1984; 5(Suppl D):101.

48. Gallucci V, Valfre C, Mazzucco A, Bortolotti U, Milano A, Chioin R, Dallas Volta S, Cevese PG. Heart valve replacement with the Hancock bioprosthesis: A 5-11 year follow-up. In Cohn LG and Gallucci V (eds): *Cardiac Bioprostheses*. Yorke Medical Books, New York 1982; p 9.

49. Duran CM, Gallo J, Ruiz B, Revuelta JM, Ochotecho A. A thousand porcine bioprostheses revisited. Do they conform with the expected pattern? In Cohn LH and Gallucci V (eds): *Cardiac Bioprostheses*. Yorke Medical Books, New York 1982; p 35.

50. Magilligan DJ, Lewis JW, Kara FM. Spontaneous degeneration of porcine bioprosthetic valves. Ann Thorac Surg 1980; 30:259.

51. Borkon AM, McIntosh CL, von Reuden TJ, Morrow AG. Mitral valve replacement with the Hancock bioprosthesis: Five to ten year follow-up. Ann Thorac Surg 1981; 32:127.

52. Deloche A, Perier P, Bourezak H, Chauvaud S, Donzeau-Gouge PG, Dreyfus G, Fabiani JH, Massoud H, Carpentier A, Dubost C. A 14-year experience with valvular bioprostheses: Valve survival and patient survival. In Cohn LH and Gallucci V (eds): *Cardiac Bioprostheses*. Yorke Medical Books, New York 1982; p 25.
53. Cohn LH, Allred EN, DiSesa VJ, Sawtelle K, Shemin RJ, Collins JJ. Early and late risk of aortic valve replacement. J Thorac Cardiovasc Surg 1984; 88:695.
54. Horstkotte D, Trampisch HJ. Long-term follow-up after heart valve replacement. Z Kardiol 1986; 75:641.
55. Grunkemeier GL, Starr A. Actuarial analysis of surgical results: rationale and method. Ann Thor Surg 1977; 24:404.
56. Kalbfleisch JD, Prentice RL. *The Statistical Analysis of Failure Time Data*. John Wiley & Sons, New York 1980.
57. Mantel N. Evaluation of survival data and two new rank order statistics arising in its considerations. Cancer Chem Rep 1966; 50:163.
58. Sage JI, van Kitert RL. Risk of recurrent stroke in patients with atrial fibrillation and non-valvular heart disease. Stroke 1983; 14:537.
59. Horstkotte D, Curtius JM, Bircks W, Loogen F. Noninvasive evaluation of prosthetic heart valves. In Rabago G and Cooley DA (eds): *Heart Valve Replacement and Future Trends in Cardiac Surgery*. Futura Publishing Company, New York 1987; p 349.
60. Horstkotte D, Loogen F. Prosthetic valve related or induced complications. In Horstkotte D and Loogen F (eds): *Update in Heart Valve Replacement*. Steinkopff Verlag, Darmstadt 1985; p 79.
61. Körfer R, Horstkotte D. Incidence, clinical findings and management of prosthetic valve malfunction. In Horstkotte D and Loogen F (eds): *Update in Heart Valve Replacement*. Steinkopff Verlag, Darmstadt 1985; p 121.
62. Horstkotte D, Haerten K, Leuner C, Pöttgen W, Kindler U, Loogen F. Chronic intravascular hemolysis following mitral valve replacement with Björk-Shiley, Lillehei-Kaster and Starr-Edwards prostheses. Z Kardiol 1978; 67:629.
63. Horstkotte D, Aul C, Seipel L, Körfer R, Budde Th, Schulte HD, Bircks W, Loogen F. Influence of valve type and valve function on chronic intravascular hemolysis following mitral and aortic valve replacement using alloprostheses. Z Kardiol 1983; 72:119.
64. Horstkotte D, Bircks W, Loogen F. Infective endocarditis of native and prosthetic valves—the case for prompt surgical intervention? A retrospective analysis of factors affecting survival. Z Kardiol 1986; 75(Suppl 2):168.
65. Horstkotte D, Körfer R, Loogen F. Prosthetic valve endocarditis: Clinical findings and management. Eur Heart J 1984; 5(Suppl C):117.
66. Horstkotte D, Schulte HD, Bircks W, Loogen F. Prothesenendokarditis: Inzidenz, Diagnostik, therapeutische Entscheidungen und Prognose. Schweiz med Wschr 1987; 117:1671.
67. Ferrans VJ, Ishihara T, Jones M, Barnhart GR, Boyce SW, Kravitz AB, Roberts WC. Pathogenesis and stages of bioprosthetic infection. In Cohn LH and Gallucci V (eds): *Cardiac Bioprostheses*. Yorke Medical Books, New York 1982; p 346.
68. Arnett EN, Roberts WC. Prosthetic valve endocarditis. Clinicopathologic analysis of 22 necropsy patients with comparison of observations in 74 necropsy patients with active infective endocarditis involving natural left-sided valves. Am J Cardiol 1976; 38:281.
69. Ferrans VJ, Boyce SW, Billingham ME, Spray TL, Roberts WC. Infection of glutaraldehyde-preserved porcine valve heterografts. Am J Cardiol 1979; 43:1123.
70. Stein PD, Sabbah HN. Measured turbulence and its effect on thrombus formation. Circ Res 1974; 35:608.
71. Myhre E, Dale J, Rasmussen K. Quantitative aspects of hemolysis in aortic valvular heart disease and ball valve prostheses. Acta Med Scand 1971; 189:101.
72. Starr A, Grunkemeier GL, Lambert LE. Aortic valve replacement: A ten-year follow-up of non-cloth-covered vs. cloth-covered caged-ball prostheses. Circulation 1977; 56(Suppl 2):133.
73. Oxman HA, Connolly DC, Ellis FM. Mitral valve replacement with the Smeloff-Cutter prosthesis. J Thorac Cardiovasc Surg 1975; 69:247.
74. Björk VO, Henze A. Ten years experience with the Björk-Shiley tilting disc valve. J Thorac Cardiovasc Surg 1979; 73:331.
75. Horstkotte D, Körfer R, Seipel L, Bircks W, Loogen F. Late complications with Björk-Shiley

and St. Jude Medical heart valve replacement. Circulation 1982; 68(Suppl II):175.

76. Marvasti MA, Markowitz AH, Eich RH, Parker FB. Late results of Lillehei-Kaster valve. Circulation 1980; 62(Suppl III):238.

77. Nicoloff DM, Emery RW, Arom KV. Clinical and hemodynamic results with the St. Jude Medical cardiac valve prosthesis: A three-year experience. J Thorac Cardiovasc Surg 1981; 82:674.

78. LeClerc JL, Wellens F, Deuvaert FE, Primo G. Long-term results with the St. Jude Medical valve. In DeBakey ME (ed): *Advances in Cardiac Valves.* Yorke Medical Books, New York 1983; p 33.

79. Janusz MT, Jamieson WRE, Allen P, Munro AJ, Miyagishima RT, Tutassura H, Burr LH, Gerein AN, Tyers GF. Experience with the Carpentier-Edwards porcine valve prosthesis in 700 patients. Ann Thorac Surg 1982; 34:625.

80. Oyer PE, Stinson EB, Reitz BA. Long-term evaluation of the porcine xenograft bioprosthesis. J Thorac Cardiovasc Surg 1979; 78:343.

81. Hetzer R, Topalidis T, Borst HG. Thromboembolism and anticoagulation after isolated mitral valve replacement with porcine heterografts. In Cohn LH and Gallucci V (eds): *Cardiac Bioprostheses.* Yorke Medical Books, New York 1982; p 172.

82. Lee SJK, Barr C, Callaghan JC, Rossall RE. Long-term survival after aortic valve replacement using Smeloff-Cutter prosthesis. Circulation 1975; 52:1132.

83. Zwart HHJ, Hicks G, Schuster B. Clinical experience with the Lillehei-Kaster valve prosthesis. Ann Thorac Surg 1979; 28:158.

84. Cheung D, Flemma RJ, Mullen DC. Ten year follow-up in aortic valve replacement using the Björk-Shiley prosthesis. Ann Thorac Surg 1981; 32:138.

85. Ionescu MI, Tandon AP, Saunders NR, Chidambaram M, Smith DR. Clinical durability of the pericardial xenograft valve: 11 years experience. In Cohn LH and Gallucci V (eds): *Cardiac Bioprostheses.* Yorke Medical Books, New York 1982; p 42.

86. Borst HG, Frank G, Frimpong-Boateng K, Bednarski P. Herz klappenprothesenwahl—1985. Z Kardiol 1986; 75:311.

87. Oyer PE, Miller DC, Stinson EB, Jamieson WRE, Shumway NE. The performance of the Hancock bioprosthetic valve over $11\frac{1}{2}$ year follow-up period: A preliminary report. In Duran C, Angell WW, Johnson AP, Oury JA (eds): *Recent Progress in Mitral Valve Disease.* Butterworth, London 1984; p 214.

88. Cohn LH. Thromboembolism after mitral valve replacement. In Duran C, Angell WE, Johnson AP, Qury JA (eds): *Recent Progress in Mitral Valve Disease.* Butterworth, London 1984; p 331.

89. Hetzer R, Hill DJ, Kerth WJ, Ansbro J, Adappa MG, Rodvien R, Kamm B, Gerbode JL. Thromboembolic complications after mitral valve replacement with Hancock xenograft. J Thorac Cardiovasc Surg 1978; 75:651.

23. COMPARATIVE ANALYSIS OF MECHANICAL AND BIOPROSTHETIC VALVES FOLLOWING AORTIC VALVE REPLACEMENT

A. M. BORKON, L. M. SOULE, K. L. BAUGHMAN, W. A. BAUMGARDNER, T. J. GARDNER, L. WATKINS, V. L. GOTT, B. A. REITZ

Abstract. *Selection of a mechanical or bioprosthetic heart valve should be based on the results of comparative long-term performance characteristics of both types of valves. In order to discern the risk-benefit ratio of mechanical and bioprosthetic valves, the follow-up of 419 patients undergoing aortic valve replacement between 1976 and 1981 was reviewed to determine late valve-related complications. Aortic valve replacement was performed with BJÖRK-SHILEY® (266) or bioprosthetic (porcine 126 and pericardial 27) aortic valves. Cumulative patient follow-up was 1705 patient-years; the mean patient follow-up was 4.1 ± 2.7 years. For all but 11 patients, survival data was obtained for up to 9 years after operation. At 5 years, survival was 81 ± 4% for all valve recipients. Valve failure in the BJÖRK-SHILEY group was predominantly due to valve-related mortality and did not result from structural failure. Patients with bioprosthetic valves experienced valve failure due to prosthetic endocarditis and intrinsic valve degeneration. While patients with bioprosthetic valves experienced a lower incidence of valve-related morbidity than mechanical valve recipients (p < 0.03), no difference between valve types could be demonstrated in the incidence of valve-related mortality or valve failure at 5 years. Mortality due to valve failure was higher for mechanical than bioprosthetic valves (p < 0.01).*

INTRODUCTION

Differences in operative techniques, patient populations, modes of follow-up, and time frames of analysis generally do not permit a meaningful comparison of single valve studies from various institutions [1]. In order to avoid these deficiencies, this study was undertaken to analyze two similar groups of patients, one undergoing mechanical and the other bioprosthetic valve replacement, during a coincident 5-year period. Computation of valve-related events and use of a comprehensive definition of valve failure were used to enable comparisons of cardiac valve substitutes with different attributes and modes of valve failure.

PATIENTS

From January 1976 to December 1981, 419 nonconsecutive adult patients underwent aortic valve replacement with either a BJÖRK-SHILEY standard spherical disc (266 patients) or a bioprosthetic valve (153 patients). Included in the bioprosthetic group were IONESCU-SHILEY® (27), CARPENTIER-EDWARDS® (37), and HANCOCK® (89) models. Patients receiving multiple valve replacements were excluded from analysis. Patients undergoing concomitant operations, such as coronary artery bypass or ascending aortic resection, were included. Selection of a particular cardiac valve substitute was determined by individual surgeon preference.

Numerous preoperative clinical characteristics were similar for patients receiving BJÖRK-SHILEY and bioprosthetic valves, except for an increased duration of cardiopulmonary bypass and total myocardial ischemia among BJÖRK-SHILEY recipients (table 23-1). A greater number of small-sized aortic valves (less than 21 mm) were present in the BJÖRK-SHILEY group (118/266; 44%) compared to the bioprosthesis group (16/153; 11%) (p < 0.001).

Warfarin anticoagulation was begun following operation for all patients and continued indefinitely for BJÖRK-SHILEY recipients unless life-threatening hemorrhage occurred, in which case antiplatelet drugs were administered. Thus, 91% of BJÖRK-SHILEY operative survivors were receiving warfarin at the time of follow-up. Patients with bioprosthetic valves received warfarin for up to 3 months after operation, after which it was usually discontinued. Only 13% of bioprosthetic recipients were receiving long-term warfarin therapy.

Valve-related complications described previously were employed [2, 3]. A thromboembolus was defined as any new focal or diffuse neurologic event, permanent or transient, appearing after operation or during the follow-up interval. Also included were emboli to visceral or extremity vessels. Patients who awoke after operation with a neurologic deficit or who did not regain consciousness were not considered to have incurred a valve-related thromboembolus. Similarly, if another source could be shown conclusively to be the cause of a neurologic event, then the episode was not considered valve-related. Valve thrombosis was confirmed at autopsy or at reoperation. Total thrombotic events were calculated by combining valve thrombosis and thromboemboli. Anticoagulant-related hemorrhage (ACH) was determined to be

Table 23-1. Preoperative clinical characteristics

	Björk-Shiley	Bioprosthesis	p value
Number of patients	266	153	—
Mean age (yrs)	57.5 ± 13.2	55.8 ± 15.4	0.53
Male/female ratio	2.3:1	4:1	0.03
Angina pectoris	64%	51%	0.01
Previous myocardial infarction	9%	15%	0.08
NYHA (CHF) Class III or IV	69%	58%	0.03
Previous aortic valve replacement	4%	2%	0.24
Endocarditis	5%	9%	0.08
Atrial fibrillation	5%	4%	0.81
Cardiothoracic ratio (%)	52 ± 6	52 ± 7	0.43
PA mean pressure (mmHg)	21 ± 11	21 ± 10	0.54
Cardiac index (L/min/M^2)	2.8 ± 1.0	2.8 ± 0.9	0.77
LVEDP (mmHg)	18 ± 9	18 ± 9	0.57
Ejection fraction (%)	59 ± 15	56 ± 16	0.17
Predominant hemodynamic lesion			0.28
Aortic stenosis	30%	39%	—
Aortic regurgitation	54%	49%	—
Mixed stenosis/regurgitation	14%	11%	—
Other	3%	1%	—
Concomitant procedure			
Coronary artery bypass	32%	24%	0.08
Aortic aneurysm resection	5%	4%	0.67
Cardiopulmonary bypass (min)	133 ± 50	111 ± 42	0.00005
Aortic cross-clamp (min)	81 ± 26	72 ± 19	0.0001

NYHA = New York Heart Association; CHF = congestive heart failure; PA = pulmonary artery;
LVEDP = left ventricular end diastolic pressure

significant, and thus valve-related, if fatal or severe enough to necessitate hospitalization. Prosthetic valve endocarditis (PVE) was defined as septicemia that could not be attributed to a source other than the prosthesis and necessitated prolonged antibiotic therapy or reoperation [4]. Structural valve failure, observed only in bioprosthetic valves, was confirmed at reoperation or autopsy and defined by the presence of characteristic leaflet calcification or cuspal disruption in the absence of PVE [5].

Composite valve-related morbidity was the sum of all patients experiencing any valve-related complication. It was not infrequent for a patient to experience more than one valve-related complication; however, only the first event was considered in this analysis. Valve-related mortality represented fatalities arising from valve-related morbidity. In the case of multiple valve-related complications resulting in death, only the precipitating event was determined to be fatal. In order to allow comparison of mechanical and bioprosthetic valves, a comprehensive definition of valve failure was employed [2, 3]. Any valve-related morbidity, such as thromboembolus, ACH, PVE, valve thrombosis, periprosthetic leak, prosthetic valve dysfunction caused by loss of structural integrity, or any other reason that necessitated reoperation or resulted in death was defined as valve failure.

Patient follow-up was achieved by contacting patients, their primary physicians, or both prior to December 1985. Follow-up information was available for all but 11 patients, 8 with BJÖRK-SHILEY valves and 3 with bioprosthetic valves, resulting in a 97% follow-up. A total of 1705 patient-years was available for analysis (1077 patient-years, BJÖRK-SHILEY; 628 patient-years, bioprosthetic valve group). Mean follow-up for all patients was 4.1 ± 2.7 years (range 0 to 9.4 years). The average follow-up for survivors was 5.1 ± 2.2 patient-years. There was no difference in mean follow-up for survivors of either valve type. In the event of reoperation for either re-replacement of the aortic prosthesis or additional valve replacement, patients were censored from analysis and considered to be withdrawn alive or dead, depending on their status 30 days after reoperation. Actuarial analysis (Kaplan-Meier) and linear statistical determination of survival rates and incidence of valve-related complications were performed [6]. Actuarial rates were expressed as percent of patients event-free. Linearized data were derived from first patient events, expressed as percent per patient-year (%/pt-yr), and compared by the Z test [7]. Continuous data are expressed as mean ±1 standard deviation; linearized rates and actuarial determinations are represented as mean ±1 standard error. Variables predictive of survival and freedom from valve-related complications were first determined individually by Kaplan-Meier actuarial analysis and their significance analyzed by the Breslow test [8]. Significant factors were then entered into a multivariate stepwise Cox proportionate hazards model to identify independent and additive variables associated with length of survival or freedom from complications [9]. The contribution of each variable entered into each model was assessed by the likelihood ratio test [10]. In addition to those variables listed in table 23-1, other dependent variables entered into univariate and multivariate analysis for all morbid and fatal events including valve type, race, duration of angina, anginal class, urgency of operation, aortic gradient, roentgenographic aortic valve calcium, aortic valve area, left ventricular systolic pressure, left ventricular systolic and diastolic volume, year of operation, valve size, and warfarin status.

RESULTS

Survival

Overall hospital mortality for both groups was 12.9% (54/419). The causes of hospital death were not different between groups (figure 23-1). Cardiac-related causes accounted for over half (32/54) of all early deaths. Valve-related deaths occurred in 2 patients, 1 with a BJÖRK-SHILEY valve who died from valve thrombosis on the sixth postoperative day, and another patient with a bioprosthetic valve who died from a cerebral thromboembolus.

Late deaths were predominantly due to cardiac causes or sudden death (figure 23-2). Valve-related complications were responsible for 24% (11/45)

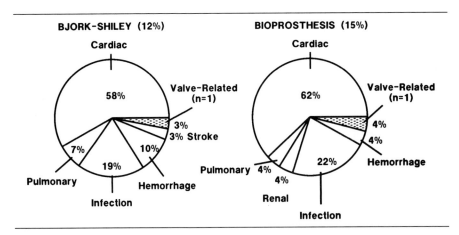

Figure 23-1. Causes of operative mortality.

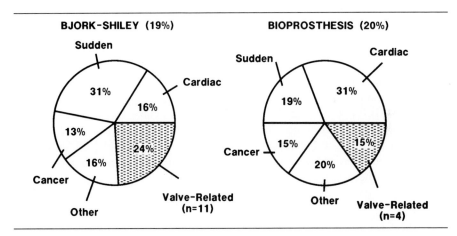

Figure 23-2. Causes of late mortality.

of late deaths in BJÖRK-SHILEY and 15% (4/26) of bioprosthetic valve patients, ACH accounted for 20% of late deaths among BJÖRK-SHILEY recipients, whereas 12% of late deaths in the bioprosthetic valve group were due to a thromboembolus. The 5-year actuarial survival rate was 81 ± 4% and was identical for operative survivors of both valve groups (figure 23-3). If operative deaths are included, the actuarial 5-year survival rate was 72 ± 3% for BJÖRK-SHILEY and 70 ± 4% for bioprosthetic valve recipients. Congestive heart failure class, endocarditis, and angina were independent preoperative risk factors predictive of an adverse outcome following operation. When operative deaths are excluded, ejection fraction less than 40%, coronary artery

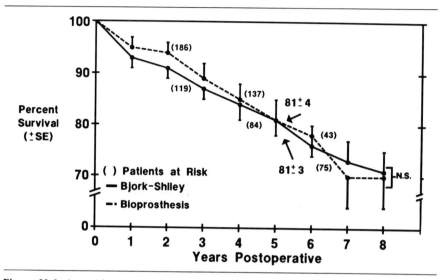

Figure 23-3. Actuarial survival depicted for operative survivors.

disease requiring coronary artery bypass, and atrial fibrillation, but not valve type, were factors independently predictive of a fatal late outcome.

Actuarial survival free from valve-related mortality was 95 ± 2% for BJÖRK-SHILEY and 97 ± 2% for bioprosthetic valve recipients at 5 years (figure 23-4). A slightly higher incidence of valve-related mortality was found in the first year (3.2 ± 1.2% per patient-year for BJÖRK-SHILEY and 1.6 ± 1.1% per patient-year for bioprosthesis), which diminished to 0.6 ± 0.3% per patient-year thereafter for both groups (p < 0.001).

Valve-related events

Linearized rates of valve-related complications are summarized and listed in table 23-2. No significant difference was found in the actuarial incidence of thrombotic events between BJÖRK-SHILEY and bioprosthetic valve recipients at 6 and 7 years (figure 23-5). For both groups, 75% of central nervous system events were permanent. The linearized incidence of fatal thrombo-embolism was 0.1 ± 0.1% per patient-year for BJÖRK-SHILEY and 0.5 ± 0.3% per patient-year for bioprosthetic recipients. The only independent predictor of thromboembolism identified for bioprosthetic valve recipients was PVE (p = 0.006). In fact, 3 of 9 patients with PVE and a bioprosthesis experienced a thromboembolus. If bioprosthetic valve recipients with PVE are excluded from analysis of thromboembolism, then the overall hazard rate for development of thromboembolism was reduced to 2.1 ± 0.6% per patient-year.

Valve thrombosis was observed in 2 patients with BJÖRK-SHILEY valves,

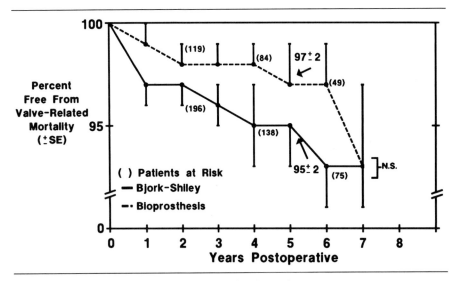

Figure 23-4. Actuarial survival free from valve-related mortality.

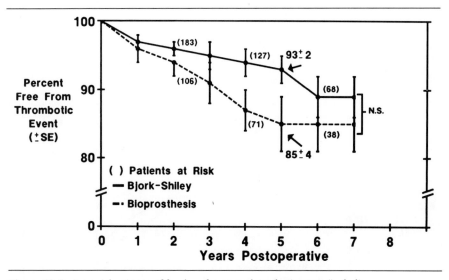

Figure 23-5. Actuarial estimate of freedom from any thrombotic event (including thromboembolus and valve thrombosis).

with 1 fatality. The overall hazard rate of valve thrombosis was $0.2 \pm 0.1\%$ per patient-year. No significant difference could be found in total thrombotic event rate between BJÖRK-SHILEY and bioprosthetic valve recipients.

Multivariate analysis disclosed valve type to be an independent predictor of

Table 23-2. Summary of rates of valve-related morbidity

	Björk-Shiley		Bioprosthesis		
	No.	Rate (%/pt-yr)	No.	Rate (%/pt-yr)	p value
Thrombotic event	16	1.6 ± 0.4	15	2.7 ± 0.7	0.05
ACH	56	6.2 ± 0.8	2	0.3 ± 0.2	0.001
PVE	3	0.3 ± 0.2	9	1.6 ± 0.5	0.03
PVL	1	0.1 ± 0.1	0	—	—
Structural failure	0	—	6	1.0 ± 0.4	0.001
Reoperation	2	0.2 ± 0.1	10	1.7 ± 0.5	0.001
Valve failure	14	1.3 ± 0.3	14	2.2 ± 0.6	0.156
Total	70	7.9 ± 0.9	27	4.9 ± 0.9	0.03

TE = thrombotic event; ACH = anticoagulant-related hemorrhage; PVE = prosthetic valve endocarditis; PVL = paravalvular leak

increased risk for ACH (figure 23-6). At 7 years, 5% of patients with BJÖRK-SHILEY valves had experienced a fatal ACH. The hazard for this complication was greatest in the first postoperative year (10.3 ± 2.3% per patient-year) compared to a relatively constant rate thereafter (5.0 ± 0.8% per patient-year; $p < 0.06$). The overall incidence of fatal ACH was 1.0 ± 0.3% per patient-year.

An increased incidence of PVE was found among bioprosthetic valve recipients. Freedom from PVE was 98 ± 1% at 5 years for BJÖRK-SHILEY

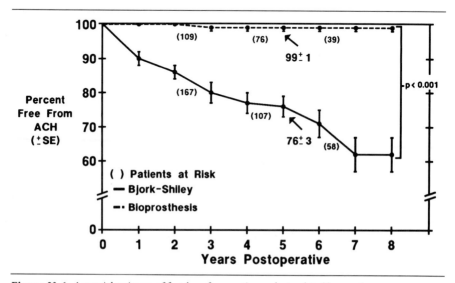

Figure 23-6. Actuarial estimate of freedom from anticoagulant-related hemorrhage.

and 92 ± 3% for bioprostheses (figure 23-7). Multivariate analysis revealed an increased risk of prosthetic valve endocarditis to be associated with the IONESCU-SHILEY valve (p = 0.002).

In the absence of PVE, structural failure was found in 6 patients with bioprosthetic valves. Reoperation was carried out in 5 patients without a fatality. One patient refused reoperation and died. The majority of bioprosthetic patients (89 ± 5%) at 7 years were free from this complication. Patients less than 36 years old had a higher risk of structural bioprosthetic failure than did older patients (p < 0.03)(figure 23-8). Multivariate analysis confirmed age as a continuous variable and both age and association of an IONESCU-SHILEY valve to be risk factors for bioprosthetic structural failure. One reoperation was carried out in a BJÖRK-SHILEY valve recipient for bland periprosthetic leak. The actuarial estimate of freedom from reoperation was greater for BJÖRK-SHILEY than bioprosthetic valves, 99 ± 1% vs. 86 ± 5% at 7 years, respectively (figure 23-9). The annual hazard of reoperation for bioprosthetic valve recipients increased with duration of follow-up, reflecting an increased number of patients with intrinsic bioprosthetic valve failure (figure 23-10). Multivariate analysis confirmed that PVE, age less than 35, and an IONESCU-SHILEY valve were associated with the need for reoperation.

Data for patients free of valve failure at 7 years is shown in figure 23-11. A broad definition of valve failure was employed to include patients who died of valve-related events (valve-related mortality) or underwent reoperation for valve failure. Figure 23-12 reveals that ACH accounted for over 64% (9/14) of valve failure in the BJÖRK-SHILEY group and was uniformly fatal. Reopera-

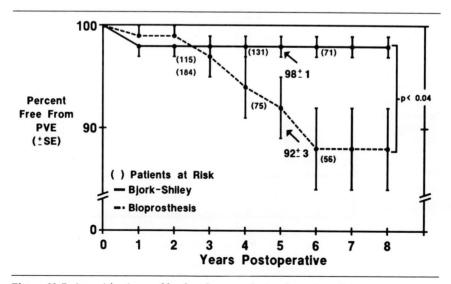

Figure 23-7. Actuarial estimate of freedom from prosthetic valve endocarditis.

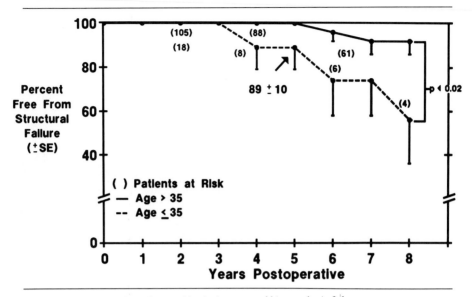

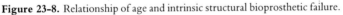

Figure 23-8. Relationship of age and intrinsic structural bioprosthetic failure.

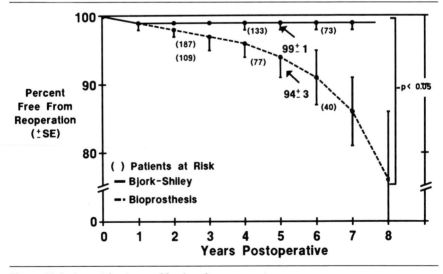

Figure 23-9. Actuarial estimate of freedom from reoperation.

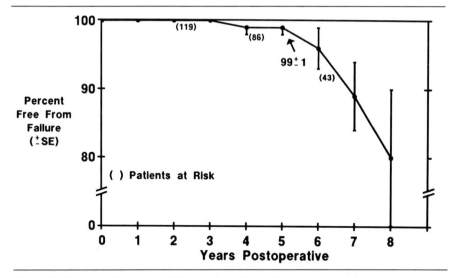

Figure 23-10. Actuarial estimate of freedom from bioprosthetic structural valve failure.

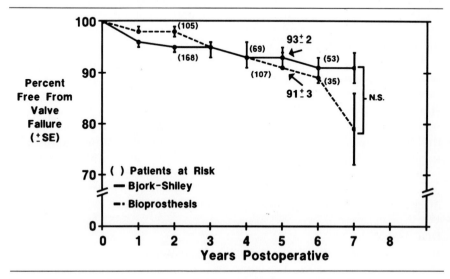

Figure 23-11. Actuarial freedom from valve failure defined in a comprehensive manner.

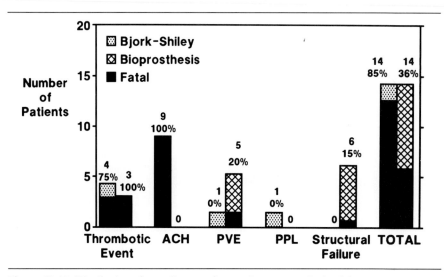

Figure 23-12. Distribution of mortality rates from various causes of valve failure.

tion was the cause of 71% (10/14) of valve failures in the bioprosthetic group due to either PVE or structural intrinsic deterioration. Overall, 86% (12/14) of BJÖRK-SHILEY patients with valve failure died compared to 36% (5/14) of patients with bioprosthetic valves (p < 0.01). The annual hazard of valve failure for BJÖRK-SHILEY valves was greatest within the first year (3.6 ± 1.3%) and diminished thereafter (0.7 ± 0.3% per patient-year, p < 0.001). On the other hand, the annual hazard rate for bioprosthetic valve failure increased from 1.6 ± 1.1% per patient-year to 6.6 ± 2.5% per patient-year for the fifth through eighth postoperative years (p < 0.001).

With regard to composite valve-related morbidity, one or more valve-related complications were observed in 70 patients with BJÖRK-SHILEY valves and 27 patients with bioprosthetic valves (figure 23-13). Overall, 17% (12/70) of patients with BJÖRK-SHILEY valves and 19% (5/27) of patients with bioprostheses succumbed from valve-related events. Actuarial survival free from any morbid valve-related event was improved for bioprosthetic valve recipients (figure 23-14). If valve-related deaths and permanent incapacitating events due to thromboemboli or ACH are analyzed and considered as patient-related failure, no difference was observed at 5 or 7 years between mechanical or bioprosthetic valve recipients (figure 23-15).

DISCUSSION
Bioprosthetic heart valves were introduced and used with increasing frequency at our institution in 1976. During a subsequent 5-year period from 1976 to 1981, two nearly identical populations of patients, one receiving mechanical BJÖRK-SHILEY and the other bioprosthetic heart valves, were available for

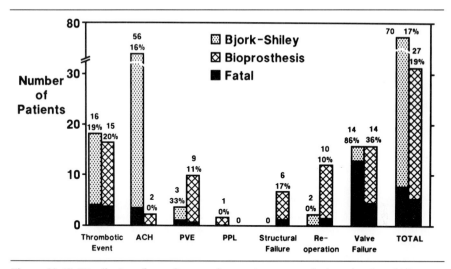

Figure 23-13. Distribution of mortality rates from various causes of valve-related morbidity.

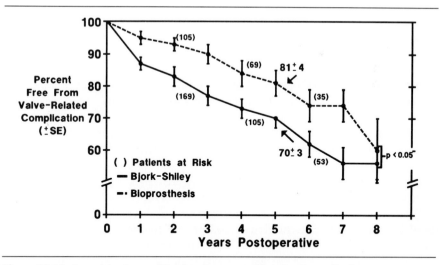

Figure 23-14. Actuarial estimate of freedom from any valve-related complication.

long-term retrospective analysis of valve-related complications. Multivariate analysis confirmed that preoperative variables differing between the two groups were not related to the risk of development of subsequent valve-related events.

Overall survival was found to be similar for bioprosthetic and BJÖRK-SHILEY valve recipients [11–21]. In our series, a majority of late deaths were

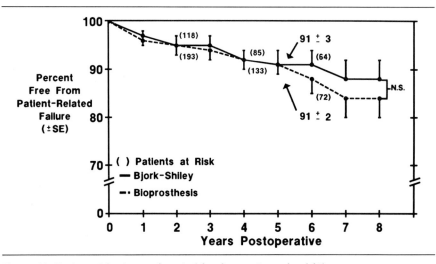

Figure 23-15. Actuarial estimate of survival free from patient-related failure.

cardiac-related [22]. Patients who died suddenly in the absence of postmortem examination were placed in the group of cardiac-related deaths, since we believe that the majority of those patients died of arrhythmia. It is possible, however, that some patients in this group may actually have died of a valve-related cause [23]. Nevertheless, computation of valve-related mortality incorporating sudden death did not yield different results.

Although the overall incidence of thrombotic events was not significantly different between groups, the incidence of thromboemboli alone was found to be greater for bioprosthetic than BJÖRK-SHILEY valves, an observation conflicting with previous reports [11–21, 23–26]. If patients with thrombo-embolism related to PVE were eliminated from the bioprosthesis group, the difference between groups does not achieve statistical significance. The lower incidence of thromboembolism in BJÖRK-SHILEY patients was offset by the relatively high rate of ACH that has been observed by others [23].

While valve thrombosis was identified in only 2 patients with BJÖRK-SHILEY valves, its presentation is abrupt and frequently associated with a high mortality rate. This valve-related complication has been widely recognized with tilting-disc mechanical valves and occurs often despite adequate anticoagulation [11–15, 27].

An ever-present risk and nearly unavoidable complication of warfarin anti-coagulation is ACH. ACH accounted for 80% of late valve-related morbidity and 75% of valve-related deaths for BJÖRK-SHILEY recipients. The high incidence of ACH detracts from the safety of all mechanical prostheses [3, 11–15, 20, 23, 24, 26, 28–31].

A slightly higher incidence of PVE was observed in bioprosthetic valve recipients and contrasts with other published reports [29, 32]. An independent risk factor for PVE was found to be the IONESCU-SHILEY valve. Bioprosthetic valves may be more predisposed to develop PVE than mechanical valves, when implanted in the setting of native valve endocarditis [33]. In the present study, the incidence of preoperative native valve endocarditis was slightly greater for bioprosthetic than BJÖRK-SHILEY valve recipients. Similarly to other reports, PVE, whether treated medically or by reoperation, was accompanied by a high mortality rate, irrespective of valve type [2, 3, 11–19].

Beyond the fifth postoperative year, structural bioprosthetic valve failure has been observed with increasing frequency [16–19, 20, 21, 26, 29]. Unlike mechanical valve failure, which is often catastrophic, structural failure of bioprosthetic valves was found to be of gradual onset, permitting safe reoperation. In the absence of severe congestive heart failure or PVE, reoperation for bioprosthetic failure may be performed with an operative mortality identical to that of the original operation [36–38]. The ability to recognize structural bioprosthetic failure by noninvasive imaging may further reduce reoperative mortality [39]. As noted by other groups, a higher rate of structural failure was observed in patients less than 36-years-old [13] and with IONESCU-SHILEY valves [34, 35]. The poor results found with the IONESCU-SHILEY valve in our study may have adversely biased the outcome of the bioprosthetic group as a whole.

Determination of the ultimate superiority of a particular valve must be based upon an overall comparison of comprehensive definitions of valve-related events including total valve-related morbidity and mortality, valve failure, and patient-related failure. In this study, the incidence of valve failure was nearly identical for BJÖRK-SHILEY and bioprosthetic valve recipients at 5 years. The mortality resulting from valve failure was much greater for patients with BJÖRK-SHILEY than bioprosthetic valves. While there was little difference in overall patient-related survival between valve types, total valve-related morbidity was found to be substantially less for bioprosthetic than BJÖRK-SHILEY valve recipients for up to 7 years following operation. Similar observations have been reported in other studies [20, 26, 28–32, 34]. Although the bioprosthetic valve appears to offer a greater margin of safety than the BJÖRK-SHILEY valve substitute for up to 7 years after operation, continued analysis will be required to determine which cardiac valve ultimately provides the greatest long-term patient safety.

REFERENCES

1. Mitchell RS, Miller DC, Stinson EB, Oyer PE, Jamieson SW, Baldwin JC, Shumway NE. Significant patient-related determinants of prosthetic valve performance. J Thorac Cardiovasc Surg 1986; 91:807.
2. Borkon AM, Soule LM, Baughman KL, Aoun H, Gardner TJ, Watkins L Jr, Gott VL, Reitz BA. Ten-year analysis of the Björk-Shiley standard aortic valve. Ann Thorac Surg, in press.
3. Miller DC, Oyer PE, Mitchell RS, Stinson ED, Jamieson SW, Baldwin JC, Shumway NE. Performance characteristics of the Starr-Edwards model 1260 aortic valve prosthesis beyond

ten years. J Thorac Cardiovasc Surg 1984; 88:193.
4. Baumgartner WA, Miller DC, Reitz BA, Oyer PE, Jamieson SW, Stinson EB, Shumway NE. Surgical treatment of prosthetic valve endocarditis. Ann Thorac Surg 1983; 35:87.
5. Spray TL, Roberts WC. Structural changes in porcine xenografts used as substitute cardiac valves. Am J Cardiol 1977; 40:319.
6. Lefrak EA, Starr A (eds). *Cardiac Valve Prostheses.* Appleton-Century-Crofts, New York 1979; p 38.
7. Snedecor GW, Cochran WG. *Statistical Methods* (7th ed). Iowa State University Press, Ames, 1980; p 41.
8. Breslow N. A generalized Kruskal-Wallis test for comparing K samples subject to unequal patterns of censorship. Biometrika 1970; 57:579.
9. Cox DR. Regression models and life tables. J Roy Stat Soc B 1972; 26:103.
10. Dixon WJ (ed). *BMDP Statistical Software.* University of California Press, Berkeley, CA 1985.
11. Karp RB, Cyrus RJ, Blackstone EH, Kirklin JW, Kouchoukos NT, Pacifico A. The Björk-Shiley valve. J Thorac Cardiovasc Surg 1981; 81:602.
12. Cohn LH, Allred EN, DiSesa VJ, Sawtelle K, Shemin RJ, Collins JJ Jr. Early and late risk of aortic valve replacement. J Thorac Cardiovasc Surg 1984; 88:695.
13. Björk VO, Henze A. Ten years' experience with the Björk-Shiley tilting disc valve. J Thorac Cardiovasc Surg 1979; 78:331.
14. Daenen W, Nevelsteen A, van Cauwelaert P, de Maesschalk E, Willems J, Stalpaert G. Nine years' experience with the Björk-Shiley prosthetic valve: Early and late results of 932 valve replacements. Ann Thorac Surg 1983; 35:651.
15. Sethia B, Turner MA, Lewis S, Rodger RA, Bain WH, Kouchoukos NT. Fourteen years' experience with the Björk-Shiley tilting disc prosthesis. J Thorac Cardiovasc Surg 1986; 91:350.
16. Magiligan DJ, Lewis JW, Tilley B, Peterson E. The porcine bioprosthetic valve: Twelve years later. J Thorac Cardiovasc Surg 1985; 89:499.
17. Cohn LH, Mudge GH, Pratter F, Collins JJ Jr. Five to eight-year follow-up of patients undergoing porcine heart-valve replacement. N Engl J Med 1981; 304:258.
18. Hartz RS, Fisher EB, Finkelmeier B, DeBoer A, Sanders JH Jr, Moran JM, Michaelis LL. An eight-year experience with porcine bioprosthetic cardiac valves. J Thorac Cardiovasc Surg 1986; 91:910.
19. Oyer PE, Miller DC, Stinson EB, Reitz BA, Moreno-Cabral RJ, Shumway NE. Clinical durability of the Hancock porcine bioprosthetic valve. J Thorac Cardiovasc Surg 1980; 80:824.
20. Hammond GL, Geha AS, Kopf GS, Hashin SW. Biological vs. mechanical valves: Analysis of 1104 valves inserted in 1012 adult patients with a 4801 patient-year follow-up. J Thorac Cardiovasc Surg, in press.
21. Janusz MT, Jamieson WR, Allen P, Munro AI, Miyagishima RT, Tutassura H, Burr L, Gerein AN, Tyers GFO. Experience with the Carpentier-Edwards porcine valve prosthesis in 700 patients. Ann Thorac Surg 1982; 34:625.
22. Gersh BJ, Fisher LD, Schaff HV, Rahimtoola SH, Reeder GS, Frater RWM, McGoon DC. Issues concerning the clinical evaluation of new prosthetic valves. J Thorac Cardiovasc Surg 1986; 91:460.
23. Tepley JF, Grunkemeier GL, Sutherland HD, Lambert LE, Johnson VA, Starr A. The ultimate prognosis after valve replacement: An assessment at twenty years. Ann Thorac Surg 1981; 32:111.
24. Martinell J, Fraile J, Artiz V, Moreno J, Rabago G. Long-term comparative analysis of Björk-Shiley and Hancock valves implanted in 1975. J Thorac Cardiovasc Surg 1985; 90:741.
25. Jamieson WRE, Janusz MT, Miyagishima RT, Munro AI, Tutassura H, Gerein AN, Burr LH, Allen P. Embolic complications of porcine heterograft cardiac valves. J Thorac Cardiovasc Surg 1981; 81:626.
26. Joyce LD, Nelson RM. Comparison of porcine valve xenografts with mechanical prostheses. J Thorac Cardiovasc Surg 1984; 88:102.
27. Wright JO, Hiratzka LF, Brandt B, Doty DB. Thrombosis of the Björk-Shiley prosthesis. J Thorac Cardiovasc Surg 1982; 84:138.
28. Douglas PS, Hirshfeld JW Jr, Edie RN, Harken AH, Stephenson LW, Edmunds LH Jr. Clinical comparison of St. Jude Medical and porcine aortic valve prostheses. Circulation 1985; 72(Suppl II):II-135.

29. Mitchell RS, Miller DC, Stinson EB, Oyer PE, Jamieson SW, Baldwin JC, Shumway NE. Perspectives on the porcine xenograft valve. Cardiol Clinics 1985; 3:371.

30. Cobanoglu A, Jamieson WRE, Miller DC, McKinley C, Grunkemeier GL, Floten HS, Miyagishima RT, Tyers GFO, Shumway NE, Starr A. A tri-institutional comparison of tissue and mechanical vlaves using a patient-oriented definition of treatment failure. Ann Thorac Surg 1987; 43:245.

31. Perier P, Bessou JP, Swanson JS, Bensasson D, Chachques JC, Chauvaud S, Deloche A, Fabiani JN, Blondeau P, D'Allaines C, Carpentier A. Comparative evaluation of aortic valve replacement with Starr, Björk and porcine valve prostheses. Circulation 1985; 72(Suppl II): II-140.

32. Rutledge R, Kim GJ, Applebaum E. Actuarial analysis of the risk of prosthetic valve endocarditis in 1598 patients with mechanical and bioprosthetic valves. Arch Surg 1985; 120:469.

33. Sweeney MS, Reul GJ Jr, Cooley DA, Ott DA, Duncan JM, Frazier OH, Livesay JJ. Comparison of bioprosthetic and mechanical valve replacement for active endocarditis. J Thorac Cardiovasc Surg 1985; 90:676.

34. Nistal F, Garcia-Satue E, Artinano E, Gomez-Duran CM, Gallo I. Comparative study of primary tissue valve failure between Ionescu-Shiley pericardial and Hancock porcine valves in the aortic position. Am J Cardiol 1986; 57:161.

35. Reul GJ Jr, Cooley DA, Duncan JM, Frazier OH, Hallman GL, Livesay JJ, Ott DA, Walker WE. Valve failure with the Ionescu-Shiley bovine pericardial bioprosthesis: Analysis of 2680 patients. J Vasc Surg 1985; 2:192.

36. Bortolotti U, Milano A, Mazzucco A, Valfre C, Talenti E, Guerra F, Thiene G, Gallucci V. Results of reoperation for primary tissue failure of porcine bioprosthesis. J Thorac Cardiovasc Surg 1985; 90:564.

37. Wideman FE, Blackstone EH, Kirklin JW, Karp RB, Kouchoukos NT, Pacifico AD. Hospital mortality of re-replacement of the aortic valve. J Thorac Cardiovasc Surg 1981; 82:692.

38. Husebye DG, Pluth JR, Piehler JM, Schaff HV, Orszulak TA, Puga FJ, Danielson GK. Reoperation on prosthetic heart valves. J Thorac Cardiovasc Surg 1983; 86:543.

39. Grenadier E, Sahn DJ, Roche AH, Valdes-Cruz LM, Copeland JG, Goldberg SJ, Allen HD. Detection of deterioration or infection of homograft and porcine xenograft bioprosthetic valves in mitral and aortic positions by two-dimensional echocardiographic examination. JACC 1983; 2:452.

24. TECHNICAL PROBLEMS IN AORTIC VALVE RE-REPLACEMENT

V. SCHLOSSER

Abstract. Between 1981 and 1986, we replaced 371 aortic valves, mainly using ST. JUDE MEDICAL® (SJM) aortic prostheses. During the same period, we had to replace the prosthetic aortic valve in 20 cases, with 1 death. Causes of reoperation were paravalvular leak in 6 patients and endocarditis in 12. In 2 patients, valve re-replacement was performed because very small prostheses had been implanted during childhood. Reoperation does not include major surgical problems, but the excision of small SJM valves from the narrow aortic anulus raises some problems. In order to prevent fracture of the leaflets during excision, we used a valve holder designed by a technician that enables traction on the valve without any risk of leaflet fracture.

INTRODUCTION

In the past 25 years, prosthetic valve replacement of the aortic valve has become a well-established and generally accepted method of treatment. Up to now, however, the ideal artificial valve prosthesis has not been found. The requirements for an optimum valve prosthesis were listed by McGoon in 1974 [1].

The double-leaflet valve from St. Jude Medical, Inc. can fulfill most of these requirements than other valves. In comparison to other mechanical heart valve prostheses, special mention should be made of the low thromboembolism rate and the excellent hemodynamic parameters. Since the valve (even in small diameters) produces low-pressure gradients, this prosthesis is especially

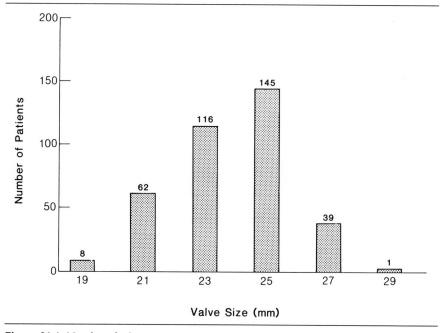

Figure 24-1. Number of valves implanted regarding valve size.

suitable in the aortic position with a narrow annulus. Smaller-sized valves were most often used in our clinic (figure 24-1). Among our own patients, when using prostheses with a diameter of 23 mm and less, prior to completion of the operation, gradient measurements have always been carried out. In all cases, results have been less than 12 mm Hg at rest. Good assessment of valve function by x-ray is an additional advantage of this prosthesis (figure 24-2).

The numerous advantages of the ST. JUDE MEDICAL (SJM) prosthesis are offset by several quite serious disadvantages. The lack of possible rotation after implantation and the high fragility of the valve mechanism are key concerns. We also see disadvantages in the possibility of the suture ring becoming loose on valves smaller than 23 mm, due to a rupture of the fixation thread.

While a lack of rotation capability can have a strong detrimental effect on considerably calcified valves (with a limited possibility of decalcification), during reoperation and prosthesis re-replacement, the high fragility is particularly problematic.

PATIENTS AND METHODS

Between 1981 and 1986 we carried out 371 aortic valve replacements using the SJM valve. Twenty of these (5.4%) were re-replacements. In 12 patients reoperation was necessary due to late infection or valve thrombosis; in 6 patients, it was due to paravalvular leak. In 2 patients, a larger prosthesis

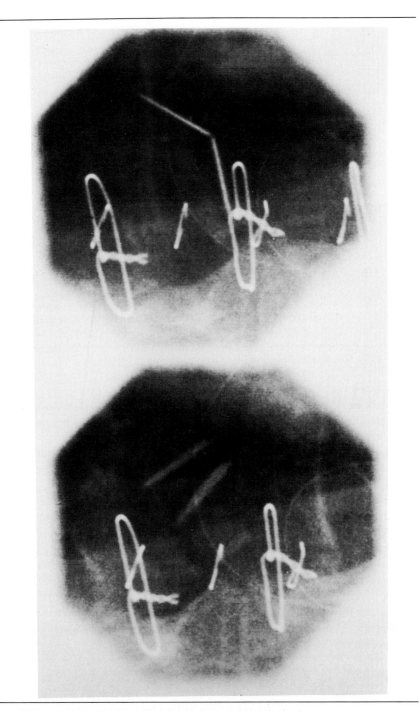

Figure 24-2. X-ray visualization of function in the St. Jude Medical valve.

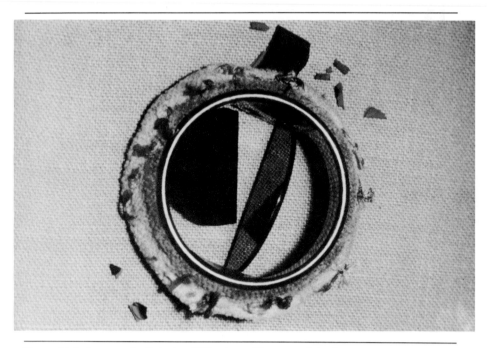

Figure 24-3. An example of a broken SJM valve and its scattered shards.

had to be implanted, since very small SJM prostheses had previously been implanted in childhood at 4 and 6 years of age, respectively. One patient died after reoperation.

During reoperation, excision of the SJM valve was found to be difficult in 8 cases. Valve breakage occurred in 5 cases, resulting in a scattering of broken pieces (figure 24-3).

The lack of working surface for holding or traction instruments easily leads to breakage of the brittle valve material. The broken pieces, some of which are frequently very small, can fall inside the left ventricle, where they are exceptionlly difficult to locate and remove.

For this reason, we have had a prototype fixation instrument developed from older devices, to secure the valve and protect it from breakage, as well as to ease the excision of the valve (figure 24-4). With this device we have carried out the last three reoperations without problems, even in patients with a very small aortic root. We see, in this instrument, a considerably easier excision of SJM prostheses in the aortic position during reoperations.

DISCUSSION

Even though the SJM valve has been known for years as an excellent prosthesis, we would be grateful for its further development so that the suture

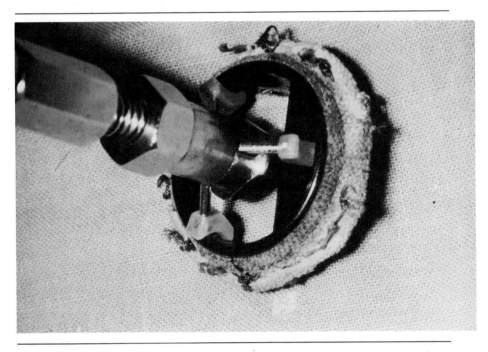

Figure 24-4. The fixation instrument developed to manipulate the SJM valve and prevent valve damage or breakage.

ring of small-sized valves will be securely fixed. The possibility of rotation after implantation, together with improved manipulation during excision, is also important.

With these improvements, the SJM valve will remain one of the best valves for the aortic position.

REFERENCES

1. McGoon DC. On evaluating valves. Mayo Clin Proc 1974; 49:233.

25. HYDRODYNAMICS OF CARDIAC VALVE PROSTHESES: IS EXCELLENCE NECESSARY?

R. J. GRAY

Abstract. Few papers have compared the hydrodynamic features of various cardiac valve prostheses with respect to surgical results. All prostheses offer resistence to blood flow and most exhibit regurgitation, but we have come to expect improvements in symptoms and survival despite widely varying hydraulic performance. When patients do not achieve the full benefits of surgery or exhibit late deterioration despite an apparently normally functioning prosthesis, we begin to suspect that the imperfections of valve substitutes are playing a role in patient outcome. Objective data, such as analysis of symptoms or sequential late studies of cardiac function, especially after 10 years, would be useful. Unfortunately, almost all surgical survivors improve postoperatively and those who deteriorate functionally die and are unavailable for late analysis. The majority of late deaths are due to congestive heart failure. Not all of these deaths can be blamed on the late timing of surgery or inadequate myocardial protection during the procedure. For these reasons and because most valve prosthesis recipients have other underlying cardiac problems, it is important to evaluate the specific impact of long-term prosthetic hydraulic performance. Contributing to poor valve performance are 1) pros- thesis-patient mismatch and 2) substantial valve area reduction, resulting in significant increases in transvalvular gradients. Most hemodynamic studies demonstrating improve- ment are reported at rest, yet many patients exhibit marked elevations of pulmonary artery pressure and transvalvular pressure gradients when exercising. Our own assess- ment of two groups of patients suggests that significant improvement in New York Heart Association (NYHA) Classification is possible with a hydraulically superior valve substitute, even in a moderate follow-up period. It is our obligation to demonstrate that new valve substitutes serve their recipients as well in the second, and even third, decade after implantation as they do in the first.

INTRODUCTION

Remarkable strides have been made during the past 25 years in the quest for a prosthetic valve with less stenosis, optimum flow characteristics, and minimum regurgitation. Unfortunately, there are little data addressing the question of whether differences in hydrodynamic function between current prostheses affect patient outcome.

Even with 25 years of development, there is no ideal valve prosthesis. All are stenotic or exhibit regurgitation to some degree. And, worsening the situation, mitral valve prosthetic implantation alters mitral annular morphology and mobility and further affects ventricular function by the removal of chordae tendineae and papillary muscles.

Despite these imperfections patient symptoms usually improve after surgery. Figure 25-1 illustrates the chest x-ray before and after successful aortic valve replacement. During the 2 years following surgery, the cardiac silhouette has dramatically returned toward normal and functional status is improved.

Thus, the high likelihood of symptomatic and cardiac functional improvement after surgery in the face of acknowledged mechanical imperfection of cardiac valve substitutes appears to be a paradox. It is the purpose of this section to examine this apparent inconsistency for evidence that hydraulically superior valve substitutes do indeed have some (possibly yet unknown) favorable impact on patient outcome.

Unfortunately, some of the available data that addresses this issue can be misleading. The analysis of symptoms in late survivors can be misleading, since those who deteriorate tend to die and are thus removed from late analysis. Conversely, those who are feeling well are likely to continue surviving and be available for late follow-up because sudden cardiac death is not a common problem. Furthermore, there is little sequential analysis of postoperative cardiac function, particularly 10 years or more after valve implantation.

DELINEATION OF THE PROBLEM

Most experienced clinicians will remember patients whose apparently normally functioning valve prostheses are simply not adequate to prevent congestive heart failure. Such a patient is R.H., a 41-year-old woman with a history of rheumatic heart disease. In 1965, she underwent mitral commissurotomy and in 1970, recurrent mitral stenosis led to mitral valve replacement using a caged discoid (Harken) prosthesis. In 1974 the prosthesis had deteriorated and was replaced with a similar Harken valve. At that time, aortic stenosis and insufficiency, as well as mild tricuspid regurgitation, were also noted. Aortic valve replacement using a BJÖRK-SHILEY® spherical disc valve and tri-

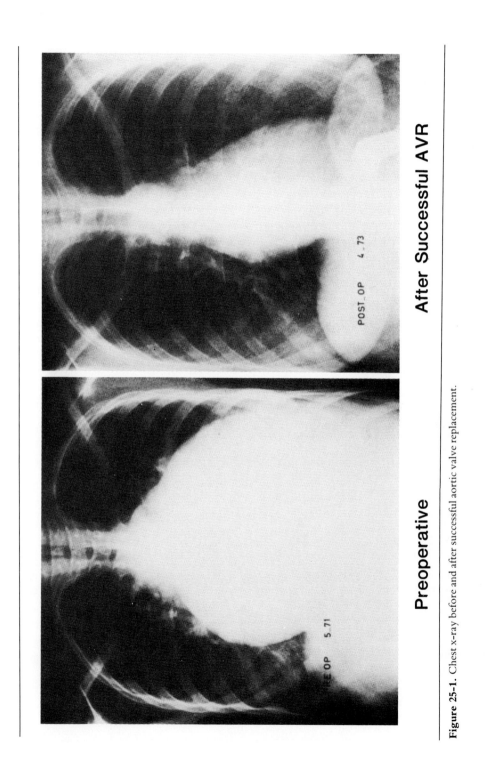

Preoperative

After Successful AVR

Figure 25-1. Chest x-ray before and after successful aortic valve replacement.

cuspid annuloplasty were performed. In 1984, the patient again presented with shortness of breath and fatigue (NYHA Class III). The sequence of hemodynamic findings is shown in table 25-1. Pulmonary arterial pressures, originally 87/40 mm Hg, were reduced in 1974 and were again further slightly reduced to 38/18 mm Hg in 1984. Pulmonary arterial wedge pressure was elevated in 1970 and 1974, but was reduced slightly to 14 mm Hg in 1984. Left ventricular ejection fraction, borderline low in 1970, improved to 66% in 1974 but was reduced to 44% in 1984. Calculated mitral valve area (Gorlin) is now 1.28 cm^2. The aortic valve area in 1974 was 0.53 cm^2, and in 1984 it is 0.62 cm^2. The appearance on fluoroscopy, as well as invasive and noninvasive testing, has revealed that both prostheses are working at expected performance levels, and yet the patient demonstrates evidence of chronic congestive heart failure and hemodynamic deterioration. The important point, illustrated by this case, is that while the prostheses may be working entirely normally, they are not serving this particular patient well from a hemodynamic standpoint.

The hemodynamic limitations of valve replacement are further illustrated in the hypothetical case seen in table 25-2. In this example, aortic valve replacement is performed for correction of severe aortic stenosis associated with a gradient of 90 mm Hg. Valve replacement reduces the gradient to 10 mm Hg (an entirely realistic expectation) and if cardiac output remains unchanged following surgery, the valve area of 0.5 cm^2 will have been increased to only 1.5 cm^2, a value still consistent with mild aortic stenosis.

Table 25-1. Hemodynamics (patient R.H.)

	1970	1974	1984
RA	8	21	14
PA	87/40 mm Hg	52/22 mm Hg	38/18 mm Hg
PAW	25 mm Hg	24 mm Hg	14 mm Hg
LVEF	50%	66%	44%
MVA	0.42 cm^2		1.28 cm^2
AVA		0.53 cm^2	0.62 cm^2
Coronaries	NL	AS/AI	TR

RA = right atrium; PA = pulmonary artery; PAW = pulmonary arterial wedge; LVEF = left ventricular ejection fraction; MVA = mitral valve area; AVA = aortic valve area; NL = normal; AS = aortic stenosis; AI = aortic regurgitation; TR = tricuspid regurgitation

Table 25-2. Hydraulic function of prostheses

	Example of AVR for aortic stenosis	
	Preoperative	Postoperative
Gradient (mm Hg)	90	10
Cardiac output (L/M)	4.75	4.75
Valve area (cm^2)	0.5	1.5

Thus, while successful surgery dramatically reduces the gradient, there is a much less dramatic increase in valve area. The long-term effects of residual, mild to moderate, aortic stenosis, especially if associated with unrepaired other valve lesions or ischemic heart disease, could be potentially deleterious. These observations should be considered in light of the fact that most patients will have cardiac dysfunction prior to surgery, on which will be superimposed the hydrodynamic limitations of currently available valve prostheses. Therefore, it is worthwhile to examine the proposition that small differences in hydraulic valve function are important to long-term outcome.

EVIDENCE LINKING PROSTHETIC PERFORMANCE TO SURGICAL OUTCOME

The remainder of this discussion will touch briefly on four types of evidence, suggesting that there may be a link between hydrodynamic valve function and the outcome after surgery.

High frequency of congestive heart failure-related death

Most late deaths are reported as cardiac non-valve-related and are most often due to congestive heart failure. For example, in a report of long-term outcome after STARR-EDWARDS® valve replacement, death was due to cardiac non-valve causes in 52% [1]. In fact, of 14 recently reported studies that list the cause of death, 10 list "cardiac non-valve" causes as the most prevalent. The incidence of death due to this cause ranges from 10% to 98% in these studies. Obviously, many factors could contribute to this extremely common cause of death, including the presence of unrepaired associated valve disease, late referral for surgery, or inadequate myocardial protection during surgery. However, it is quite unlikely that these factors alone could explain the very large proportion of deaths.

Prosthesis-patient mismatch

Virtually all patients have "prosthesis-patient mismatch." This term, coined by Dr. Shahbudin Rahimtoola several years ago, means that the effective orifice area of implanted prostheses rarely, if ever, approaches that of the normal valve [2]. This is illustrated in figure 25-2, which shows effective orifice area data obtained in patients with various prostheses. In the upper panel, data from representative 25 mm aortic valve prostheses are shown. The bars depict data compiled from several published studies and indicate that no type of prosthesis results in an effective orifice area within the normal range, as indicated by the dotted line. In the lower panel, similar data for representative 29 mm mitral valves is shown, and with the exception of one type of prosthesis, none of them reach well into the expected normal zone. Figure 25-3 further illustrates a shortcoming of valve prostheses when effective orifice area calculations are normalized for body surface area. The average valve area of 1.8 cm^2 is reduced to 1.0 cm^2/m^2, a 44% decrease. Of interest are 2 patients

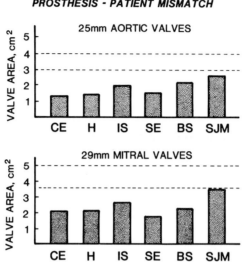

Figure 25-2. Effective orifice area with various prostheses. CE = Carpentier-Edwards; H = Hancock; IS = Ionescu-Shiley; SE = Starr-Edwards; BS = Björk-Shiley; SJM = St. Jude Medical.

with widely differing effective orifice areas, seen at the top of the left side of this figure, who have similar effective orifice area indices, indicating the marked difference in hydrodynamic character resulting from differing flow demands.

Normal cardiac valves have little, if any, transvalvular gradient, even under conditions of markedly enhanced flow. This flow reserve allows a several-fold increase in cardiac output such as with vigorous exercise, without any substantial resistance to flow. Conversely, with development of disease, resting blood flow is initially well maintained with minimum resistance to flow despite considerable reduction in orifice area. However, in the progressively diseased state, modest further decreases in flow orifice size result in large increases in transvalvular gradient. Illustrating this is the data in figure 25-4, which was obtained from an in vitro pulse duplicator experiment in which pulsatile flow of fixed volume was forced through an orifice progressively restricted in size. The flow characteristics and orifice size were designed to simulate the aortic valve position as it is reduced from the normal (> 3 cm^2) to that often seen in critical aortic stenosis (0.5 cm^2). The transvalvular gradient remains close to zero until the orifice area is approximately 2 cm^2, and then striking increases in gradient are associated with further relatively small increments in orifice reduction [2]. The shaded zone reflects the calculated effective orifice area often seen with aortic valve replacement.

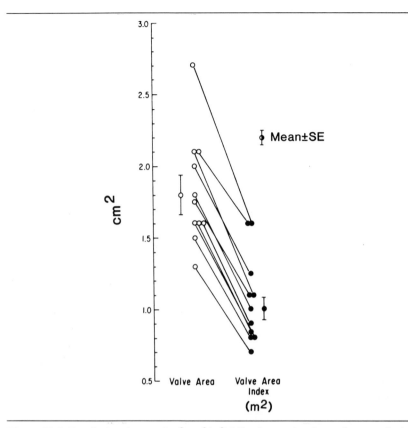

Figure 25-3. Prosthetic valve area (cm²; cm²/m²) following aortic valve replacement for isolated aortic incompetence. [Reproduced by permission of the American Heart Association, Inc. from Rahimtoola SH. The problem of valve prosthesis-patient mismatch. Circulation 1978; 58(1):21.]

Relationship to postoperative cardiac function

The third line of evidence indicating the importance of hydrodynamic function is that linking postoperative hemodynamic data to cardiac performance. Dr. Viking Björk reported rest and exercise mean pulmonary pressures in patients before and after successful mitral valve replacement [3]. He demonstrated the expected decrease in resting pulmonary arterial pressure as a result of surgery as seen in the left panel of figure 25-5. In the right panel of that figure, surgery has also reduced the exercise mean pulmonary arterial pressure. What has not been changed, however, is the relative increase in pulmonary arterial pressure from rest to exercise, both before and after surgery, as indicated by the similar slope of the two dotted lines. In one of the few studies of aortic prostheses during exercise, Dr. Michael Rothkopf [4] demonstrated striking increases in mean prosthetic valve gradient from rest to

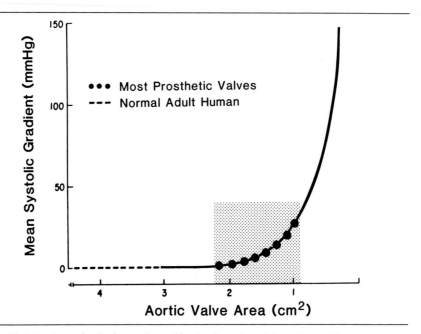

Figure 25-4. In vitro pulse duplicator flow of fixed volume forced through an orifice progressively restricted in size. [Reproduced by permission of the American Heart Association, Inc. from Rahimtoola SH. The problem of valve prosthesis-patient mismatch. Circulation 1978; 58(1):22.]

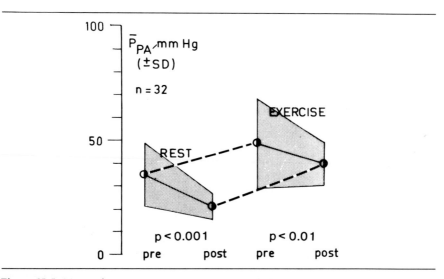

Figure 25-5. Mean pulmonary artery pressure in patients before and after mitral valve replacement. Ppa = pulmonary artery mean pressure. [Reproduced by permission of the Journal of Thoracic and Cardiovascular Surgery from Björk V, Henze A. Ten years experience with the Björk-Shiley tilting disc valve. J Thorac Cardiovasc Surg 1979; 78(3):337.]

Table 25-3. Summary of rest and exercise data in three patients

Case no.	Cardiac output (liters/min)		Mean prosthetic valve gradient		Prosthetic aortic valve area (cm^2)	
	Rest	Ex	Rest	Ex	Rest	Ex
6	3.8	5.5	17	38	1.0	0.9
8	5.4	10.8	26	46	1.2	1.5
12	5.4	7.2	11	15	1.5	1.5

Ex = exercise
(Reproduced with permission from Rothkopf M, et al. Am J Cardiol 1979; 44:211.)

exercise in 2 patients whose prosthetic valve areas were 1.0 cm^2 and 1.2 cm^2, respectively (table 25-3). In a third patient exhibiting a more modest increase, the valve area was 1.5 cm^2, a response that would have been predicted by the pulse duplicator study of Rahimtoola [2].

Dr. Dieter Horstkotte's data [5] begins to link postoperative hemodynamics to cardiac function and exercise duration. Figure 25-6 shows a group of

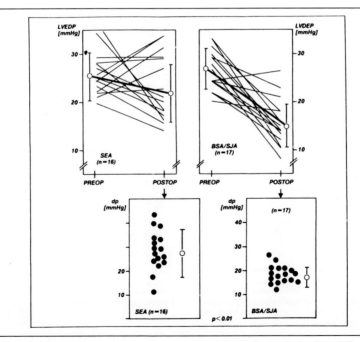

Figure 25-6. Left ventricular end-diastolic pressure (LVEDP) before and after Starr–Edwards (SEA) and St. Jude Medical or Björk–Shiley aortic valve replacement (SJM/BSA) versus the postoperative transaortic gradients in both groups. [Reproduced by permission of Steinkopff Verlag Darmstadt from Horstkotte D, Loogen F (eds). *Update in Heart Valve Replacement.* Springer-Verlag, New York 1986; p 66.]

patients with STARR-EDWARDS aortic valve replacement and another group with BJÖRK-SHILEY or ST. JUDE MEDICAL® aortic valve replacement. The transvalvular gradient is higher with the STARR-EDWARDS valve and is associated with, and possibly responsible for, a lesser degree of left ventricular end-diastolic pressure (LVEDP) reduction, as seen in the upper panels. These data suggest a link between correction of gradient and improvement of LV performance.

The decrease in pulmonary arterial pressure after mitral valve replacement can be related to the level of subjective functional improvement (i.e., NYHA Class). Patients who have less than one NYHA Class improvement are contrasted to patients having one or two NYHA Class improvements in figure 25-7. The patients who have the most dramatic fall in pulmonary arterial pressures are those patients who have the greatest improvement in symptomatology after surgery. A similar trend for the mitral prosthesis gradient is also demonstrated in figure 25-8 (i.e., the lowest transmitral gradient, both at rest and with exercise, is seen in patients with the greatest postoperative improvement in symptoms). Lastly, exercise capacity, measured by a stair-climbing test, is greatest in patients having the greatest postoperative decrease in mean pulmonary artery pressure (figure 25-9).

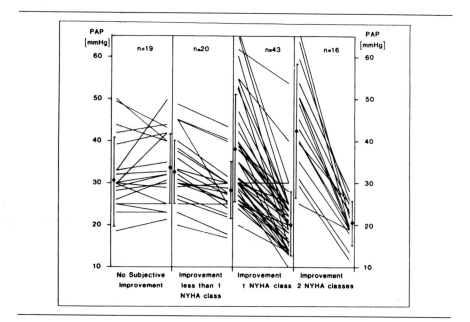

Figure 25-7. Correlation between clinical improvement (NYHA) and mean pulmonary artery pressure (PAP) before and after mitral valve replacement. [Reproduced by permission of Steinkopff Verlag Darmstadt from Horstkotte D, Loogen F (eds). *Update in Heart Valve Replacement.* Springer-Verlag, New York 1986; p 56.]

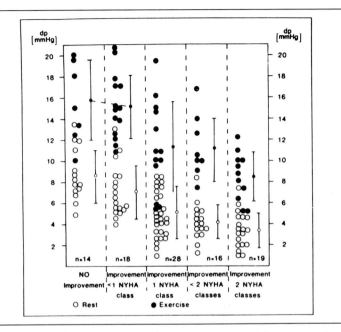

Figure 25-8. Correlation between clinical improvement (NHYA) and the transmitral gradient measured as diastolic pressure (dp) after mitral valve replacement. The open circles represent the measurements at rest; the closed circles, under 30 watts bicycle exercise in the supine position. [Reproduced by permission of Steinkopff Verlag Darmstadt from Horstkotte D, Loogen F (eds). *Update in Heart Valve Replacement.* Springer-Verlag, New York 1986; p 57.]

Relationship to postoperative functional status

The fourth line of data to be presented is that of enhanced postoperative improvement in functional status, which appears related to the use of a hydraulically superior valve prosthesis. In this study, the late clinical outcome in patients receiving porcine valves was compared to those receiving the ST. JUDE MEDICAL bileaflet tilting disc prosthesis [6]. Both in vitro and in vivo data suggest that the ST. JUDE MEDICAL prosthesis functions with geater hydraulic efficiency than either currently available porcine valve. These differences are greater in smaller valve sizes. The postoperative status of 696 valve recipients (363 ST. JUDE MEDICAL, 293 bioprostheses) was determined. The majority of the porcine valves (256 patients) were CARPENTIER-EDWARDS®. Equal numbers of patients received mitral and aortic ST. JUDE MEDICAL valves (155 and 156, respectively), and a somewhat greater proportion of bioprosthetic recipients were aortic (154) than mitral (116). Certain preoperative baseline characteristics were different. Left atrial size and end-diastolic volume were larger, and stroke volume and prosthetic size were smaller, in ST. JUDE MEDICAL recipients. In the mitral position, regurgitation, and in the aortic position, stenosis, were more common preoperative

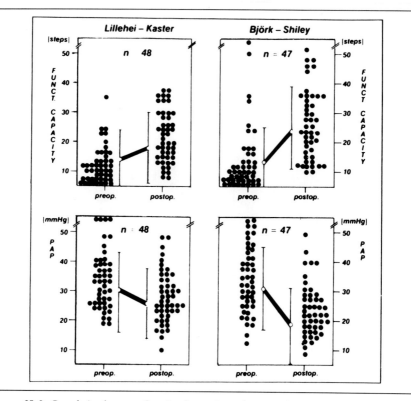

Figure 25-9. Correlation between functional capacity and mean pulmonary artery pressure (PAP) preoperatively and postoperatively. Functional capacity was evaluated by a stair-climbing test. Björk-Shiley and Lillehei-Kaster mitral valve replacement. [Reproduced by permission of Steinkopff Verlag Darmstadt from Horstkotte D, Loogen F (eds). *Update in Heart Valve Replacement*. Springer-Verlag, New York 1986; p 59.]

diagnoses in ST. JUDE MEDICAL recipients, as was the presence and extent of coronary disease. Bypass grafts and intra-aortic balloon use were also more common in ST. JUDE MEDICAL recipients. Preoperatively, more ST. JUDE MEDICAL recipients were of advanced Functional Classification (Class III or IV) than porcine valve recipients (96% versus 89%; $p < .05$). Figure 25-10 shows the actuarial survival status to be virtually identical at 5 years (ST. JUDE MEDICAL 72% versus porcine 71%). In spite of a more advanced preoperative Functional Classification, a greater preponderance of ischemic-related disease and general use of smaller prosthetic valve sizes, ST. JUDE MEDICAL patients tended to fare better postoperatively than did porcine recipients, as more are asymptomatic (Class I, 60% versus 39%) and fewer have advanced symptom status (Class III and IV, 14% versus 24%; $p < .05$).

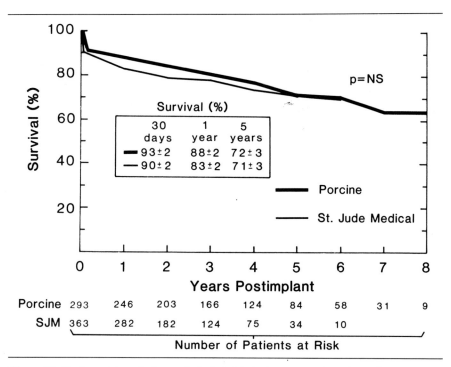

Figure 25-10. Actuarial survival curve in St. Jude Medical versus porcine valve replacement patients.

CONCLUSION

Progress in the surgical treatment of valve disease must keep pace with several other trends. Namely, active longevity is increasing in most segments of the population, cardiovascular deaths are reduced, and the surgical risk of valve implantation is progressively lower than before. For these reasons, we are obligated to demonstrate that newer valve substitutes serve their recipients as well in their second and third decade as they do in their first. This underscores the potential impact of even small differences in valve performance noted during traditionally short follow-up periods.

REFERENCES

1. Rahimtoola SH. Valvular heart disease: A perspective. JACC 1983; 1:199–215.
2. Rahimtoola SH. The problem of valve prosthesis–patient mismatch. Circulation 1978; 58: 20–24.
3. Björk V, Henze A. Ten years experience with the Björk-Shiley tilting disc valve. J Thorac Cardiovasc Surg 1979; 78:331–342.
4. Rothkopf M, Davidson T, Lipscomb K, Narahara K, Hillis LD, Willerson JT, Estrera A, Platt M, Mills L. Hemodynamic evaluation of the Carpentier-Edwards bioprosthesis in the aortic position. Am J Cardiol 1979; 44:209–214.

5. Horstkotte D, Loogen F (eds). *Update in Heart Valve Replacement.* Springer-Verlag, New York 1986.
6. Czer LSC, Matloff JM, Chaux A, DeRobertism, Gray RJ. Comparative clinical experience with porcine bioprosthetic and St. Jude valve replacement. Chest 1987; 91:503–514.

26. SURGICAL TREATMENT OF PROSTHETIC VALVE ENDOCARDITIS

M. SLIWINSKI, M. HOFFMAN, A. BIEDERMAN, W. SITKOWSKI, M. SZUFLADOWICZ

Abstract. Between 1982 and 1986, 31 patients with prosthetic valve endocarditis were operated upon. Indications for operation were progressive heart failure, prosthetic valve dysfunction, and sepsis. The hospital mortality was 35%. The most important factors influencing hospital mortality were cardiogenic shock, timing of operation, and experience of the operating team.

INTRODUCTION

Paravalvular endocarditis after valve replacement is not uncommon and is responsible for high mortality.

PATIENTS AND METHODS

Between 1982 and 1986, 819 patients had valve replacement. Thirty-one patients were operated on because of paravalvular endocarditis. Seventeen had early and 14 had late onset of this complication. The overall incidence was 3.8%. In the literature, the incidence of this complication varies between 1% and 9.5%. The latter figure relates to the era before correct antibiotic prophylaxis. Mortality is very high, especially for paravalvular endocarditis developing early after operation.

Thirty-one patients underwent 36 operations; 23 had aortic valve replacement, 9 had mitral valve replacement, and 5 patients had two operations.

Patients operated for paravalvular endocarditis were quite often in critical condition; more than half of them were in heart failure (NYHA Class IV) or had sepsis. Some had cardiogenic shock. One fourth presented systemic complications such as kidney or liver failure or embolus.

It took time to develop routine management of this complication. Patients with a diagnosis of paravalvular endocarditis are treated with two or three broad spectrum antibiotics, according to blood culture. Early operation, in this case, does not mean a specific period of time, but rather indicates that operation could be done before deterioration of the clinical condition of the patient. In cases with a positive blood culture, a decision concerning the treatment is rather simple. However, the clinical picture of endocarditis usually is not very clear and is changed by the antibiotics. Most often, the only symptom of the beginning of endocarditis is an elevation of temperature, but elevation of temperature after operation is not the same as with diagnosis of endocarditis. Therefore, in some cases, the diagnosis is not easy and gives a delay in treatment.

RESULTS AND DISCUSSION

The operative results depend on several factors, such as condition of the patient, duration of symptoms, type of bacteria, and extent of inflammatory process around the valve. The majority of the patients had severe local changes, so during the operation extensive debridement was performed, abscessed cavities were closed, and pledgets were used. In all cases, the prostheses were placed in the anatomical position.

The results indicate high hospital mortality and late mortality in patients with early paravalvular endocarditis. This is particularly true of the patient reoperated on within 2 months of initial operation. All patients who died after reoperation were in heart failure or shock, and had twice the number of systemic complications as patients who survived the operation.

Mortality rates were significantly reduced in these patients by utilizing a more aggressive approach and, we believe, better surgical technique. Mortality decreased from 50 in 1982 to 17 in 1986. The same is true of the incidence of paravalvular endocarditis, which decreased from 6.1 in 1982 to 2.4 in 1986. However, even with very strict aseptic technique and with prophylactic use of broad spectrum antibiotics, paravalvular endocarditis was not eradicated and still is a potential danger for patients with valve replacement.

27. PERFORMANCE OF FOUR DIFFERENT TYPES OF MECHANICAL AND TWO BIOPROSTHETIC VALVES IN THE TRICUSPID POSITION

F. WELLENS, G. VAN NOOTEN, J. GOLDSTEIN, F. DEUVAERT, J. L. LECLERC, G. PRIMO

Abstract. Experience with tricuspid valve replacement (TVR) was reviewed in 145 patients, operated on from June 1967 until December 1981 (28 single VR, 101 double VR, 21 triple VR). Eighty-five mechanical valves (15 KAY-SHILEY®, 23 BJÖRK-SHILEY®, 31 SMELOFF-CUTTER®, and 16 ST. JUDE MEDICAL®) and 65 bioprostheses (29 HANCOCK®, 36 CARPENTIER-EDWARDS® porcine) were implanted. Overall early mortality was 16.6% and late mortality 7.5% per patient-year. Minimum follow-up was 5.5 years; maximum 16 years. In the mechanical valve group, valve thrombosis occurred in 6 patients at 18-months postimplantation and was fatal in 5 cases. Late pannus formation occurred in 9 patients at 90-months postimplantation and was fatal in 5. Reoperation was performed in 7 patients receiving mechanical valves and was fatal in 2. The bioprosthesis group (implantation between 1975 and 1980) was free from thrombotic complications, except in 1 patient who had a reoperation for mitral valve replacement (MVR) and acute thrombosis of the tricuspid bioprosthesis, treated successfully by thrombectomy. Six other MVR/TVR patients needed MVR for primary valve dysfunction. One patient presented with tricuspid bioprosthetic valve degeneration with subsequent TVR. Following tricuspid valve replacement, actuarial survival is 60% at 9 years for bioprostheses and 75% at 6.5 years for ST. JUDE MEDICAL valves. Functional status is satisfactory. The actuarial probability of freedom of valve thrombosis is 96% for CARPENTIER-EDWARDS and 100% for HANCOCK at 8 and 9 years, respectively, and 92% for ST. JUDE MEDICAL valves at 6.5 years. We conclude that late survival is strongly influenced by the type of prosthesis used. The bioprosthesis performs best in the tricuspid position, and primary valve failure is of much lesser concern than in the mitral position. Of the mechanical substitutes used, only the ST. JUDE MEDICAL prosthesis has an adequate performance and a lower thrombosis occlusion rate at up to 6.5 years.

INTRODUCTION

This retrospective study is an update of a series of 145 patients with tricuspid valve replacement (TVR), operated upon from June 1967 until December 1981. Eighty-five mechanical valves (15 KAY-SHILEY, 23 BJÖRK-SHILEY, 31 SMELOFF-CUTTER, 16 ST. JUDE MEDICAL) and 65 bioprostheses (29 HANCOCK, 36 CARPENTIER-EDWARDS porcine) were implanted. Patient data and early results have been previously published [1, 2].

RESULTS

Late follow-up has been recently updated. The 125 early survivors were followed for a minimum of 5.5 years and a maximum of 16 years (mean 6.7 years) for a total of 831 patient-years. Only 2 patients were lost to follow-up (1 HANCOCK and 1 CARPENTIER-EDWARDS).

Overall late mortality was 7.5% per patient-year and was strongly influenced by the prosthesis implanted (table 27-1). Progressive myocardial failure was the main cause of death in this series.

The most common valve-related problem was acute valve thrombosis and progressive pannus formation (table 27-2). Reoperation was carried out in 7 patients receiving mechanical prostheses, with 2 fatalities. The bioprosthesis group was relatively free from thrombotic complications, except in 1 patient who had a reoperation for primary mitral valve degeneration and acute thrombosis of the tricuspid valve.

Table 27-1. Incidence of late death in 62 patients after tricuspid valve replacement as a function of the prosthesis implanted

Prosthesis	%/pt-yr
KS	12.9
BS	4.4
SC	13.5
SJM	5.5
H	6.6
CE	5.1
Overall	7.5

KS = Kay-Shiley; BS = Björk-Shiley; SC = Smeloff-Cutter; SJM = St. Jude Medical; H = Hancock; CE = Carpentier-Edwards

Table 27-2. Incidence of valve thrombosis and pannus formation after tricuspid valve replacement as a function of the prosthesis implanted

Prosthesis	No. at risk	No. of thromboses	Incidence (%/pt-yr)	Death	Reoperation
KS	13	2	3.5%	1	1
BS	19	5	3.2%	3	3
SC	23	8	6.1%	6	3
SJM	14	1	1.4%	1	–
H	23	–	–	–	–
CE	33	1	0.5%	–	1

KS = Kay-Shiley; BS = Björk-Shiley; SC = Smeloff-Cutter; SJM = St. Jude Medical; H = Hancock; CE = Carpentier-Edwards

Successful treatment consisted of mitral valve replacement with a ST. JUDE MEDICAL prosthesis and tricuspid valve thrombectomy.

The problem of bioprosthetic valve degeneration is of lesser concern in the tricuspid than in the mitral position. In the bioprosthetic valve group, a cohort of 45 patients could be identified with simultaneous bioprosthetic valve implantation in the mitral and tricuspid positions.

Primary valve failure occurred in 8 instances in the mitral position (3.07% per patient-year) and once in the tricuspid position (0.38% per patient-year). Mitral valve re-replacement was carried out in 7 patients, with 1 perioperative death. Tricuspid valve re-replacement was successful in the only patient with right-sided valve degeneration.

Functional status of the actual survivors (table 27-3) is far from excellent, with only 11 of the 53 survivors in New York Heart Association (NYHA)

Table 27-3. New York Heart Association (NYHA) Classification of 53 actual survivors after tricuspid valve replacement as a function of the prosthesis implanted

| Prosthesis | NYHA Class | | | |
	I	II	III	IV
KS	–	1	–	–
BS	2	2	3	1
SC	1	2	–	–
SJM	1	7	2	–
H	3	5	2	–
CE	4	13	3	1
Total	11	30	10	2

KS = Kay-Shiley; BS = Björk-Shiley; SC = Smeloff-Cutter; SJM = St. Jude Medical; H = Hancock; CE = Carpentier-Edwards

Class I. Myocardial dysfunction and possible malfunction of the prosthetic valves in the tricuspid position could be responsible for these results.

Ten-year actuarial survival is 60% for BJÖRK-SHILEY, 22% for SMEL-OFF-CUTTER, and 12% for KAY-SHILEY valves. For bioprosthetic tricuspid valve replacement, actuarial survival is 60% at 9 years, with good functional status. Actuarial probability of freedom from valve thrombosis is 96% for CARPENTIER-EDWARDS and 100% for HANCOCK valves at 8 and 9 years, respectively.

Actuarial survival is 75% at 6.5 years for ST. JUDE MEDICAL tricuspid valve replacement, with an actuarial probability of freedom from valve thrombosis of 92%.

DISCUSSION

The following conclusions can be drawn from this retrospective study:

1. Tricuspid valve replacement has a high perioperative risk and low long-term survival rates in patients with rheumatic heart disease.
2. Late survival and functional status are influenced by the prosthesis implanted.
3. Acute thrombosis is most frequent in the BJÖRK-SHILEY disc valve and late pannus is frequent in the SMELOFF-CUTTER ball valve.
4. Thrombosis is very low in bioprosthetic tricuspid valve replacement.
5. Bioprosthetic primary valve failure is very low in the tricuspid position, even in children.
6. The ST. JUDE MEDICAL valve performs relatively well up to 6.5 years.
7. In view of the current results, a bioprosthesis remains the valve of choice in the tricuspid position.

REFERENCES

1. Wellens F, Van Dale P, Deuvaert F, LeClerc JL, Primo G. The role of porcine heterografts in a 14-year experience with tricuspid valve replacement. In Cohn LH, Gallucci V (eds): *Cardiac Bioprostheses*. Yorke Medical Books, New York 1982; pp 502–515.
2. Wellens F, LeClerc JL, Deuvaert F, Van Nooten G, Goldstein J, Primo G. Tricuspid valve replacement. A comparative experience with different valve substitutes. In Matloff JM (ed): *Cardiac Valve Replacement*. Martinus Nijhoff Publishing, Boston 1985; pp 91–97.

28. COMPARISON OF REOPERATION AND COMPLICATIONS IN DOUBLE VALVE (MITRAL AND AORTIC) IMPLANTS WITH MECHANICAL OR BIOLOGICAL PROSTHESES

G. DE RÁBAGO, J. FRAILE, J. MARTINELL, V. ARTIZ

Abstract. A total of 1160 patients received a double valve implant, in the mitral and aortic positions, between January 1970 and December 1986. Either mechanical (984 patients) or biological (176 patients) valves were implanted. Operative mortality was 8%. Patients were followed-up for a total of 4641 patient-years (mean 5.12) in the mechanical valve group and a total of 1106 patient-years (mean 6.86) in the biological valve group. There was a significantly higher incidence of reoperation (p < 0.001) in the biological valve compared to the mechanical group because of a high number of primary tissue failures. An analysis of the actuarial data shows no significant difference in long-term survival. In conclusion, we think that the indications for double (mitral and aortic) biological valve implantation should be analyzed carefully. Given the freedom from reoperation after 12 years of only 28%, only very specific cases should be considered for biological valve implantation.

INTRODUCTION

During the last 20 years, we have implanted almost 6000 valves in 4500 patients. The results of double implants in the mitral and aortic positions in 1160 patients will be discussed.

METHODS

Between 1970 and 1986, we implanted double mechanical valves in 984 patients and double biological valves in 176 patients. Operative mortality was

8%. Patients were followed-up for a total of 4641 patient-years (mean 5.12) in the mechanical valve group and a total of 1106 patient-years (mean 6.86) in the biological valve group.

RESULTS AND DISCUSSION

The linearized complication rates are shown in table 28-1. There was no significant difference in late mortality or in the incidence of thromboembolic complicatons between the mechanical and biological valve groups. Of course, there was a significant difference in the incidence of hemorrhagic complications, because we do not use any type of anticoagulant after 6 months postoperation in the biological valve group. There was no significant difference in the incidence of late infective endocarditis.

The principal significant difference between the mechanical and biological valve groups was in the linearized incidence of reoperation, with only 1.5% per patient-year for the mechanical group, but 5.7% per patient-year for the biological valve group.

Comparing the etiology of reoperation in the mechanical and biological valve groups (table 28-2), most of the reoperations in the biological valve group were due to primary tissue failure. There were few cases of primary mechanical failure, so there was a very high significant difference between both groups for this parameter. There was no, or a very small, significant difference between mechanical and biological valves in the incidence of dehiscence or paravalvular noninfective leak. There was no significant difference in the indication for reoperation due to the incidence of infective endocarditis. Thrombosis was one of the main reasons to reoperate in the mechanical group. Nonthrombotic obstruction showed no difference between both groups due to the growth of tissue pannus. There was a very significant incidence of total indications for reoperation in both groups.

In all cases of valve failure in the biological group, both valves were not

Table 28-1. Incidence of complications following double implantation with mechanical or biological valves

| Complication | Mechanical | | Biological | | p value |
	No.	Percent per patient-year	No.	Percent per patient-year	
Late mortality	91	1.9 ± 0.2	22	1.9 ± 0.4	NS
Thromboembolism	86	1.8 ± 0.1	14	1.2 ± 0.3	NS
Infective endocarditis	26	0.5 ± 0.1	10	0.9 ± 0.2	NS
Hemorrhage	102	2.1 ± 0.2	11	0.9 ± 0.2	< .001
Reoperation	74	1.5 ± 0.1	64	5.7 ± 0.7	< .001

NS = Not significant

Table 28-2. Cause of reoperation following double valve implantation

Reoperative cause	Mechanical		Biological	
	No.	Operative mortality	No.	Operative mortality
Nonrelated prosthesis	4	1	–	–
Primary tissue failure	–	–	54	6
Primary mechanical failure	2	2	–	–
Noninfected dehiscence	29	4	3	1
Infective endocarditis	19	7	5	2
Valve thromobis	18	3	–	–
Nonthrombotic obstruction	2	1	2	1

always affected. However, the indication to remove both valves, even if one of them was working well, was systematically followed: we removed both valves at reoperation.

Another of the main reasons for reoperation was to improve hospital mortality. If we operated on an emergency basis, the mortality was higher in both groups, either mechanical or biological, than when we operated on a programmed basis. It should be noted that in the biological group, the incidence of emergency surgery was less than in the mechanical group.

Another factor that influenced hospital mortality is the learning curve. When we divide the curve into three periods, the first period had high mortality at reoperation, it decreased in the second period, and significantly decreased in the third period. This was not only because of the learning curve of the technical surgical team, but due to the learning curve for the diagnosis of valve malfunction, showing that we learned the early indications for reoperation.

An analysis of the actuarial data shows that the survival rate for both groups of patients was quite similar; approximately 70% at 13 years. There was no significant difference between the groups with respect to long-term survival.

However, the difference in the actuarial freedom from reoperation was very high. In the mechanical valve group at 13 years, approximately 15% of the patients required reoperation. In contrast, in the group with double biological valves, 70% of the patients have been reoperated upon, mainly because of primary tissue failure.

In conclusion, when we studied our large number of patients, there was a significant difference in the incidence of reoperation between mechanical and biological valves (table 28-1). Primary tissue failure was the main cause for reoperation in biological valves. The main reasons for reoperation on mechanical valves were valve thrombosis, noninfected dehiscence, and infective endocarditis (table 28-2). Operative mortality at reoperation was related to emergency surgery and to the decrease in the learning curves for the surgical team and for diagnosis of valve malfunction. Given the low freedom from reoperation with biological valves, we believe only very specific cases should be considered for double valve implantation with these prostheses.

29. QUALITY OF LIFE IN PATIENTS WITH MECHANICAL HEART VALVES: INFLUENCE OF ANTICOAGULATION THERAPY AND VALVE NOISE

L. I. THULIN, C. L. OLIN

Abstract. There are two significant drawbacks with mechanical heart valves: the need for long-term anticoagulation and valve noise. To study these aspects with respect to patients' quality of life, a follow-up was made of all patients receiving mechanical valves in our institution between 1981 and 1983. All patients were traced. Early and late mortality was 11.2%. A questionnaire was sent to the surviving patients and 281 (99%) responded. Two hundred forty-three had BJÖRK-SHILEY® 70° Convexo-Concave valves and 38 had ST. JUDE MEDICAL® valves. Mean age at follow-up was 63 years. Mean follow-up time was 2.5 years. Nine percent of patients experienced bleeding complications; 3% were major, 6% minor. This corresponds to 3.2% per patient-year. Thromboembolic complications, including TE and TIA, were experienced by 3.2% of the patients. Only 1 patient had sequelae. There were no instances of valve thrombosis. Ninety-seven percent of the patients did not feel restricted by the anticoagulation therapy; 6% felt as if they were on a special diet. The therapy was well regulated in 90% of the patients. Sixty percent of the patients used alcohol without restrictions and 25% traveled abroad without problems. Twenty-five percent of the patients were sometimes disturbed by valve noise and 8.5% were more regularly disturbed. There were no statistically significant differences between the BJÖRK-SHILEY and the ST. JUDE MEDICAL valves or due to age, valve location, or valve size. In order to study and compare noise of various heart valves during standardized conditions, an in vitro study was carried out. The results suggest that the anticoagulation therapy in the majority of patients was well regulated and associated with a *low incidence of complications. In spite of advanced age, most patients lived active lives and were not restricted. Some patients were occasionally disturbed by the valve noise, and this problem deserves further attention.*

INTRODUCTION

Quality of life means different things for the patient and the doctor, since side effects are experienced by the patient, while the surgeon often only looks to the benefits of his intervention. Quality of life after heart valve replacement with a mechanical prosthesis does not only include freedom from valve- or anticoagulation-related complications, but also includes a number of factors related to the patient's ability to live a "normal" life without restrictions and special considerations. Thus, the aim of surgical treatment of valvular diseases is to improve total patient function and to reduce the degree of illness, adding quality to the remaining year.

METHODS

There are two major drawbacks with mechanical heart valves: the need for long-term anticoagulation and valve noise. To study these aspects with respect to patient's quality of life, we performed a follow-up study on consecutive patients receiving mechanical valves in our institution between 1981 and 1983. All patients were traced. Early and late mortality was 11.2%. Questionnaires were answered by 281 or 99% of the 283 surviving patients (243 with BJÖRK-SHILEY 70° CC valves and 38 with ST. JUDE MEDICAL valves). The mean age at the time of follow-up was 63 years and mean follow-up time was 2.5 years.

RESULTS AND DISCUSSION

Bleedings and thromboembolism

Nine percent of the patients (all were in the BJÖRK-SHILEY group) had experienced bleeding complications, corresponding to an incidence of 3.2% per patient-year. Three percent were major bleedings necessitating hospital care, transfusions, etc, and 6% were minor bleedings treated in outpatient care. In only 2 patients with cerebral hemorrhage was the anticoagulation therapy thought to be responsible for the fatal outcome. There were no deaths due to thromboembolism. Only 3.2% (9 patients in the BJÖRK-SHILEY group and 1 in the ST. JUDE MEDICAL group) had experienced thromboembolic complications including thromboembolism, transient ischemic attacks, and amaurosis fugax. This corresponded to an incidence of 1% per patient-year. Only 1 patient had permanent sequelae and there was no valve thrombosis.

There was no early thromboembolism (within 30 days postoperatively). We attribute this to our aggressive initiation of anticoagulation. Warfarin is normally given intravenously from the day after operation, then continued by oral medication as shown in table 29-1. We have not found any disadvantages

Table 29-1. Initiation of anticoagulation therapy

Day 1	Operation		
Day 2		Warfarin IV (dose dependent on actual TT-value, usually 10–15 mg given)	
Day 3	Chest tubes removed	Warfarin orally	Heparin IV (if TT-values not within therapeutic range)
Day 4	Ambulation	Warfarin orally	Heparin IV (if TT-values not within therapeutic range)

giving warfarin intravenously. On the contrary, the effect comes earlier and is more reliable than with early oral administration.

Additional heparin is given according to a special protocol from day 3 if thrombotest values are not within the therapeutic range of 5%–15%, which corresponds to an International Normalized Ratio (INR) of 2.1–4.8. The heparin protocol is based on bedside determination of the clotting time, as shown in table 29-2.

Regarding long-term anticoagulation therapy, patients should not be discharged from the hospital before they are fully instructed concerning anticoagulation therapy and until their cardiologist or home physician has taken over the responsibility for the treatment. Increased doses of anticoagulation medication are usually required when the patient returns home, due to improvement of liver and kidney function, mobilization, and normalization of food intake. Therefore, during this period, frequent checkups of the prothrombin time are needed.

We found some patients to be unstable and out of the therapeutic ranges of anticoagulation. In a number of cases, this was due to known reasons such as dental treatment, minor operations, etc. However, in 40% of these patients, there were no explanations as to why they were not well regulated. In patients who had encountered spontaneous bleedings, anticoagulation was found to be inadequate (thrombotest below 5%) in 55% of cases at the time of the event.

Table 29-2. Heparin protocol (based on bedside determinations of clotting time by nurses)

Clotting time	Heparin dosage (Q 6 H)
< 10 min.	5000 IU IV
10–20 min.	2500 IU IV
> 20 min.	No heparin given

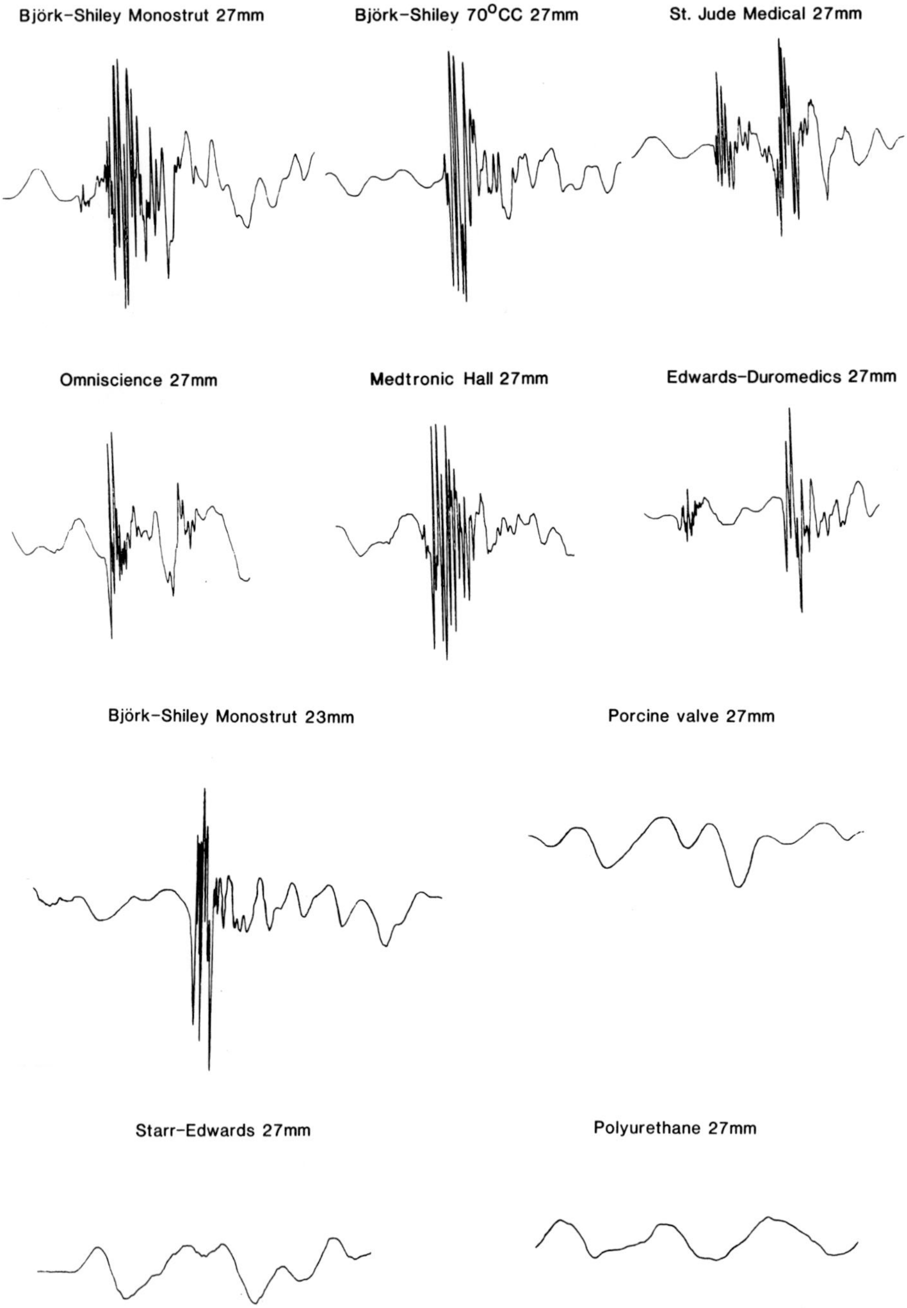

Figure 29-1. Closing noise patterns of various mechanical heart valves in a pulse duplicator. Note the double closing sound of bileaflet valves.

Corresponding figures for thromboembolic complications were 35% (thrombotest values above 15%).

Concerning patient acceptance and compliance to the compulsory anticoagulation therapy, 97% claimed that they did not feel restricted by it. Only 6% said that they felt as if they were on a special diet due to restrictions in their food intake. As judged from the laboratory tests during a 3-month period prior to this investigation, 90% of the patients were found to be well regulated (i.e., within therapeutic range). Sixty percent of the patients used alcohol without restrictions; 2% admitted restrictions. Twenty-five percent had traveled abroad for up to 3 months without problems.

In 25 patients on chronic anticoagulation therapy, 32 major and minor cardiac and noncardiac surgical procedures had been performed without any mortality or complications related to the valves or the anticoagulant treatment.

Valve noise

Twenty-five percent of the patients were sometimes, and 8.5% were more regularly, disturbed by the valve noise. Atrial flutter was more common among those who complained of noise. It was noted that in some positions valve noise was more frequently and strongly heard. The magnitude of sounds seemed increased especially when the patient was lying on the left side. Patient age, valve position, valve size, and valve type did not seem to significantly influence the perception of the noise. Some patients did not hear valve noise at all, while others felt safe hearing the valve clicking, indicating that it was functioning as expected. There was no significant difference between the BJÖRK-SHILEY and ST. JUDE MEDICAL valves.

The influence of mechanical heart valve noise on quality of life seems to be overlooked by both surgeons and physicians, and is manifested by the lack of patient-related literature on this matter. To study and compare the noise of different heart valves during standardized conditions (valve size, stroke volume, frequency, and pressure), we performed an in vitro study using a pulse duplicator. Recordings were made with a microphone 10 cm from the valve. Each type was found to have its own closing noise pattern, depending on the construction of the valve. These are illustrated in figure 29-1. Size of the valve also seemed to influence the amount of noise generated.* There are, however, great difficulties in transferring these results into clinical use, since the generation and perception of valve noise in the individual patient is very dependent on patient-related factors such as heart rate, blood pressure, configuration of the thorax, and hearing. Nevertheless, we consider it important to be aware of valve noise as a factor affecting quality of life. Improved patient information about mechanical valve noise, both preoperatively and postoperatively, is essential for better patient acceptance.

---

* A large-size valve produced more noise than a small-size valve.

30. VALVED CONDUITS AND CONDUIT EXCHANGE: LONG-TERM FOLLOW-UP

E. R. DE VIVIE, H. KORB. W. RUSCHEWSKI

Abstract. Due to unsatisfactory long-term results with porcine valved conduits, the selection of material for extracardiac conduit surgery remains an unsolved problem. Between 1972 and 1987, 103 patients ranging from less than 1 year to 21 years of age underwent surgical repair of various types of complex congenital heart defects using an extracardiac valved conduit. The follow-up period ranged from 2 months to 10 years and included data of multiple catheterization and cross-sectional echocardiography. The probability of event-free conduit performance after 5 years was 80% and after 8 years was only 12%. Twenty-three conduits had to be replaced due to severe stenosis of the porcine valve. For the pericardial valved conduits, late results only up to 5 years are available. Four dysfunctions occurred (i.e., valvular stenosis and/or insufficiency) at 27 months (2 dysfunctions), 36, and 54 months after implantation. One death occurred during conduit exchange surgery. Since 1983 we have preferred to use antibiotic-preserved fresh aortic root homografts as conduit material in anticipation of better long-term results. However, the availability of homografts is limited, especially in the small sizes. In conclusion, the durability of porcine and bovine pericardial valved conduits in infants and children is limited. The early results with pericardial valved conduits in these patients is also limited. However, the early results with pericardial valved conduits are better than with comparable porcine valved conduits. The exchange of a malfunctioning conduit is a low-risk procedure. Therefore, the use of a valved conduit can be recommended for infants and small children whenever an aortic homograft is not suitable or available. Superior long-term results (i.e., more than 10 to 15 years) with aortic root homografts remain to be proven. The ideal conduit has not yet been found.

INTRODUCTION

An external valved conduit was first used at our institution in 1972. A 5-year-old girl with ventricular septal defect (VSD) and pulmonary atresia received a surgeon-made woven DACRON® conduit with a size 14 LILLEHEI-KASTER® valve. Despite good early results with 2 other cases, since 1974 we have been using porcine valved conduits to avoid anticoagulation in children. Since 1980 we have preferred the IONESCU-SHILEY® bovine pericardial valved conduit, because of unsatisfactory late results due to degenerative calcification in the HANCOCK® porcine valve. Since 1984, we have used 5 CARPENTIER-EDWARDS® porcine valved conduits in infants and small children. After 1983 we implanted fresh aortic root homografts in children. Although we intended to use homografts more often, this was not possible because of supply problems.

PATIENTS AND METHODS

The cardiac lesions that required cardiac surgery most often were Tetralogy of Fallot or VSD with pulmonary atresia, transposition of the great arteries, truncus, and tricuspid atresia (table 30-1, figure 30-1). Most of the patients already had one to four previous palliative operations, as listed in table 30-2. From 1972 to 1979, porcine valve HANCOCK conduits (n = 45), DACRON prostheses with tilting disc prosthetic valves (n = 3), and DACRON prostheses without valves were used (n = 17). We have implanted 22 pericardial valve IONESCU-SHILEY conduits since 1980, 5 porcine valve CARPENTIER-

Table 30-1. Distribution of conduit operations

Diagnosis	No. of patients	Hospital mortality	
		No. cases	(%)
Fallot, PA	24	4	
TGA, VSD, PS	15	3	
Truncus arteriosis communis	8	2	
DORV, PS/PA	6	1	
DOLV, PS	1	–	
TA/SV, PS	26	4	
Total	80	14	17.5
Conduit exchange	23	1	4.3

PA = pulmonary atresia; TGA = transposition of the great arteries; VSD = ventricular septal defect; PS = pulmonary stenosis; DORV = double outlet right ventricle; DOLV = double outlet left ventricle; TA = tricuspid atresia; SV = single ventricle

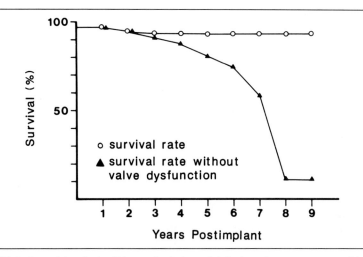

Figure 30-1. Actuarial analysis of bioprosthesis + conduit in the pulmonary artery position in 64 patients.

Table 30-2. Palliative procedures before conduit operation in 51 of 80 patients

Operation	No. of procedures
Blalock–Taussig shunt	46
Glenn shunt	7
Waterston–Cooley shunt	15
Blalock–Hanlon procedure	2
Pulmonary artery banding	4
Aorticopulmonary window	1
Systemico-pulmonary shunt (Teflon, Dacron)	7
Total	82

EDWARDS conduits since 1984, and 11 aortic root homografts since 1983 (table 30-3). Among the patients who survived the insertion of a HANCOCK porcine valved conduit more than 9 years, 16 (38%) have already had conduit exchange. Another 10 patients are experiencing severe conduit dysfunction, 4 of whom will require a second operation in the near future.

The mean age of the 11 patients at the first operation was 7.6 ± 3.1 years (range 2 to 14 years) and at the second operation it was 13.4 ± 4.0 years (range 6 to 21 years). The mean interval between implantation and exchange of the 16 explanted HANCOCK conduits was 66.2 ± 17 months (table 30-4). It was striking that the two exchanged mechanical valved conduits were explanted only after 104 and 128 months because of outgrown prosthetic valves, without failure of the DACRON graft or the valves. A third patient with a mechanical

Table 30-3. Extracardial conduit operation

Type of prosthesis	No. of patients	Reoperation
Hancock	45	16
Ionescu-Shiley	22	1
Carpentier-Edwards	5	–
Dacron without valve	17	3
Dacron with valve	3	3
Homograft	11	–
Total	103	23

Table 30-4. Age and time interval in 23 children with conduit exchange

Age at first operation		Mean 7.6 years (range 2–14 years)
Age at second operation		Mean 15.4 years (range 6–22 years)

Type of original conduit	Number of exchanges	Mean interval between implantation and exchange (months)
Valveless	3	29.7 ± 9
Hancock	16	66.2 ± 17
Mechanical valve	3	112.0 ± 8
Ionescu-Shiley	1	63

valved conduit is now in the twelfth postoperative year and is in good physical condition without failure of the conduit or the size 21 BJÖRK-SHILEY® valve.

The most frequent cause for conduit exchange was valve degeneration (table 30-5). Two of the 8 outgrown conduits were 18-mm DACRON grafts with size 14 LILLEHEI-KASTER valves. One was a pericardial conduit with a size 16 HANCOCK valve implanted in a 2-year-old girl 5 years ago.

Valved conduit exchange was indicated whenever: 1) systemic pressure was found in the right ventricle in combination with congestive heart failure, a decrease in vitality, and an increase in rhythm disturbances; 2) when the right ventricle pressure was higher than the left ventricle pressure; or 3) shunt inversion could be observed at a residual VSD.

The complications of conduit exchange procedures included surgical injuries of the aorta from cross-clamping (n = 2) and intraoperative (n = 1) or postoperative (n = 1) bleeding due to severe scarring. Renal failure (n = 1) and cerebral disturbances (n = 1) have been sequelae of postoperative low-output syndrome. Most of these complications can be avoided by arterial cannulation of the iliac or femoral artery before thoracotomy, limited preparation of the retro-sternal space, and optimal myocardial protection. Only 1 patient with conduit exchange died. This 15-year-old boy had the reoperation as a fifth

Table 30-5. Indications for conduit exchange

	No. of patients
Outgrown prosthesis	8
Proximal stenosis	–
Peripheral stenosis	3
Valve degeneration	10
Compression	1
RVOT aneurysm	1
Total	23

Combination of indication with other condition	No. of patients
With rest VSD	5
Persistent Blalock shunt	2
Persistent PDA	1
Unroofed CS	1
Total	9

RVOT = right ventricular outflow tract; VSD = ventricular septal defect; PDA = persistent ductus arteriosus; CS = coronary sinus

procedure. He died as a result of surgical problems needing the use of extra-corporeal circulation for 334 minutes.

The preparation of the conduit itself is a low-risk procedure because the separation of the scar tissue and the woven DACRON is easy. A second exchange of a malfunctioning conduit after another 7 years, however, will bear a much higher risk. We have not yet performed such a procedure but have much experience with similar procedures in conventional valve surgery. Therefore, the use of a conduit with a two-component detachable, screw-in porcine bioprosthesis does not seem very promising to us, since the problem of a second or third procedure is not the exposure of the conduit itself, but rather the scarring of the natural surrounding structures. The results of using thin TEFLON® membranes to prevent tissue adhesion by reconstruction of the pericardial sac remain to be seen.

Between 1980 and 1984, we implanted 22 IONESCU-SHILEY valved conduits. Ten of them (44%) were exchanges of other malfunctioning conduits, including 9 HANCOCK conduits and 1 outgrown mechanical valved conduit. The mean age of patients with IONESCU-SHILEY conduits was about 12 years old. Since the first implantation occurred in January 1980, the longest observation period was not much more than 6 years, which does not reach the critical period of approximately 7 to 8 years. Fifteen (65%) of the patients with IONESCU-SHILEY valved conduits underwent hemodynamic studies, including right and left ventricular catheterization, within 2 years postoperatively.

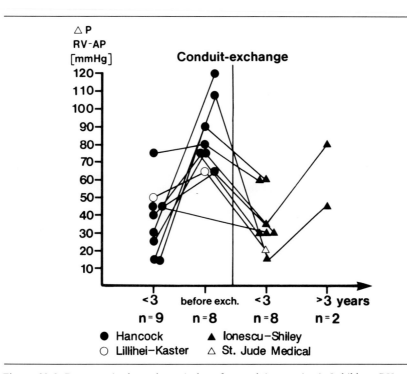

Figure 30-2. Postoperative hemodynamic data after conduit operation in 9 children. RV = right ventricle; AP = pulmonary artery.

Twelve (80%) of them had no gradient or a small gradient of 5 to 20 mm Hg and only 1 had a gradient of 50 mm Hg. These early hemodynamic results were much better than those of 18 HANCOCK conduits of similar size. Some of the latter showed early gradients in excess of 50 mm Hg (figure 30-2).

Six patients with IONESCU-SHILEY conduits received second catheterizations at 27 to 42 months after operation. Two patients showed no gradient after 29 and 38 months. Two other patients who had no gradient at their first catheterization 12 and 15 months postoperatively, had significant gradients of 45 mm Hg and 65 mm Hg after 41 and 42 months, respectively. The 2 patients with high gradients are now in poor clinical condition with congestive heart failure and rhythm disturbances. Both had HANCOCK conduits implanted (at the ages of 4 and 5) prior to implantation of the IONESCU-SHILEY conduits (at the ages of 11 and 12). The patients are now 15- and 17-years-old, respectively, and need a third surgical procedure. Three other patients in the IONESCU-SHILEY group displayed clinical signs of valvular stenosis and insufficiency at 33, 34, and 54 months after implantation. They had not received a second postoperative catheterization.

RESULTS AND DISCUSSION

In summary, our data showed that, like the porcine valved conduit, the bovine pericardial valved conduits also have very limited durability in children [1–4]. Although the early hemodynamic results with the bovine pericardial valves were better, the late results were equally unsatisfactory [5–7]. Therefore, we no longer recommend the use of bioprosthetic valved conduits in children [6, 7]. We prefer the use of fresh antibiotic sterilized aortic root homografts. Unfortunately, in Germany, and especially in small cities like Goettingen, it is very difficult to maintain an adequate supply of homografts (particularly in small sizes). Therefore, we cannot use a homograft as often as we would like. Thus, we still use bioprosthetic valved conduits, whenever homografts are unavailable, in infants and in small children.

In searching for the ideal valved conduit, the advantages and disadvantages of the different conduits have been summarized in figure 30-3. Biological valved conduits are available in all sizes and do not need anticoagulation. They are especially suitable for infants and small children [5, 8, 9], but a second or third procedure is necessary every 4 to 8 years [6, 7]. The mechanical valved conduits, retrospectively, have had better long-term results than expected [8–10]. There were no valve-related complications or thromboembolic events, even without anticoagulation. However, the number of patients was very limited. This system might be recommended for older children and adults, especially for exchange procedures [9]. A readily fabricated composite conduit with a mechanical ST. JUDE MEDICAL® valve is available in all sizes except 19 mm. At present, the aortic homograft seems to be the best conduit available [6, 7, 11–15]. It has demonstrated good long-term results (up to 15 years) but,

Criteria \ Conduit	Conduit + Bioprosthesis	Conduit + Mech. Prosth.	Homograft
Valve degeneration	+++	(+)	+
Anticoagulation	O	O	O
Age < 2a	+	O	O
Age > 2a	O	+	+
Availability	+	(+	(+)

Which conduit is the best?

+ = good/marked
0 = no
shading = remarkable

Figure 30-3. A comparison of advantages of various conduits.

even in fresh homografts, degeneration and calcification have to be expected after that period [12, 15].

The other component of the valved conduit, the prosthetic or biological graft, is also of great importance with respect to hemodynamic performance and late results. Low-porosity woven DACRON reduces intraoperative bleeding problems but produces a high incidence of late complications including thickening, calcification, and peeling of the neointima [1, 2]. Another disadvantage is the stiffness of the graft, especially for the construction of smooth, nonundulated proximal and peripheral anastomoses [6, 7]. Malfunction of mechanical valves in woven DACRON grafts has been caused by peeling and obstruction by the neointima [1, 2]. These disadvantages can be avoided by the use of high porosity knitted double velour DACRON grafts presealed with human fibrin glue. We have already had good experience with these grafts in the replacement of descending aortas, even with complete heparinization and use of extracorporeal circulation.

A valved PTFE conduit with a ST. JUDE MEDICAL mechanical valve would be the best composition, but it may be difficult to fix the valve in the graft. A ST. JUDE MEDICAL® pulmonic valved graft prosthesis is available in all sizes. A disadvantage in creating nonangulated anastomoses with this prosthesis may be the stiffness of the nontrimmed, thick wall.

Autologous pericardium has the same advantages as the aortic homografts [16]. Calcification may occur, but probably to a lesser extent and later than in homografts. The phrenic to phrenic pericardium might not always be large enough to create a complete tube, or it may be of inferior quality following pericarditis. However, the main problems with the pericardial conduits are their durability (especially with high pressures in the right ventricle) and the suture line holding the valve. Experience with this type of valved conduit is very limited [16]. Our only 2-year-old patient who received a pericardial conduit with a porcine valve developed a right ventricular aneurysm and underwent conduit exchange 5 years later.

Summarizing the results in the literature and analyzing our own experience, we have drawn the following conclusions:

1. The use of valved extracardiac conduits has significantly improved the poor prognosis of several complex congenital heart defects.
2. The durability of porcine and bovine pericardial valved conduits is limited to about 4 to 8 years.
3. The early results with pericardial valved conduits are better than those with the compared porcine valved conduits.
4. The exchange of a malfunctioning conduit is a low-risk procedure, but probably cannot be repeated several times.
5. The aortic homograft seems to have better long-term results, but is not always suitable or available, especially in small sizes.

6. The use of a biological valved conduit, therefore, is still indicated in small infants and children.
7. The use of mechanical valves in pericardial, knitted DACRON or PTFE tubes should be reconsidered because of limited, but promising, results even without anticoagulation.

REFERENCES

1. Agrawal KC, William DE, Feldt RH, Danielson GK, Puga FJ, McGoon DC. Clinipathological correlates of obstructed right-sided porcine-valved extracardiac conduits. J Thorac Cardiovasc Surg 1981; 81:591–601.
2. Bailey WW, Kirklin JW, Bargeron LM, Pacifico AG, Kouchoukos NT. Late results with synthetic valved external conduits from venous ventricle to pulmonary arteries. Circulation 1977; 56(suppl II): II-73–79.
3. Rupprath G, Vogt J, Kirchhoff PG, de Vivie ER, Beuren AJ. Spätergebnisse nach Korrekturoperationen bei Transposition der großen Gefäße nach Rastelli. Z Kardiol 1980; 69:515–519.
4. Rupprath G, Vogt J, de Vivie ER, Beuren AJ. Conduit repair for complex congenital heart disease with pulmonary atresia or right ventricular outflow tract obstruction. Part II: Early and late hemodynamic and echocardiographic findings. Thorac Cardiovasc Surg 1981; 29:337–344.
5. Rupprath G, Thürer O, Vogt J, Weber H, Hellberg K, de Vivie ER, Beuren AJ. The durability of bioprosthesis in young people. Long-term results with intra- or extracardiac implanted porcine valves. J Cardiovasc Surg 1985; 26:251–257.
6. de Vivie ER, Rupprath G, Kirchhoff PG, Beuren AJ, Koncz J. Extracardial conduit operations with TGA, Fallot's Tetralogy and Truncus Arteriosus. First World Congress Pediatric Cardiology, London 1980; abstract 230.
7. de Vivie ER, Hellberg K, Kutzner DD, Rahlf G, Rupprath G, Beuren AJ. Conduit repair for complex congenital heart disease with pulmonary atresia or right ventricular outflow tract obstruction. Thorac Cardiovasc Surg 1981; 29:329–336.
8. Ciaravella JM, McGoon DC, Danielson GK, Wallace RB, Mair DD. Experience with the extracardiac conduit. J Thorac Cardiovasc Surg 1979; 78:920–930.
9. Marceletti C, Mair DD, McGoon DC, Wallace RB, Danielson GK. The Rastelli operation for transposition of the great arteries. J Thorac Cardiovasc Surg 1976; 72:427–434.
10. Cartmill TB, Celermajer JM, Stuckey DS, Bowdler JD, Johnson DC, Hawker RE. Use of Björk-Shiley tilting disc prosthesis in valved conduits for right ventricular outflow reconstruction. Br Heart J 1974; 36:1106–1108.
11. Brawley RK, Gardner TJ, Donahoo JS, Neill CA, Rowe RD, Gott VL. Late results after right ventricular outflow tract reconstruction with aortic root homografts. J Thorac Cardiovasc Surg 1972; 65:314–321.
12. Moodie DS, Mair DD, Fulton RE, Wallace RB, Danielson GK, McGoon DC. Aortic homograft obstruction. J Thorac Cardiovasc Surg 1976; 72:553–561.
13. Ross DN, Sommerville J. Correction of pulmonary atresia with a homograft aortic valve. Lancet 1966; II:1446–1447.
14. Shabbo FP, Ross DN. Right ventricular outflow reconstruction with aortic homograft conduit: Analysis of the long-term results. Thorac Cardiovasc Surg 1980; 28:21–25.
15. Sommerville J, Ross DN. Long-term results of complete correction with homograft reconstruction in pulmonary outflow tract atresia. Br Heart J 1972; 34:29–36.
16. Macartney FJ, Tandon AP, Ionescu MI. Right ventricular outflow tract reconstruction with pericardial patch and valved conduit. In Ionescu MI (ed): Tissue Heart Valves. Butterworth, London 1979; p 261–273.

PART IV. DISCUSSION

MARKO TURINA, MODERATOR

VALVES IN ARTIFICIAL HEARTS

JACK KOLFF: Four valves are needed for an artificial heart. Which brand of valve would the panelists put into an artificial heart when, for example, they want to use it as a bridge to transplantation?

MARKO TURINA: There have been some disastrous experiences with the valves in the mechanical artificial heart because they are subjected to much higher stresses. Dr. Reul, what are you using?

GEORGE REUL, JR.: We've used the Jarvik heart, but at the present time, we are mostly using left ventricular assist devices as a bridge to transplantation.

MARKO TURINA: A bridge is needed for a very short time, around 3 days on average. Therefore, I think the consideration of valve longevity is very secondary. I'm all for bioprostheses.

GEORGE REUL, JR.: I would disagree with that. In our experience, all patients with these devices have had thromboembolic events, mostly relating to the lining of the device, but some relating to the valves. So I think it is important to have valves that last a long time and have good flow dynamics.

DIETER HORSTKOTTE: The most important consideration is matching the valvular prosthesis to the type of heart driver being used. Some devices produce very high positive and negative pressures and accelerations, and, therefore, the valves can break. A standard mechanical BJÖRK-SHILEY® valve can break under the stresses in the artificial heart.

271

CECIL VAUGHN: We elected to use the ST. JUDE MEDICAL® valve in an artificial heart. In our bench testing we found that the ST. JUDE MEDICAL valve functioned quite well, despite the admonitions of the FDA, which advocated that we could only use the MEDTRONIC HALL™ valve.

VALVE SELECTION

MARKO TURINA: Dr. Horstkotte, at what age do you recommend a biological rather than a mechanical valve?

DIETER HORSTKOTTE: If you consider the increasing life expectancy in our general population, and if you agree to a 50% reoperation rate, you can use biological valves in women older than 67 or 68 years. If you only want a reoperation rate of 10%, you have to increase the age by 10 years, to 76. The surgeon's opinion must also be considered.

MARKO TURINA: If you have a very active man who does a lot of skiing, a lot of sports, and he needs a valve replacement, what would be the youngest age that you would consider the biological prosthesis still acceptable?

DIETER HORSTKOTTE: I would prefer using a biological valve in patients who want to be independent of anticoagulation at the age of 40, if the patients request it. I would tell them they will have to be reoperated upon at the age of 50 or 55. At that time I would put in a mechanical valve, rather than being faced with implanting bioprosthetic valves in patients between 60 and 65.

MARKO TURINA: Can I ask the panel, do you intensively discuss valve choice with each patient before surgery, and is it the surgeon or the cardiologist who points the patient in the right direction?

FRANCIS WELLENS: I always try to avoid discussing it with the patient. I don't know much reason to bother the patient with our problems.

A. MICHAEL BORKON: I'll take the opposite point of view. We are clearly in an age of consumerism and, as a surgeon or a cardiologist, we have an obligation to our patients to choose a prosthesis, whether it is mechanical or biological, based upon the quality of life and the lifestyle that the patient anticipates. I do not think we can justifiably place a mechanical substitute in a patient who represents a high risk for anticoagulant-related bleeding, which is a major deterrent for mechanical valves. I sit with all of my patients and very objectively discuss the pros and cons. I think that is very important. The reality of reoperation is one that has to be faced by all patients receiving biological prostheses, but yet I do not think, as a surgeon, that it is a major deterrent for selecting a bioprosthesis. I do not view age, necessarily, as an indication or contraindication for one type of valve or another. It is the patient who should be allowed to participate in that decision.

E. RAINER DE VIVIE: In my experience, most of the patients are not willing to make the decision about what type of valve they should receive, so we normally don't discuss this point extensively. We have rules and make the decision together with our cardiologists from year to year. We are very restrictive in selecting which patients are implanted with tissue valves.

ENDOCARDITIS

MARKO TURINA: Given a patient with acute endocarditis, on whom you have to operate, is there any preference for a biological or a mechanical valve, all other factors being equal? Is anybody preferentially putting in a biological or a mechanical valve in the presence of acute infection? Dr. Horstkotte?

DIETER HORSTKOTTE: There are some papers that indicate that the reinfection rate or the recurrence rate is greater with biological valves, but we have never seen that in our experience with more than 100 patients having infective endocarditis.

A. MICHAEL BORKON: I agree. Our population of endocarditis-infected patients is heavily skewed towards drug abusers, and that population is relatively noncompliant with COUMADIN® therapy. Recently I have been impressed with the reports that bioprostheses have an increased incidence of reinfection.

MARKO TURINA: One of the problems, which has not received enough attention, is that of left ventricular function prior to valve replacement. Dr. Gray, does infection enter into your consideration when selecting a valve if you have a patient with poor ventricular function or a patient who is young, and has a well-contracting ventricle but has a stenotic or incompetent valve?

RICHARD GRAY: Of course it does. In a patient who has an excellent ventricle, I think you have the opportunity to make the decision to use a bioprosthesis or a mechanical prosthesis on any number of grounds. It may be a patient's personal preference to take or not to take anticoagulants; but it may be a surgeon's preference for one valve or another. In our experience at Cedars-Sinai, the patient with a poorly contracting ventricular function or a patient who is young, and has a well-contracting ventricle but has a stenotic or incompetent valve?

VENTRICULAR FUNCTION

MARKO TURINA: In patients who are oligosymptomatic, but the heart is somewhat larger, do you go to greater lengths to evaluate left ventricular function when determining an indication for valve replacement for an incompetent aortic valve? In other words, do you perform echocardiography or do serial follow-up? Do you make gated blood pool studies? Do you do biopsies? We have tried biopsies for a number of years because the dilated heart does develop a certain fibrosis, but the biopsies have not proved to be of value. The left ventricular biopsy does not help in making the choice.

RICHARD GRAY: In our experience, aortic insufficiency clearly presents the biggest problem in determining when to operate. These patients are very often asymptomatic late into the course of disease; the first presentation may be pulmonary edema or cardiac death. Very often there is no clue to aortic insufficiency, except for an enlargement of the heart. While there are a variety of criteria that may be used, we generally use echocardiographic criteria in the presence of an asymptomatic patient. Patients are usually followed at 6-month intervals; however, we do not strictly adhere to the end-systolic 5.5 cm diameter.

MARKO TURINA: The patients can deteriorate even when the prosthesis might be functioning normally. Given a patient about 50-years-old who is still a candidate for transplant, with a small or residual gradient across the reconstructed valve or a small gradient across a number 19 prosthesis, would you opt for a transplantation or would you try to replace the prosthesis, although you know that he has a cardiomegaly and a poorly functioning ventricle?

RICHARD GRAY: We don't actively do transplantation at our center, but we have the opportunity to refer patients on occasion, but not specifically, with that indication. We would still attempt a reoperation, perhaps to replace the valve with a better prosthesis, if we felt that a severe patient-prosthesis mismatch was responsible. If the patient had severe deterioration, beyond that which we could explain based on the prosthesis alone, and such that we wouldn't expect improvement, we probably would refer that patient for transplantation. I should add that the age for transplantation seems to be going up; 55 is no longer a critical age.

CRAIG SMITH: If the valve doesn't appear to be causing the problem, I think that the patient might be a candidate for transplant, but I would add that patients with primary valvular pathology have not been transplanted frequently. We have transplanted as many valve patients as anybody (150) and results have not been great in that small specific subgroup (about 15 patients). We're not sure whether it's because of their distorted atrial anatomy, but there's some reason that these patients have not done well. Because of this experience, we might hesitate to transplant.

GEORGE REUL, JR.: At Texas Heart Institute the major problems are pulmonary vascular resistance and pulmonary hypertension. In these patients, Dr. Frazier has done approximately 15 piggyback transplants to manage the situation. These patients have a very poor time if they have pulmonary hypertension, but transplantation is not necessarily contraindicated if you use the piggyback heart.

ACQUIRED IMMUNE DEFICIENCY SYNDROME (AIDS)

NICO G. MEIJNE: I would like to ask Dr. Smith, as far as infection is concerned, do you have a special policy for drug addicts, and do you take any measures as far as AIDS is concerned?

CRAIG SMITH: Drug addicts are a group of patients in which we do not discuss valve choice; they get a porcine prosthesis, almost regardless of their age. As far as AIDS is concerned, that is a tougher question. Right now, personally, I am insisting that the patient have a preoperative HIV titer. That is not to say I refuse to operate on them. I generally will, but I do not insist that an anesthesiologist, perfusionist, and others operate on them, without the knowledge that this patient is at high risk for infecting them. Certainly that group of patients puts us all at risk.

RICHARD GRAY: At our center in California, all patients, regardless of whether we think they are at high risk, have an HIV test. On the other side, the patients are more concerned about the risk of blood transfusion-associated AIDS than they have been before. It is rare that, when asked about transfusion, a patient has no opinion. Most patients say, "Yes, I want to have blood that my family has donated or [that] I know the sources of," even though they are told that all blood is tested for HIV at the donor level. This is also true in the postoperative period. We have a donor-directed program to deal with the situation, and it is a very sensitive issue.

CRAIG SMITH: Parenthetically, at Massachusetts General, in New York, and in several other places around the country, the distribution of HIV, CMV, and hepatitis antigen in the designated donor pool has been the same as in the general blood donor pool. Patients thinks it is their friends who are clean, but obviously there are some who are not. There has not been a perfect solution.

RICHARD GRAY: That has been our experience too. An excellent letter to the editor, which addresses this issue, appeared in the *New England Journal of Medicine* in early 1989 from the blood bank director at the Mayo Clinic. There is immense pressure placed on family members to declare their cleanliness and to donate blood, neither of which may be entirely safe.

PROPHYLACTIC REOPERATION

MARKO TURINA: Coming back to the question of reoperations, I have a question for Dr. Smith. You introduced the term, "prophylactic reoperation." What is the operative risk for these patients? Is it 6%?

CRAIG SMITH: Rather than introducing the term, maybe I should retire it, because it refers to a group of patients that were operated on in the late 1970s or early 1980s and received Braunwald–Cutter prostheses. They were thought to be at such high risk that the prostheses should be removed. Maybe we will encounter the same thing in the future, if some new valve design runs into similar problems, but the patients in the Columbia series have all been treated and had their valves replaced.

MARKO TURINA: The same question was posed when the problem developed in the BJÖRK-SHILEY 70° valve. It is very difficult to recommend elective surgery to a completely asymptomatic patient, purely on statistical grounds. Has anyone on the panel prophylactically exchanged those valves? We have calculated the risk of reoperation to be higher than the risk of valve failure, and they have a 40% or 50% chance of surviving a catastrophic failure.

CRAIG SMITH: Twenty to 25 of our patients were operated on for prophylactic reasons or systemic complications. That is not a large number; however, there was zero mortality in that group. If we were to enlarge the group, I am sure that more mortality cases would appear. However, the risk in the prophylactic group is smaller.

DIETER HORSTKOTTE: The Shiley company has calculated the risk of strut fracture in the 70° valve to be about 1.5%, which is lower than the reoperation risk, and the incidence is decreasing with the time the valve has been implanted. In most of these cases the fractures occurred within the first 4 years, and, because these years have passed, I think there is now no indication to make a prophylactic change of the valve.

MARKO TURINA: You would take this position knowing that the breakages happened after implantation?

DIETER HORSTKOTTE: Yes.

MARKO TURINA: [Repeating a barely audible question from the audience.] What would the panelists do in this case: You have a patient with a valve that may have a potential problem; you have been informed by the manufacturers, and you have heard about it in meetings. The potential is at an extremely low statistical level, let's say 1.5%. Do you make the patient nervous, or do you withhold the information? Will you warn the patient or not?

DIETER HORSTKOTTE: Every implanted valve has a risk, maybe it is 0.1% or 1% or it is 2%. Every patient has to know that when something goes wrong, for example, when he has rhythm disturbances that he did not have before, if he has shortness of breath, and so on, he has to immediately see his doctor or come to his clinic. It doesn't matter whether he has a ST. JUDE MEDICAL valve, a biological valve (which can suddenly tear), or a BJÖRK–SHILEY valve. Every patient should leave the clinic with this information.

MARKO TURINA: And you would make no special note to the patient if he has a BJÖRK-SHILEY 70° valve?

DIETER HORSTKOTTE: No, we haven't done it. We have 100 patients who are at risk; we have had 3 strut fractures, but we did not indicate this risk to the patient.

CRAIG SMITH: In my experience, it has usually worked the other way. The patients read about it in *The New York Times* and call us up. No matter what kind of valve they have in, they want to know what the risk is. Sometimes, patients are almost more informed than we are.

MARKO TURINA: There is a potential legal problem here. I almost had a lawsuit brought by the family of a patient. She suddenly collapsed, was brought to another hospital, and from there transferred to another, and by the time she came to us, it was too late. The family asked why she was not specifically warned about the risk. It was settled by long conversations.

V. LONG-TERM CLINICAL FOLLOW-UP

31. SEVEN-YEAR EXPERIENCE AND FOLLOW-UP WITH ST. JUDE MEDICAL® PROSTHESES

L. C. D'ALESSANDRO, A. PUCCI, P. MAMONE, R. CINI

Abstract. At the Division of Cardiac Surgery of St. Camillo Hospital, 1411 patients were operated on for valve replacement with ST. JUDE MEDICAL® prostheses from November 1978 through June 30, 1986. Six hundred eighty patients had mitral valve replacement (MVR), 468 had aortic valve replacement (AVR), 5 had tricuspid valve replacement (TVR), 246 had MVR + AVR, 8 had MVR + TVR, 1 had AVR + TVR, 3 had MVR + AVR + TVR, and 1 had MVR + AVR as well as ascending aorta replacement with a ST. JUDE MEDICAL aortic valved graft. The total number of implanted prostheses was 1672. Associated procedures were: left atrium thrombectomy 98, tricuspid valve repair 92, coronary artery bypass grafting 52, subaortic membrane repair 19, and atrial septal defect closure 16. The operative mortality rate was 9.3% for MVR, 5.8% for AVR, 40% for TVR, 6.8% for MVR + AVR, 14% for MVR + TVR, 66.6% for MVR + AVR + TVR, and 0% for AVR + TVR. The 7-year actuarial survival rate was 78% for MVR, 86% for AVR, and 80% for MVR + AVR. At 7 years, the actuarial rate of freedom from thromboembolism was 82% for the complete series, and the actuarial rate of freedom from major events (prosthesis failure and prosthesis thrombosis) was 92%. Seven-year actuarial survival in patients with concomitant coronary artery bypass grafting was similar to that for patients without coronary artery disease. Clinical improvement was observed in 97% of patients.

INTRODUCTION

Since the first clinical application of the ST. JUDE MEDICAL prostheses in 1977 [1] for diseased valve replacement, many reports have been published emphasizing its excellent hemodynamic properties (especially in small sizes) and its low incidence of thromboembolic events and valve-related mechanical complications [2–5]. Our experience with the ST. JUDE MEDICAL prosthesis began at St. Filippo Hospital in Rome in November 1978 and proceeded to St. Camillo Hospital in January 1982. Our complete experience and follow-up with this valve from November 1978 through June 30, 1986 is reported here.

PATIENTS AND METHODS

From November 1978 through June 30, 1986, 1411 patients aged 6 to 74 years (mean 48 years) had valve replacement with the ST. JUDE MEDICAL prosthesis. The patient population, with age and sex distribution, is detailed in table 31-1. The total number of prostheses was 1672, and the number of prostheses for each size implanted are described in figure 31-1. The 309 associated procedures are described in table 31-2. In 73 patients with a small aortic anulus, a size 21 prosthesis was implanted. The patient population in this group, with age distribution and other surgical data, is shown in table 31-3.

Of 13 patients ages 6–12, 9 had mitral valve replacement and 4 had mitral and aortic valves replaced (table 31–4). It was possible to implant an adult-sized prosthesis in either the mitral or aortic position.

Cardiopulmonary bypass was performed with moderate hypothermia of 25 °C to 28 °C with bubble oxygenators in the majority of patients; in a few cases, membrane oxygenators were used. Myocardial protection was achieved with cold hyperpotassic crystalloid solution (St. Thomas Solution N.I.) and topical hypothermia with iced saline in the pericardial well.

Table 31-1. Patient population

Operation	No. of patients	Age (mean)	Male	Female
MVR	680	6–73 (46)	245	435
AVR	468	15–74 (50)	337	131
TVR	5	22–36 (29)	3	2
MVR + AVR	246	12–70 (49)	128	118
MVR + TVR	8	34–66 (48)	2	6
AVR + TVR	1	26	1	0
MVR + AVR + TVR	3	37–52 (45)	3	0
Total	1411			

AVR = aortic valve replacement; MVR = mitral valve replacement; TVR = tricuspid valve replacement

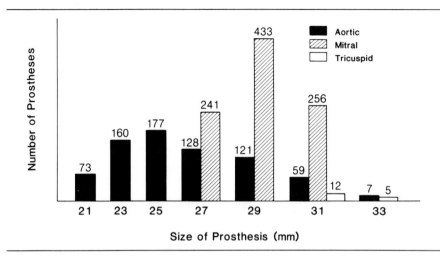

Figure 31-1. Number and size of implanted prostheses in 1672 cases.

Table 31-2. Associated procedures

Procedure	No. of patients
Mitral valve repair	28
Tricuspid valve repair	92
CABG	52
ASD repair	16
ASC.AO. replacement	1
Left atrium thrombectomy	98
Subaortic membrane resection	19
Aortic annuloplasty (Konno)	2
Resection of left atrium mixoma	1
Total	309

CABG = coronary artery bypass graft; ASD = atrial septal defect;
ASC.AO. = ascending aorta

Table 31-3. Small aortic anulus group

Number of patients	72 (6 male, 66 female)
Size of prosthesis	21 mm
Age (years)	25–70 (mean 53)
BSA (m²)	1.3–1.7 (mean 1.5)
Associated procedures	MVR: 45; other: 18
Preoperative TVPG	80–160 mm Hg (mean 98)
Postoperative TPPG	0–20 mm Hg (mean 8)
Operative mortality rate	5 patients (6.8%)

BSA = body size area; TVPG = transvalvular pressure gradient;
TPPG = transprosthetic pressure gradient

Table 31-4. Pediatric age group

Number of patients	13
Age (years)	6–12 (mean 10.5) years
Operation	MVR: 9 patients (1 exitus) MVR + AVR: 4 patients
Prosthesis size	Mitral: 27 mm (7); 29 mm (6) Aortic: 21 mm (1); 23 mm (3)
Follow-up	7 patients; 54%; mean 56 months

AVR = aortic valve replacement; MVR = mitral valve replacement

Interrupted sutures were used in the majority of patients. Valve orientation was in the anatomical position for mitral valve implantation and for the aortic position, with one of the pivot guards placed at the commissure between the right and noncoronary sinuses.

Anticoagulation was begun on the second postoperative day. Operative mortality was recorded when death occurred within 30 days of operation.

Follow-up was carried out by examining the patients or by contacting them or their relatives by telephone. Major events strictly related to the prostheses were considered when valve thrombosis and mechanical valve failure occurred. Survival and event-free evaluations were performed using the actuarial method [6, 7].

RESULTS

The overall operative mortality rate was 7.8% (111 patients) (table 31-5). No hospital death was found to be valve-related. In the small aortic anulus group

Table 31-5. Operative mortality

Operation	No. of patients	Operative mortality*	
		No. of cases	%
MVR	680	63	9.3
AVR	468	26	5.8
TVR	5	2	40.0
MVR + AVR	246	18	6.8
AVR + TVR	1	0	0.0
MVR + TVR	8	1	12.5
MVR + AVR + TVR	3	2	66.6
Total	1411	112	7.8

AVR = aortic valve replacement; MVR = mitral valve replacement; TVR = tricuspid valve replacement
* No hospital death was found to be valve-related.

Table 31-6. Causes of late death

Heart failure	11
Arrhythmia	3
Cerebral hemorrhage	4
Cerebral thromboembolism	2
Bacterial endocarditis	1
Prosthetic thrombosis	1
Paravalvular leak	1
Noncardiac	16
Unknown	13
Total	52

(table 31-3), the transprosthetic pressure gradient was measured before sternal closure; the mean value was 8 mm Hg. The operative mortality rate was 6.8% (5 patients); 1 pediatric patient died (table 31-4). Of the 1285 survivors, 964 (75%) were followed for a mean of 54 months (range 3–84 months). Fifty-two late deaths were observed; causes of death are summarized in table 31-6. The 7-year actuarial survival was 86% for aortic valve replacement, 78% for mitral valve replacement, and 80% for aortic and mitral valve replacement (figure 31-2).

Systemic embolism was found in 11 cases (table 31-7), with a linearized rate of 0.48 per patient-year for all patient groups. The 7-year actuarial freedom

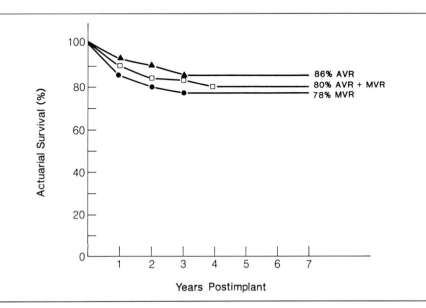

Figure 31-2. Seven-year actuarial survival. AVR = aortic valve replacement; MVR = mitral valve replacement.

Table 31-7. Follow-up of cases of systemic embolism

Operation	No. of cases	Site	
MVR	3	Cerebral	2
		Omeral	1
AVR	4	Cerebral	1
		Femoral	2
		Omeral	1
MVR + AVR	4	Femoral	2
		Omeral	1
		Abdominal	1
Total	11		
Overall rate	(0.48 pt/yr)		

AVR = aortic valve replacement; MVR = mitral valve replacement

from thromboembolism was 82% (figure 31-3). Paravalvular leak occurred in 14 cases (table 31-8). Among them, valve re-replacement was performed in 8 cases (including 1 case of aortic plus mitral valve replacement), and valve repair was performed in 6 cases. The mortality rate was 14.3% (2 patients). Occurrences of hemolysis were always related to paravalvular leak. No mechanical valve failure was observed. Three patients were reoperated on for

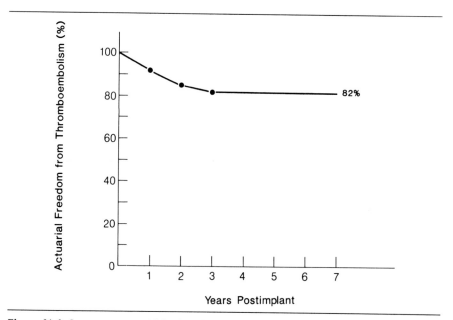

Figure 31-3. Seven-year actuarial freedom from thromboembolism.

Table 31-8. Follow-up of cases involving paravalvular leak

Initial valve replacement (position)	No. of cases	Re-replacement or repair	No. of cases	Operative mortality
MVR	7	MVR replacement★	5	0
		MVR repair	2	1
AVR	6	AVR replacement	2	1★★
		AVR repair	4	0
MVR + AVR	1	MVR + AVR replacement	1	0
Total	14		14	2
Overall	(0.98% per pt/yr)	8 re-replacements 6 repair		(14.3%)

AVR = aortic valve replacement; MVR = mitral valve replacement
 ★ One patient operated on in another institution
★★ Postoperative bacterial endocarditis

Table 31-9. Follow-up of cases involving mitral valve thrombosis

Case number	Time (days)	Operation	Result
1	184	MVR★★	OK
2★	75	MVR★★	Exitus
3	35	MVR★★	OK

MVR = mitral valve replacement; AVR = aortic valve replacement; TV = tricuspid valve
 ★ Previous operation: AVR + MVR + TV commissurotomy
★★ Heterograft valve

mitral valve thrombosis. All 3 patients were taking warfarin sodium for anticoagulation; 1 patient died after reoperation (table 31-9). Seven-year actuarial freedom from major events related to the valve was 92% (figure 31-4).

Clinical improvement, as evaluated by New York Heart Association (NYHA) Functional Class, was reached in 97% of patients (figure 31-5). Preoperatively, 90% of patients were in Class III or IV; postoperatively, 94.2% of patients were in Class I or II.

DISCUSSION

Our experience with 1411 patients operated on for valve replacement with the ST. JUDE MEDICAL prosthesis is in agreement with the results of others

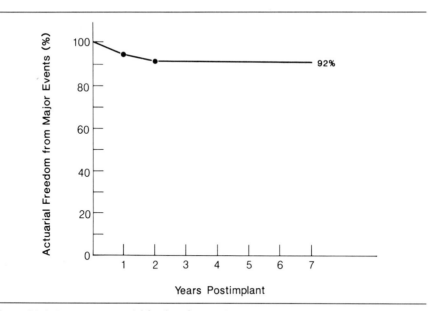

Figure 31-4. Seven-year actuarial freedom from major events.

who emphasize excellent hemodynamic performance, low thrombogenicity, and absence of mechanical failure of this prosthesis [1–5]. These properties are attributed to the large orifice in relation to the sewing ring; the central, laminar, and nonturbulent flow; and to the total pyrolytic carbon construction of the valve.

Low transvalvular pressure gradients have been observed, particularly with small-sized valves applied in the small aortic anulus [8]. In this group of

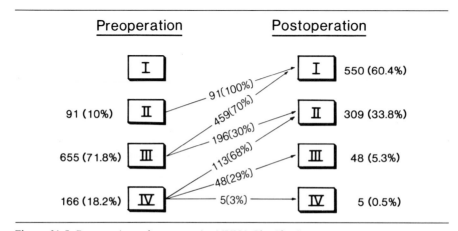

Figure 31-5. Preoperative and postoperative NYHA Classification.

patients, an aortic annuloplasty (Konno's procedure) [9] was used in only 2 patients with severe aortic anulus hypoplasia. In 72 adult patients, a small-sized valve (21 mm) was applied, with good hemodynamic results.

Mechanical valve failure and thrombosis of the prosthesis are considered to be major events strictly related to the valve. While no case of mechanical failure occurred in our experience, 3 cases of severe valve thrombosis were observed. In all cases, because only one of the leaflets was blocked, sufficient time was available to reoperate before critical clinical conditions could occur. Anticoagulation is advisable in patients with ST. JUDE MEDICAL valves, especially in adult patients with mitral valve replacement, atriomegaly, or atrial fibrillation [4, 5]. Our policy has been to place all patients on a regimen of anticoagulation with warfarin sodium, except for cases in which some contraindication was present. This policy accounts for the low incidence of thromboembolism and valve thrombosis observed in our patients.

Concern has been raised in the past about the ideal valve for the pediatric age group. This is because of the necessity to match the largest possible prosthesis with a small sewing ring, to have the most durable valve, and to not require an obligatory anticoagulation regimen. The ST. JUDE MEDICAL valve is in accord with these requirements. In our limited experience with valve replacement in pediatric-age patients, we were able to implant an adult-sized valve either in the mitral or aortic position. No late complications were observe, but follow-up was available only in half of the patients.

In conclusion, the ST. JUDE MEDICAL prosthesis can be considered to be an effective valve, with a low rate of valve-related complications, particularly in pediatric patients and in patients with a small aortic anulus.

REFERENCES

1. Emery RW, Mettler E, Nicoloff DM. A new cardiac prosthesis: The St. Jude Medical cardiac valve: In vivo results. Circulation 1979; 60:48.
2. Duncan JM, Cooley DA, Livesay JJ, Ott DA, Reul GJ, Walker WE, Frazier OH. The St. Jude Medical valve: Early clinical results in 253 patients. Texas Heart Inst J 1983; 10:11.
3. Horstkotte D, Haerten K, Herzer JA, Seipel L, Bircks W, Loogen F. Preliminary results in mitral valve replacement with the St. Jude Medical prosthesis: Comparison with the Björk-Shiley valve. Circulation 1981; 64(Suppl II):II-203.
4. Baudet EM, Oca CC, Roques XF, Laborde MN, Hafez AS, Collot MA, Ghidoni IM. A $5\frac{1}{2}$ year experience with the St. Jude Medical cardiac prosthesis. Early and late results of 737 valve replacements in 671 patients. J Thorac Cardiovasc Surg 1985; 90:137.
5. Duncan JM, Cooley DA, Reul GJ, Ott DA, Hallman GL, Frazier OH, Livesay JJ, Walker WE, Adams PR. Durability and low thrombogenicity of the St. Jude Medical valve at 5-year follow-up. Ann Thorac Surg 1986; 42:500.
6. Grunkemeier GL, Starr A. Actuarial analysis of surgical results: Rationale and method. Ann Thorac Surg 1977; 24:404.
7. Kaplan EL, Meier P. Nonparametric estimation from incomplete observations. Am Stat Assoc J 1958; 53:457–481.
8. Wortham DC, Tri TB, Bowen TE. Hemodynamic evaluation of the St. Jude Medical valve in the small aortic anulus. J Thorac Cardiovasc Surg 1981; 81:615.
9. Konno S, Imai Y, Iida Y, Nakajima M, Tatsuno K. A new method for prosthetic valve replacement in congenital aortic stenosis associated with hypoplasia of the aortic valve ring. J Thorac Cardiovasc Surg 1975; 70:909–917.

32. DURABILITY AND LOW THROMBOGENICITY OF THE ST. JUDE MEDICAL® HEART VALVE: LONG-TERM FOLLOW-UP

D. A. COOLEY

Abstract. From November 1978 through December 1986, 1953 patients under-went valve replacement at the Texas Heart Institute with the ST. JUDE MEDICAL® cardiac valve prosthesis. Aortic valve replacement (AVR) was done in 1203 patients, mitral valve replacement (MVR) in 572 patients, and double valve replacement (AVR + MVR) in 178 patients. Of the total patients, 65.1% were men and 34.9% were women. The mean age of patients was 52.8 years (range 1–88 years): 52.2 years for patients having AVR, 54.0 years for patients having MVR, and 53.4 years for patients having AVR + MVR. There were 619 associated procedures performed. Eighty-three percent of patients were in New York Heart Association (NYHA) Functional Classes III or IV preoperatively. Total follow-up was 3106 patient-years with a maximum of 99 months (mean 19 months). The early mortality rate (within 30 days) for the entire series of patients was 7.5%. The early mortality rate was lowest in patients undergoing isolated procedure. The total early mortality rate for AVR was 5.7%; for MVR, 8.9%; and for AVR + MVR, 14.6%, reflecting the severity of disease in patients requiring double valve replacement. The 7-year actuarial survival rate was 84.9% for AVR, 81.0% for MVR, and 78.7% for patients who underwent AVR + MVR. Few valve-related complications occurred. There were no instances of structural valve failure. Postoperatively, 98.3% of patients were in NYHA Functional Classes I or II, compared with only 17.1% in these two classes preoperatively. In all respects, the ST. JUDE MEDICAL valve proved superior to other mechanical valves. The valve has good hemodynamic characteristics, has a low incidence of thromboembolism, and is durable. It has a low profile and is easily inserted, even in the small aortic root. We currently favor this valve in all patients unless there is a specific contraindication to long-term anticoagulation.

INTRODUCTION

The ST. JUDE MEDICAL valve, which was first used clinically in 1977, has unique design features compared to other available prostheses. Because of its bileaflet, central-flow design, lower transvalvular pressure gradients can be obtained with this valve than with other mechanical valves. Because of its pyrolytic carbon-coated components, the valve offers durability and thrombo-resistance. Early reports [1–3] have indicated that the valve is performing well, with a low incidence of valve-related problems.

Our experience with the ST. JUDE MEDICAL valve began on a limited basis in November 1978. Our initial favorable results were reported in 1983 [4]. We were impressed with the ease with which the valve could be implanted in patients with a small aortic root, the low incidence of thromboembolic events in patients who were anticoagulated, and the low pressure gradients found even with the smaller-sized valves. Thus, the more we investigated the ST. JUDE MEDICAL valve, the more it became the most commonly used prosthesis in our surgical program. This report summarizes our most recent experience with the ST. JUDE MEDICAL valve.

PATIENTS AND METHODS

Standard surgical techniques including cardiopulmonary bypass with bubble oxygenation are used in our institution for valve replacement. Mild systemic hypothermia (30°C), cold crystalloid KCl cardioplegia, and topical hypo-thermia (saline solution, 4°C) are used routinely to provide myocardial pro-tection. Usually valve implantation is performed with everting, interrupted, pledget-supported sutures.

From November 1978 through December 1986, 1953 patients underwent valve replacement with the ST. JUDE MEDICAL cardiac valve prosthesis (figure 32-1). The majority of valves were implanted after 1982. Aortic valve replacement (AVR) was done in 1203 patients, mitral valve replacement (MVR) was done in 572 patients, and double valve replacement (AVR + MVR) was done in 178 patients. Of the total patients, 65.1% were men and 34.9% were women. More AVRs were done in men (77.4%) and more MVRs were done in women (57.7%) (table 32-1). Most patients were between 40 and 69 years of age (figure 32-2), although 254 patients (13%) were between 70 and 79 years of age. The mean age of patients was 52.8 years, with a range of 1–88 years (AVR 52.2 years; MVR 54.0 years; AVR + MVR 53.4 years). There were 619 procedures performed in association with valve replacement, the most common being coronary artery bypass grafting in 389 patients and repair of ascending aortic aneurysm in 90 patients. Associated procedures most often occurred in conjunction with AVR (table 32-2). Eighty-three percent of the

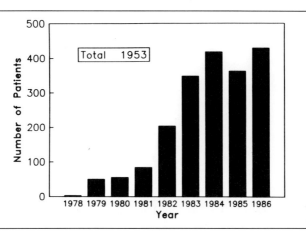

Figure 32-1. Number of patients by year who underwent valve implantation with the St. Jude Medical valve at the Texas Heart Institute (1978–1986).

Table 32-1. Age and sex distribution using the St. Jude Medical valve

	Age (years)		Sex (no. of patients; %)	
	Range	Mean	Male	Female
AVR	4–88	52.2	931 (77%)	272 (23%)
MVR	1–81	54.0	242 (42%)	330 (58%)
AVR + MVR	10–81	53.4	99 (56%)	79 (44%)
Total	1–88	52.8	1272 (65%)	681 (35%)

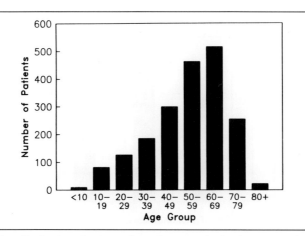

Figure 32-2. Age distribution of patients who underwent valve implantation with the St. Jude Medical valve.

Table 32-2. Associated procedures by valve position using the St. Jude Medical valve

	AVR		MVR		AVR + MVR	
	No. of patients	%	No. of patients	%	No. of patients	%
CAB	273	22.7	97	17.0	19	10.7
AATA	87	7.2	0	0	3	1.7
ADTA	3	0.2	1	0.2	0	0
AARC	12	1.0	1	0.2	0	0
ASD	4	0.3	9	1.6	0	0
ASV	8	0.7	0	0	1	0.6
VSD	18	1.5	3	0.5	0	0
M annuloplasty	16	1.3	1	0.2	0	0
T annuloplasty	1	0.1	22	3.8	9	5.1
M commissurotomy	22	1.8	1	0.2	0	0
T commissurotomy	1	0.1	2	0.3	1	0.6
Valvotomy	2	0.2	2	0.3	0	0

CAB = coronary artery bypass; AATA = aneurysm ascending thoracic aorta; ADTA = aneurysm descending thoracic aorta; AARC = aneurysm arch; ASD = atrial septal defect; ASV = aneurysm sinus Valsalva; VSD = ventricular septal defect; M = mitral; T = tricuspid

patients were in New York Heart Association (NYHA) Functional Class III or IV preoperatively (figure 32-3).

Anticoagulation was begun after the chest drainage tubes were removed, usually on the second postoperative day. The dosage of anticoagulation was adjusted to keep the prothrombin time between 1.5 to 2 times the control value. Follow-up was obtained either by direct patient contact or by questionnaires sent to the patient or referring physician. Total follow-up was 3106 patient-years with a maximum of 99 months (mean 19 months). Partial or

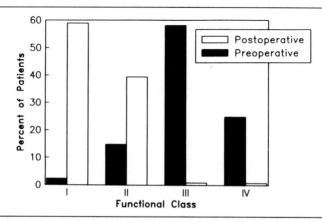

Figure 32-3. Preoperative and postoperative New York Heart Association (NYHA) Functional Classification of patients.

complete follow-up was obtained for 90% of patients. Because of the wide referral base at the Texas Heart Institute (28% foreign patients), 10% of the patients were lost to follow-up.

Statistical analysis

All survival data and freedom-from-event percentages were calculated using standard Kaplan-Meier actuarial methods [5]. Whenever necessary, the Gehan-Wilcoxon test was used to compare actuarial curves [6].

RESULTS

Mortality rate

The early mortality rate (within 30 days) for the entire series of patients was 7.5%. The early mortality rate was lowest in patients undergoing isolated procedures: AVR alone 2.7%, MVR alone 3.9%, and AVR + MVR alone 7.1%. Reoperation was associated with a higher early mortality, especially in the MVR group (8.9%) and the AVR + MVR group (17.1%), as shown in tables 32-3 through 32-5. Most of these patients had a previously implanted

Table 32-3. Aortic valve replacement with the St. Jude Medical valve

	No. of patients	% Mortality	
		Early	Total
AVR	561	2.7	5.5
AVR with other procedure	367	7.6	13.6
Reoperation			
AVR	193	7.3	16.1
AVR with other procedure	82	14.6	29.3
Total	1203	5.7	11.3

AVR = aortic valve replacement

Table 32-4. Mitral valve replacement with the St. Jude Medical valve

	No. of patients	% Mortality	
		Early	Total
MVR	233	3.9	10.7
MVR with other procedure	102	15.7	20.6
Reoperation			
MVR	158	8.9	19.0
MVR with other procedure	79	15.2	27.9
Total	572	8.9	17.1

MVR = mitral valve replacement

Table 32-5. AVR + MVR with the St. Jude Medical valve

	No. of patients	% Mortality	
		Early	Total
AVR + MVR	99	7.1	12.1
AVR + MVR with other procedure	29	17.2	24.1
Reoperation			
AVR + MVR	35	17.1	31.4
AVR + MVR with other procedure	15	53.3	60.0
Total	178	14.6	21.9

AVR = aortic valve replacement; MVR = mitral valve replacement

bioprosthesis that had calcified or degenerated. The early mortality rate was higher when reoperation was combined with other procedures. The total early mortality for AVR was 5.7%, for MVR 8.9%, and for AVR + MVR 14.6%, reflecting the severity of disease in the patients requiring double valve replacement. The linearized mortality rate was 3.32% for AVR, 5.80% for MVR, and 4.81% for AVR + MVR. Most late deaths in our series that could be determined resulted from worsening of patients' heart disease and were not valve-related (table 32-6). The total mortality rate was 11.3% per patient-year for AVR, 17.1% for MVR, and 21.9% for AVR + MVR, for a total mortality

Table 32-6. Causes of late death with the St. Jude Medical valve

Causes of late death	Frequency	Percent
Myocardial failure	8	6.3
Prosthetic valve infection	1	0.7
Thromboembolus	1	0.8
Arrhythmia	7	5.5
Myocardial infarction	1	0.8
Infection	3	2.4
Cardiac arrest	14	11.0
Hemorrhage	4	3.1
Respiratory insufficiency	1	0.8
Malignancy	6	4.7
Trauma	2	1.6
Arteriosclerotic heart disease	2	1.6
Congestive heart failure	11	8.7
Cerebrovascular insufficiency	6	4.7
Diabetic acidosis	1	0.8
Pump failure	1	0.8
Multi-system organ failure	2	1.6
Other cardiac	2	1.6
Other noncardiac	5	3.9
Undetermined	49	38.6

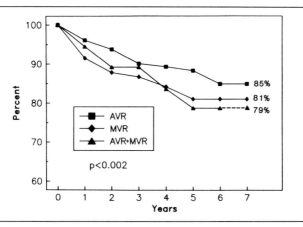

Figure 32-4. Actuarial survival rate by valve position. Dashed line indicates too few patients to be statistically significant.

rate of 14.0%. The 7-year actuarial survival was 84.9% for AVR, 81.0% for MVR, and 78.7% for patients who underwent AVR + MVR (p < 0.002) (figure 32-4).

Valve-related complications

Few valve-related complications occurred. There were no instances of structural valve failure. The linearized incidence of systemic embolism was 0.55% per patient-year for AVR (11 events), 0.50% for MVR (4 events), and 0.37% for AVR + MVR (1 event) (table 32-7). For infective endocarditis, there was a 0.40% incidence in AVR but none in MVR or AVR + MVR. Freedom from endocarditis (AVR) was 99% (figure 32-5). Paravalvular leakage occurred at a linearized incidence of 0.25% in AVR (5 events), 0.25% in MVR (2 events),

Table 32-7. Morbidity and mortality rates (% per patient-year) with the St. Jude Medical valve*

Cause	AVR		MVR		AVR + MVR	
	Events	%	Events	%	Events	%
Endocarditis	8	0.40	0	0.00	0	0.00
Paravalvular leak	5	0.25	2	0.25	1	0.37
Systemic embolism	11	0.55	4	0.50	1	0.37
Anticoagulant complications	8	0.40	0	0.00	1	0.37
Other**	0	0.00	1	0.12	0	0.00
Late mortality	67	3.32	47	5.8	13	4.81

 * Three patients had more than one valve problem
** Poor hemodynamics or hemolysis

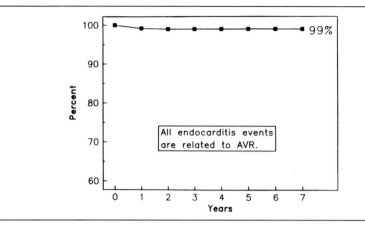

Figure 32-5. Actuarial rate for freedom from endocarditis.

and 0.37% in AVR + MVR (1 event). There were 9 anticoagulant complications: 8 with AVR (0.40%) and 1 with AVR + MVR (0.37%). The actuarial rate for freedom from thromboembolism at 7 years was 98.4% for AVR, 98.1% for MVR, and 98.7% for AVR + MVR (figure 32-6).

In a recent study of ours (data through 1983) [7], 93% of all AVR patients and 98% of all MVR patients were on a regimen of anticoagulation with warfarin during the follow-up period. Nine patients had suspected or confirmed thromboembolic episodes, and the embolic rate varied with valve position. Of these 9 patients, 5 were taking warfarin at the time of the embolic episode and were considered to be adequately anticoagulated. All except 2 patients (1 MVR reoperation, 1 AVR + MVR) had AVR either alone or with

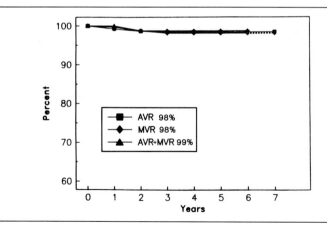

Figure 32-6. Actuarial rate for freedom from thromboembolism. Dashed line indicates too few patients to be statistically significant.

an associated procedure. The time of occurrence from operation to thrombo-embolic episode ranged from 32 to 720 days. Five of the 9 patients were left with a residual neurological deficit (1 AVR reoperation, 1 AVR with ascending aneurysm, 3 AVR). Follow-up for our current series revealed that 89.3% of AVR, 92.4% of MVR, and 96% of AVR + MVR patients were on anticoagulant therapy. Seven thromboembolic episodes occurred during the additional 3 years of the study, with 2 of these 7 patients suffering residual deficits.

Functional class

Postoperatively, 98.3% of patients were in NYHA Functional Class I or II, compared with only 17.1% in these two classes preoperatively (figure 32-3).

DISCUSSION

The low-profile ST. JUDE MEDICAL valve offers certain advantages over other types of prostheses that have a much higher profile [8, 9]. In our series, aortic replacements predominated, partly because of our practice of doing valve repair on mitral valve lesions whenever the pathologic process permits.

In all respects, the ST. JUDE MEDICAL valve proved superior to other mechanical valves, and our results are consistent with those of others [10–14]. As was determined in our previous study [7], early mortality increased in each valve position when associated procedures were necessary or when the patient was undergoing a reoperation for a valve-related problem. Patients having reoperation or associated procedures made up 53.4% of the AVR group, 59.2% of the MVR group, and 44.4% of the AVR + MVR group. The early mortality for patients having isolated first-time valve replacement was only 4.5% (2.7% AVR, 3.9% MVR, 7.1% AVR + MVR). Only 1 death was valve-related, and that occurred in a patient undergoing a second reoperation, following a reoperation elsewhere for prosthetic valve endocarditis.

The ST. JUDE MEDICAL valve has excellent mechanical properties, in-cluding lower transvalvular pressure gradients and a larger effective orifice area when compared with tilting disc valves or bioprostheses [12–15]. More-over, as a result of the lower pressure gradients, the surgeon can implant even the smaller 19 mm or 21 mm valves in patients with small aortic roots and obtain satisfactory hemodynamics, often without enlarging the anulus. Chandran [14] reported that pressure drop, percent regurgitation, and turbulent normal stresses immediately downstream from the valve were better than those with other prosthetic mechanical valves and bioprostheses.

Thromboembolism remains the major threat in implantation of valve pros-theses, and adequate anticoagulation is necessary to prevent thromboembolism in patients with mechanical valves. In our series, 92.5% of all patients were on anticoagulants at follow-up. In 1985, Czer [13] reported a threefold increase in the incidence of thromboembolic complications in patients not adequately anticoagulated with warfarin. In 1986, Ribeiro [16] reported that antiplatelet drugs alone (aspirin and dipyridamole) were not sufficient to prevent thrombosis of ST. JUDE MEDICAL aortic valves. Thus, all patients with this valve should be anticoagulated indefinitely.

Recently, Baudet et al. [12] found that valve orientation and adequate anticoagulation were both important in lowering the incidence of thromboembolism and increasing hemodynamic function. We analyzed our previous series of patients, and although we did not find any correlation, there are theoretical advantages. Thus, we have begun to implant valves according to the technique Baudet describes, i.e., when the valve is in the aortic position, the long axis should be oriented perpendicular to the septum, and when the valve is in the mitral position, it should be oriented perpendicular to the natural leaflets.

Another threat in implantation of prosthetic valves is active endocarditis. We studied 185 patients who underwent valve replacement for active valvular endocarditis during the past 5 years in an effort to determine whether bioprosthetic or mechanical valves should be used in patients who have active endocarditis [17]. In the study, Group I patients had replacement with the IONESCU-SHILEY® pericardial valve, and Group II had replacement with the ST. JUDE MEDICAL valve. The early mortality was not significantly different between the groups. Of the survivors in Group I, 15 underwent valve reoperation: 10 because of recurrent endocarditis and 5 because of sterile paravalvular leakage. The frequency of reoperation was significantly different ($p < 0.01$) from that in Group II, in which only 5 patients underwent valve reoperation: 4 for recurrent endocarditis and 1 for sterile paravalvular leakage. The actuarial rate for freedom from reoperation was also significantly higher in Group II patients; 94.6% were free from reoperation at 4 years compared to 75% at 4 years in Group I ($p < 0.01$). The actuarial survival rate, which also differed significantly between groups, was 78.7% at 4 years in Group I and 87.4% at 4 years in Group II ($p < 0.05$). Patients receiving a bioprosthesis for active endocarditis had a significantly higher reoperation rate and a significantly greater incidence of recurrent endocarditis ($p < 0.01$). Since this study, we have used mechanical valves for replacement in most of our patients with active endocarditis.

CONCLUSION

The results with the ST. JUDE MEDICAL valve are excellent. The valve has good hemodynamic characteristics, has a low incidence of thromboembolism, and is durable with no instances of valve failure recorded in our series of patients. Because of its low profile, the ST. JUDE MEDICAL valve can be easily inserted, even in the small aortic root. This is in contrast to our results with the IONESCU-SHILEY valve, where there was definitely a higher incidence of complications, mainly calcification (3.0%) and leaflet disruption (2.5%), leading to reoperation (7.3% or 2.13% per patient-year) with a subsequent mortality of 9.2%. Thus, we currently use the ST. JUDE

MEDICAL valve in all patients unless there is a specific contraindication to long-term anticoagulation.

REFERENCES

1. Emery RW, Mettler E, Nicoloff DM. A new cardiac prosthesis: The St. Jude Medical cardiac valve: In vitro results. Circulation 1979; 60:48.
2. Emery RW, Nicoloff DM. St. Jude Medical cardiac valve prosthesis: In vitro studies. J Thorac Cardiovasc Surg 1979; 78:269.
3. Nicoloff DM, Emery RW. Current status of the St. Jude cardiac valve prosthesis. Contemp Surg 1979; 15:11.
4. Duncan JM, Cooley DA, Livesay JJ, et al. The St. Jude Medical valve: Early clinical results in 253 patients. Texas Heart Inst J 1983; 10:11.
5. Kaplan EL, Meier P. Nonparametric estimation from incomplete observations. Am Stat Assoc J 1958; 53:457–481.
6. Gehan EA. Generalized Wilcoxon test for comparing arbitrary single-censored samples. Biometrika 1965; 52:203.
7. Duncan JM, Cooley DA, Reul GJ Jr, et al. Durability and low thrombogenicity of the St. Jude Medical valve at 5-year follow-up. Ann Thorac Surg 1986; 42:505.
8. Gray RJ. Hemodynamic function of St. Jude aortic valves: Comparison with a porcine and Björk-Shiley prosthesis. In DeBakey ME (ed): *Advances in Cardiac Valves*, Proceedings of the Third International Symposium on the St. Jude Medical Heart Valve. Yorke Medical Books, New York 1983; pp 247–258.
9. Wortham DC, Tri TB, Bowen TE, Hemodynamic evaluation of the St. Jude Medical valve prosthesis in the small aortic anulus. J Thorac Cardiovasc Surg 1981; 81:615.
10. Nicoloff DM, Emery RW, Arom KV, et al. Clinical and hemodynamic results with the St. Jude Medical cardiac valve prosthesis: A three-year experience. J Thorac Cardiovasc Surg 1981; 82:674.
11. Horstkotte D, Haerten K, Herzer JA, et al. Preliminary clinical and hemodynamic results after mitral valve replacement using St. Jude Medical prostheses in comparison with the Björk-Shiley valve. Thorac Cardiovasc Surg 1981; 29:93.
12. Baudet EM, Oca CC, Roques XF, et al. A $5\frac{1}{2}$ year experience with the St. Jude Medical valve: Hemodynamic performance, surgical results, biocompatibility and follow-up. JACC 1985; 6:904.
13. Czer LSC, Matloff JM, Chaux A, et al. A 6-year experience with the St. Jude Medical valve: Hemodynamic performance, surgical results, biocompatibility and follow-up. JACC 1985; 6:904.
14. Chandran KB. Pulsatile flow past St. Jude Medical bileaflet valve: An in vitro study. J Thorac Cardiovasc Surg 1985; 89:743.
15. Kawachi Y, Tokunaga K, Watanabe Y, et al. In vivo hemodynamics of prosthetic St. Jude Medical and Ionescu-Shiley heart valves analyzed by computer. Ann Thorac Surg 1985; 39:456.
16. Ribeiro PA, Al Zaibag M, Idris M, et al. Antiplatelet drugs and the incidence of thromboembolic complications of the St. Jude Medical aortic prosthesis in patients with rheumatic heart disease. J Thorac Cardiovasc Surg 1986; 91:92.
17. Sweeney MS, Reul GJ Jr, Cooley DA, et al. Comparison of bioprosthetic and mechanical valve replacement for active endocarditis. J Thorac Cardiovasc Surg 1985; 90:676.

33. AORTIC AND MITRAL VALVE REPLACEMENT WITH THE ST. JUDE MEDICAL® PROSTHESIS: A NINE-YEAR UPDATE REPORT

K. V. AROM, D. M. NICOLOFF, W. G. LINDSAY, W. F. NORTHRUP,
T. E. KERSTEN, R. W. EMERY

Abstract. *Records of 614 patients (393 AVR, 221 AVR + CAB—Group A) and 421 patients (291 MVR, 130 MVR + CAB—Group B) were reviewed 9 years after the first ST. JUDE MEDICAL® valve was implanted in 1977.* ★ *Mean age was 63 years in Group A (410 males and 204 females) and 59 years of age in Group B (173 males and 248 females). The operative mortality was 6.5% (3% AVR, 4.5% AVR + CAB, 8.5% MVR, 16% MVR + CAB). Follow-up was completed in 97.7% of the patients (1450 patient-years in AVR, 786 in AVR + CAB, 1105 in MVR, and 403 in MVR + CAB). Significant improvement in New York Heart Association (NYHA) Functional Classification was seen in Group A but not in Group B, particularly in the MVR + CAB. Actuarial estimates (including operative deaths) showed the same survival of 74.1 ± 6.4% in AVR and AVR + CAB, but only 57.4 ± 8.8% in MVR and 52.3 ± 14.4% in MVR + CAB. AVR and AVR + CAB patients are doing well, however, the ratio of anticoagulant-related hemorrhage to thromboembolism is high in the isolated AVR group (3:1). Therefore, reduction of the COUMADIN® dose is suggested. MVR + CAB patients are not doing well; the LVR group is not quite improved after surgery and incidence of all complications (including deaths) remains high, in spite of the benefits from better hemodynamics of the ST. JUDE MEDICAL prosthesis.*

★ AVR = aortic valve replacement; MVR = mitral valve replacement; CAB = coronary artery
bypass

INTRODUCTION

Since October 1977, we have implanted approximately 1200 ST. JUDE MEDICAL prostheses. In this series, however, we would like to present only data for valves in the aortic and mitral positions. Double valve replacement and valves with associated procedures were excluded from this study.

METHODS

In this series we had a total of 1035 patients (583 males, 452 females), who were operated upon from October 1977 through October 1986 (table 33–1). Ages ranged from 9 months to 84 years. There were 614 aortic valve replacements (AVR) and 421 mitral valve replacements (MVR). Severe calcific aortic stenosis comprised the major part of the aortic valve group and approximately two-thirds of the mitral valve group had mitral regurgitation, either from floppy mitral valve or ischemic rupture of the papillary muscle. In the aortic valve group, slightly more than 50% had concomitant coronary artery bypass (CAB) surgery (table 33-2). Slightly less than 50% in the mitral valve group also had this type of surgery.

RESULTS AND DISCUSSION

Operative mortality, shown in figure 33-1, was 6.5%, with 68 deaths among these patients. Mortality was 3% in the AVR group, 4.5% for AVR + CAB, 8.5% for MVR, and 16% for MVR + CAB. The majority of the MVR +

Table 33-1. Study parameters

Number of patients	1035
Period	October 1977–October 1986
Sex	583 males, 452 females
Age	9 months–84 years
Pathology	Aortic valve disease: 614 patients Mitral valve disease: 421 patients

Table 33-2. Number of prostheses

Procedure	Number of patients
AVR	393
AVR + CAB	221
MVR	291
MVR + CAB	130
Total	1035

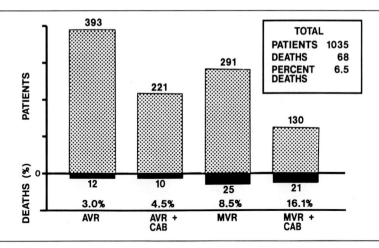

Figure 33-1. Operative mortality. AVR = aortic valve replacement; MVR = mitral valve replacement; CAB = coronary artery bypass.

CAB patients were operated upon on an urgent basis following acute rupture of the papillary muscle from the ischemic mitral valve.

We followed these patients from a minimum of 3 months to a maximum of 108 months, with a mean of 44 months (table 33-3). Nine hundred sixty-seven patients (98%) were available for follow-up; 105 patients had died at the time of follow-up, for a late mortality of 10.8%. As figure 33-2 illustrates, in the AVR group 7.8% patients had died at the end of 9 years; 11% in AVR + CAB; 12% in the MVR group; and 18.3% in MVR + CAB. The majority of these deaths were due to ongoing congestive heart failure.

If we look at the cause of late mortality in the AVR and MVR groups, three areas are interesting: myocardial infarction, cardiac failure, and valve-related deaths (table 33-4). In the AVR group, approximately 25% of patients died from myocardial infarction. We believe that, in spite of valve replacement and coronary artery bypass surgery, the residual concentric aortic left ventricular hypertrophy still remained, and the blood supply per gram of tissue of myocardium was still inadequate. Therefore, the majority of these people probably died from ischemic problems. In congestive heart failure, only 13%

Table 33-3. Patient follow-up

Number of patients	967
Percent complete	98%
Patients lost to follow-up (late mortality)	105
Percent lost to follow-up (late mortality)	10.8%
Length of follow-up (months)	3–108
Mean follow-up (months)	44

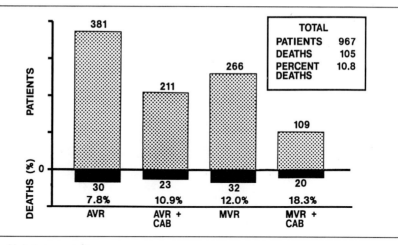

Figure 33-2. Late mortality.

of the AVR patients died in comparison to 29% in the MVR group. The majority of these people had ischemic mitral valve disease and chronic long-term mitral regurgitation. In spite of the benefits from better hemodynamics of the ST. JUDE MEDICAL prosthesis, inability to improve left ventricular function in the long term played a major role in the course of congestive heart failure. Valve-related deaths occurred in 10% of the AVR group and 20% of the MVR group.

If we look more closely at valve-related death and complications, there are two areas of concern in our experience. Thromboembolic episodes occurred in 5% of the entire series, and 1% of these patients died (table 33-5). When one evaluates the incidence of thromboembolic phenomena, one should know how many of these patients discontinued COUMADIN use for a certain period of time during the postoperative stage. In this series, 21% of patients discontinued COUMADIN use at some time for various reasons. During the survey period, patients were asked to answer a question on significant thrombo-

Table 33-4. Causes of late mortality

		Deaths
Myocardial infarction	AVR	25%
Cardiac failure	AVR	13%
	MVR	29%
Valve-related deaths	AVR	10%
	MVR	20%

AVR = aortic valve replacement; MVR = mitral valve replacement

Table 33-5. Valve-related deaths and complications

	No. episodes	No. deaths
Thromboembolism	48 (5%)	10 (1.0%)
Anticoagulant-related bleeding	87 (9%)	
Major: 41 patients		2 (0.2%)
Minor: 46 patients		0 (0.0%)
Valve thrombosis	6 (0.5%)	3 (0.3%)
Paravalvular leak	9 (0.9%)	1 (0.1%)
Prosthetic endocarditis	6 (0.6%)	1 (0.1%)
Reoperation	8 (0.8%)	0 (0.0%)
Mechanical failure	0 (0.0%)	0 (0.0%)
Total	164 (16.9%)	17 (1.75%)

embolic or bleeding episodes they were experiencing. They were asked to report either major, minor, transient, or permanent emboli and/or any major or minor bleeding. An incident of major bleeding was one requiring transfusion. An example of minor bleeding would be bleeding from the gums. Eighty-seven people suffered from anticoagulant hemorrhage; 41 of them required transfusion and 2 of these patients died.

Valve thrombosis occurred only in the MVR group. Paravalvular leaks also occurred in the mitral valve group, and, in our experience, the inability to remove all the calcium along the posterior ring of the mitral valve played a significant role in this complication. Eight out of 9 paravalvular leaks were operated upon; 1 patient died because of congestive heart and multi-organ failures. There were 6 incidents of prosthetic endocarditis, all within the first year after implantation. No prosthetic endocarditis occurred after the first year. This low incidence of late infective endocarditis may be due to the design of the ST. JUDE MEDICAL valve. Reoperation was only related to paravalvular leak. The total valve complication rate was 17%. In the entire series 1.75% of the patient deaths were related to the prosthesis. There were no mechanical failures whatsoever.

The linearized rate of complications in both the aortic and mitral groups was calculated in order to make a more meaningful comparison with the other series. Data are shown in table 33-6. Anticoagulant hemorrhage developed in 3.1% of the AVR group, which is about 3 times higher than the incidence of thromboembolism in AVR patients. This is in contrast with the MVR group, which had a 2.5% incidence of anticoagulant-related hemorrhage. We feel that perhaps we made the prothrombin time longer than it should have been in the aortic valve group. We recommend keeping it less than 20 seconds in the AVR group. The rate of prosthetic endocarditis was 0.1% per patient-year in the AVR group and 0.3% for the MVR group. There was no valve thrombosis, reoperation, or valve failure in the aortic position and no valve failure in the

Table 33-6. Valve-related complications shown as percent per patient-year with standard error

Complications	AVR	MVR
Anticoagulant-related bleeding	3.1 (.42)	2.5 (.46)
Thromboembolism	1.3 (.28)	2.0 (.41)
Prosthetic endocarditis	0.1 (.06)	0.3 (.14)
Valve thrombosis	–	0.1 (.08)
Reoperation	–	0.5 (.20)
Valve failure	–	–
All complications (including all deaths)	9.0 (.72)	13.6 (1.1)

AVR = aortic valve replacement; MVR = mitral valve replacement

Table 33-7. Thromboembolism shown as percent per patient-year with standard error

	AVR	AVR + CAB	Aortics	MVR	MVR + CAB	Mitrals
Transient/minor	.7 (.25)	1.0 (.40)	.8 (.22)	.8 (.29)	1.6 (.73)	1.0 (2.9)
Transient/major	–	–	–	–	–	–
Permanent/minor	–	.2 (.16)	.1 (.06)	.2 (.16)	.3 (.33)	.3 (.14)
Permanent/major	.2 (.13)	.5 (.28)	.3 (.13)	.5 (.22)	1.0 (.57)	.6 (.22)

Years of follow-up:
  AVR = 1144; AVR + CAB = 612; aortics (combined) = 1726
  MVR = 897; MVR + CAB = 306; mitrals (combined) = 1203

AVR = aortic valve replacement; MVR = mitral valve replacement; CAB = coronary artery bypass

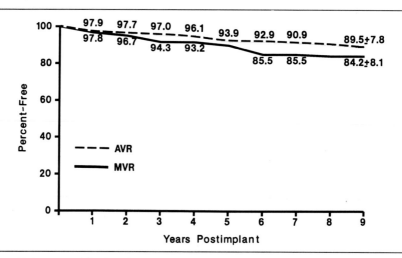

Figure 33-3. Actuarial freedom from thromboembolism. AVR = aortic valve replacement; MVR = mitral valve replacement.

mitral position. The overall complication rate, including death, was 9.0% per patient-year AVR and 13.5% per patient-year MVR.

In table 33-7 thromboembolic episodes are classified into transient minor, transient major, permanent minor, and permanent major episodes. In AVR, the transient minor rate is 0.8% per patient-year, which is more than the combined permanent minor and permanent major episodes. In MVR as well, the majority of patients experienced transient and minor emboli.

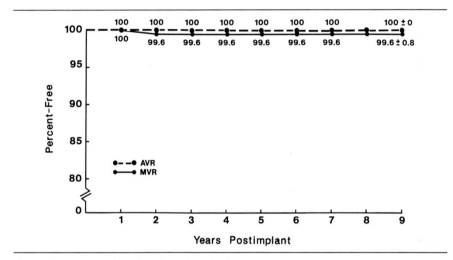

Figure 33-4. Actuarial freedom from thrombosis.

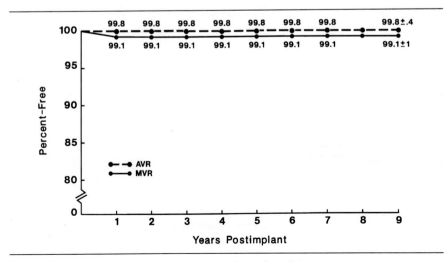

Figure 33-5. Actuarial freedom from prosthetic valve endocarditis.

Actuarial freedom from thromboembolism at 9 years (figure 33-3) was 89.5% for AVR and about 84.2% for MVR. Valve thrombosis occurred only in the mitral valve group and the actuarial freedom at 9 years (figure 33-4) was 99.6% for MVR. Freedom from endocarditis (figure 33-5) has also been very stable during the past 8 years; infective endocarditis occurred after 2 months and before the first year. At the end of 9 years, freedom from endocarditis was 99.8% AVR and 99.1% MVR. Actuarial freedom from reoperation (figure 33-6) was 100% in the AVR group and 98.1% for MVR. Reoperation was related only to paravalvular leak. There was no mechanical failure (figure 33-7).

Actuarial freedom from all complications including death was 74.1 ± 6.4% for AVR and 57.4 ± 8.8% for MVR (figure 33-8). At the end of 9 years, approximately three-fourths of the aortic valve patients are still doing well. This is also true for the AVR + CAB group. In the mitral valve group, however, approximately 60% of the MVR patients were free from all complications and death at this time, but only 52.3 ± 14.4% of the MVR + CAB patients were free from death and all complications.

Patients receiving the ST. JUDE MEDICAL valve have done very well in our experience. They have shown significant improvement in New York Heart Association (NYHA) Functional Classification, mainly in AVR and MVR. At the time of follow-up, the majority of patients were in Functional Class I and II, regardless of age.

We feel that the valve has very low thrombogenicity. The reoperation rate is related to paravalvular leak. The incidence of prosthetic endocarditis is negligible after the first year. Significant hemolysis does not occur with normally functioning ST. JUDE MEDICAL valves. Thromboembolism and anticoagu-

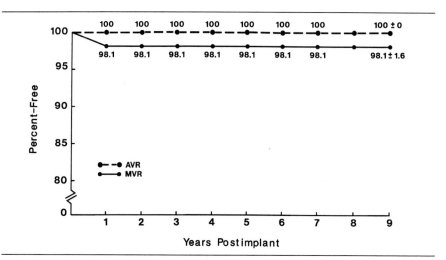

Figure 33-6. Actuarial freedom from reoperation.

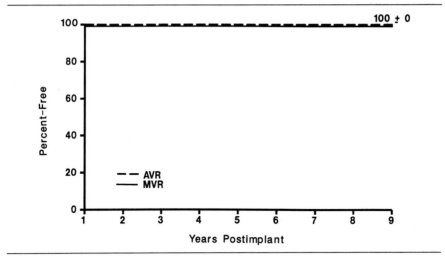

Figure 33-7. Actuarial freedom from valve failure.

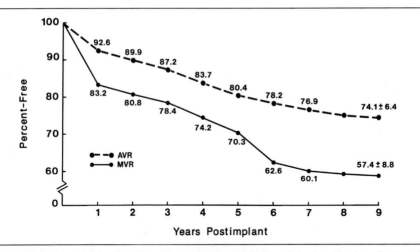

Figure 33-8. Actuarial freedom from all complications including all deaths. (The dates for 2 aortic TE events, 1 aortic death, and 1 mitral death were not available.)

lant hemorrhage still remain our major concerns at this point. With time and longer follow-up, we hope to show better results for these complications.

We feel that the ST. JUDE MEDICAL prosthesis is the best mechanical valve available at the present time due to its freedom from mechanical failure, low thromboembolism rates, minimal obstruction in the valve orifice area, and the lack of hemolysis with normally functioning valves.

34. EIGHT-YEAR CLINICAL EXPERIENCE WITH THE ST. JUDE MEDICAL® CARDIAC PROSTHETIC VALVE

E. D. MUNDTH, R. S. BOOVA, I. P. GOEL, A. H. HAKKI, F. T. HOPKINS, L. HILL, J. B. MUNDTH

Abstract. This clinical study reviews 683 patients who had 744 ST. JUDE MEDICAL® cardiac valves implanted over 8.2 years. Beginning in October 1978, 226 patients had isolated aortic valve replacement (AVR), 222 patients had isolated mitral valve replacement (MVR), 53 patients had aortic and mitral valve replacement (AVR + MVR), 115 patients had aortic valve replacement combined with coronary artery bypass (AVR + CAB), 59 patients had mitral valve replacement combined with coronary artery bypass (MVR + CAB), and 8 patients had AVR + MVR + CAB. Follow-up ranged from 2 months to 98 months (8.2 years). The overall operative mortality for the series was 6.3%. One hundred nine patients were lost to follow-up; the remaining 531 patients (83%) were followed for a mean period of 45 months (3.75 years). The overall late death occurrence over the 8-year period was 15.6% among the 531 patients. The mean late death rate was 4.2% per year. Major complications occurred postoperatively in 8% of the patients and minor complications in 6%. Valve-related complications occurred in 11.7% of the patients. Thromboembolic complications (TE) of cerebrovascular accident (CVA) occurred in 3.8% overall, for an incidence of 1.0% per patient-year. Bleeding complications relating to anticoagulation occurred in 3.0% overall for an incidence of 0.8% per patient-year. Prosthetic endocarditis occurred in 1.7%, with reoperative replacement of the infected valve required in 2 patients. The incidence of documented paravalvular leak was 1.9%, with 1 patient requiring reoperation. Significant hemolysis occurred in 0.4%, relating to a paravalvular leak in both patients. The functional status of 448 patients followed for a *mean of 45 months was evaluated; 77% were in New York Heart Association (NYHA) Class I, 20% in NYHA Class II, and only 3% in NYHA Class III. The majority of patients were relieved of symptoms of failure and angina. There were no documented instances of primary valve failure. This continued excellent clinical experience makes us consider this prosthesis our valve of choice.*

INTRODUCTION

Follow-up of a previously reported clinical study of 376 patients [1] with an additional 307 patients constitutes the basis of this current clinical report, which analyzes the results of patients undergoing cardiac valve replacement utilizing the ST. JUDE MEDICAL cardiac prosthetic valve. Reports of valve replacement using the ST. JUDE MEDICAL valve have been most encouraging, with overall excellent results in terms of postoperative functional status, valvular hemodynamic performances, valve durability, and an acceptably low incidence of valve-related complications [1–5].

MATERIALS AND METHODS

This clinical study reviews 683 patients who had 744 ST. JUDE MEDICAL cardiac valve implants over 8.2 years, beginning in October 1978. The distribution of patients undergoing valve replacement is shown in table 34-1. Follow-up ranged from 2 months to 98 months (8.2 years) with a median of 45 months (3.75 years) for 531 patients, reflecting an 83% follow-up postoperatively. The loss of follow-up in 109 patients was primarily due to patients moving to other locales without leaving forwarding addresses.

Operative mortality was analyzed in relation to preoperative risk category (table 34-2). High-risk category patients were primarily in NYHA Functional Class III or IV preoperatively.

Major postoperative complications were defined as those resulting in serious morbidity delaying hospital discharge, adversely affecting long-term func-

Table 34-1. Distribution of valve replacement procedures in 8.2 years (98 months)

Patients	683
Valve implants	744
Isolated AVR	226
Isolated MVR	222
AVR + MVR	53
AVR + CAB	115
MVR + CAB	59
AVR + MVR + CAB	8

AVR = aortic valve replacement; MVR = mitral valve replacement; CAB = coronary artery bypass

CORR.23

Table 34-2. High-risk clinical parameters

1. Preoperative left ventricular ejection fraction less than 30%

2. Cardiac index of less than 2.0 L/min/M; associated with left ventricular segmental wall contractile abnormalities

3. Systolic pulmonary artery pressure over 60 mm Hg; associated with a significantly lowered cardiac output

4. Acute myocardial infarction less than 3 weeks preoperatively

tional results, or necessitating further surgical intervention. These included re-exploration for bleeding, cerebrovascular accident (CVA), renal failure requiring dialysis, perioperative myocardial infarction causing significant left ventricular dysfunction, respiratory failure requiring reintubation and/or prolonged ventilatory support, severe infection resulting in mediastinal sepsis or prosthetic endocarditis, etc.

Minor complications were characterized as complications not resulting in delayed hospital discharge or having an adverse influence on late functional results and included minor wound infection, transient azotemia, transient arrhythmias, post-pericardiotomy syndrome, etc.

Valve-related complications were characterized as primary and included: 1) thromboembolic complications; 2) anticoagulant bleeding complications; 3) prosthetic endocarditis; 4) periprosthetic valvular leak; and 5) significant hemolysis.

The late functional status of 448 surviving patients was assessed by direct interview or questioning 2 to 98 months postoperatively, with a median of 45 months. Functional classification was based upon the NYHA Functional Classification system.

Hospital mortality (operative mortality) was defined as postoperative death occurring within 30 days of surgery, prior to discharge. Late mortality and cumulative survival was analyzed using the Kaplan-Meier method [6].

RESULTS

The overall operative mortality was 6.3%, with an operative mortality of 3.5% for low-risk patients and 12.0% for high-risk patients. Major postoperative complications occurred in 8% and minor complications in 6%. Valve-related complications occurred in 11.7% of the overall group of 531 patients. The incidence of thromboembolic CVA was 1.0% per patient-year, and the rate of anticoagulant-related complications was 0.8% per patient-year (table 34-3). Late survival follow-up was achieved in the 531 patients (83%) for a median 45 months, with late death (> 30 days) of 15.6% for the entire study period, or 4.2% annually.

The functional status of 448 surviving patients followed for a median of 45

Table 34-3. Valve-related complications in 531 patients followed for mean of 45 months

	Number of incidents	% per patient-year
Thromboembolic (CVA)	20	3.8%
Incidence per patient-year		1.0%
Anticoagulant-related	16	3.0%
Incidence per patient-year		0.8%
Prosthetic endocarditis	9	1.7%
Significant paravalvular leak	10	1.9%
Hemolysis	2	0.4%
Valve thrombosis	1	0.2%
Total	62	11.7%

CVA = cerebrovascular accident

months revealed that 77% were NYHA Functional Class I (asymptomatic), 20% were NYHA Class II (moderately symptomatic), and 3% were NYHA Class III (severely symptomatic). There were no patients in Functional Class IV. The great majority of patients were relieved of symptoms of congestive heart failure and angina. There were no documented instances of primary valve failure.

Isolated aortic valve replacement (226 patients)

The overall operative mortality for 226 patients was 0.9%, with 0% operative mortality for 181 patients in the low-risk category and 4.4% for 45 high-risk patients. Of 205 patients followed (91% follow-up rate) for a median of 42 months, the incidence of late death was 8.9%, with an annual rate of 2.4% per year. Valve-related complications occurred in 8.0%, and 81% of patients were asymptomatic at follow-up. The incidence of thromboembolic CVA was 0.6% per patient-year, and the incidence of significant anticoagulant-related complications was 0.7% per patient-year (table 34-4).

Isolated mitral valve replacement (222 patients)

The overall operative mortality for 222 patients was 5.9%, with 3.7% operative mortality for 134 patients in the low-risk category and 9.0% for 88 high-risk patients. Of 172 patients followed (82% follow-up rate) for a median of 47 months, the incidence of late death was 19.8%, with an annual rate of 5.1% per year. Valve-related complications occurred in 7.5%, and 73% were asymptomatic at follow-up. The incidence of thromboembolic CVA was 1.0% per patient-year, and the incidence of significant anticoagulant-related complications was 0.6% per patient-year (table 34-5).

Table 34-4. Results of isolated aortic valve replacement in 226 patients

Operative mortality		0.9%
Low-risk		0%
High-risk		4.4%
Follow-up 205 patients (mean 42.4 months)		91.0%
Late death incidence		8.9%
Late death annual rate		2.4%
Valve-related complications		8.0%
Thromboembolic (CVA)	2.0%	0.6% per patient-year
Anticoagulant-related	2.4%	0.7% per patient-year
Prosthetic endocarditis	2.0%	0.6% per patient-year
Paravalvular leak	1.5%	0.4% per patient-year
Postoperative NYHA Classification		
Class I		81%
Class II		18%
Class III		1%
Class IV		0%

Table 34-5. Results of isolated mitral valve replacement in 222 patients

Operative mortality		5.9%
Low-risk		3.7%
High-risk		9.0%
Follow-up 172 patients (mean 47.2 months)		82.0%
Late death incidence		19.8%
Late death annual rate		5.1%
Valve-related complications		7.5%
Thromboembolic (CVA)	4.0%	1.0% per patient-year
Anticoagulant-related	2.3%	0.6% per patient-year
Prosthetic endocarditis	0.6%	0.2% per patient-year
Paravalvular leak	1.1%	0.3% per patient-year
Postoperative NYHA Classification		
Class I		73%
Class II		25%
Class III		2%
Class IV		0%

Aortic and mitral valve replacement (53 patients)

The operative mortality for 53 patients was 13.2%, with 6.7% operative mortality for 30 low-risk patients and 21.7% for 23 high-risk patients. Forty-three patients were followed for a median of 44 months, with a 26.0% late death incidence corresponding to an annual mortality rate of 7.0% per year.

Table 34-6. Results of aortic and mitral valve replacement in 53 patients

Operative mortality		13.2%
Low-risk		6.7%
High-risk		21.7%
Follow-up 43 patients (mean 44.3 months)		93.5%
Late death incidence		26.0%
Late death annual rate		7.0%
Valve-related complications		11.5%
Thromboembolic (CVA)	4.6%	1.2% per patient-year
Anticoagulant-related	4.6%	1.2% per patient-year
Prosthetic endocarditis	0%	0.0% per patient-year
Paravalvular leak	2.3%	0.6% per patient-year
Postoperative NYHA Classification		
Class I		74%
Class II		26%
Class III		0%
Class IV		0%

Complications related to the valve occurred in 11.5%, with an incidence of thromboembolic CVA of 1.2% per patient-year and, similarly, an incidence of anticoagulant-related complications of 1.2% per patient-year. Seventy-four percent were asymptomatic at follow-up (table 34-6).

Aortic vavle replacement combined with coronary artery bypass (115 patients)

The operative mortality in this group was 16.5%, with 8.0% operative mortality for 59 low-risk patients and 25.0% for 56 high-risk patients. Of 60 patients followed (61% follow-up rate) for a median of 42.6 months, the incidence of late death was 15.0%, with an annual rate of 4.2% per year. There were 6.7% valve-related complications with no documented thromboembolic CVA and a 0.9% per patient-year incidence of anticoagulant-related complications. Seventy-six percent were asymptomatic at follow-up (table 34-7).

Mitral valve replacement combined with coronary artery bypass (59 patients)

The operative mortality was 3.4%, with no deaths in 35 low-risk patients and 8.3% in 24 high-risk patients. Of 30 patients followed (53% follow-up rate) for a median of 40 months, the late death incidence was 23.0%, for an annual rate of 7.4% per year. Valve-related complications occurred in 13.4%, with a 2.2% per patient-year incidence of thromboembolic CVA. There were no anticoagulant-related complications in this group. Sixty-one percent of the patients were asymptomatic at follow-up (tabler 34-8).

    Aortic and mitral valve replacement combined with coronary artery bypass was carried out in 8 patients in this series, with 1 operative death. This number of patients is considered too small for meaningful statistical analysis.

Table 34-7. Results of aortic valve replacement combined with coronary artery bypass in 115 patients

Operative mortality		16.5%
Low–risk		8.0%
High–risk		25.0%
Follow–up 60 patients (mean 42.6 months)		61.0%
Late death incidence		15.0%
Late death annual rate		4.2%
Valve–related complications		6.7%
Thromboembolic (CVA)		0% per patient-year
Anticoagulant–related	3.3%	0.9% per patient-year
Prosthetic endocarditis	1.7%	0.5% per patient-year
Paravalvular leak	1.7%	0.5% per patient-year
Postoperative NYHA Classification		
Class I		76%
Class II		18%
Class III		6%
Class IV		0%

Table 34-8. Results of mitral valve replacement combined with coronary artery bypass in 59 patients

Operative mortality		3.4%
Low–risk		0%
High–risk		8.3%
Follow–up 30 patients (mean 40 months)		53.0%
Late death incidence		23.0%
Late death annual rate		7.4%
Valve–related complications		13.4%
Thromboembolic (CVA)	6.7%	2.2% per patient-year
Anticoagulant–related		0% per patient-year
Prosthetic endocarditis		0% per patient-year
Paravalvular leak	6.7%	2.2% per patient-year
Postoperative NYHA Classification		
Class I		61%
Class II		35%
Class III		4%
Class IV		0%

Cumulative survival

Cumulative survival (CS) for isolated aortic valve replacement for patients discharged following surgery was 89% entering the eighth year postoperatively (figure 34-1). Cumulative survival for isolated mitral valve replacement

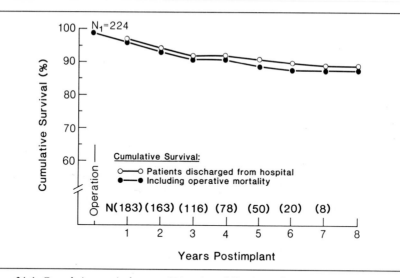

Figure 34-1. Cumulative survival among 226 patients following isolated aortic valve replacement. Operative mortality was 0.9%.

entering the eighth year postoperatively was significantly less at 77%. When cumulative survival included operative mortality, the corresponding CS was 73% (figure 34-2). For double valve replacement of the aortic and mitral valves, the CS entering the seventh year postoperatively was 70% for hospital

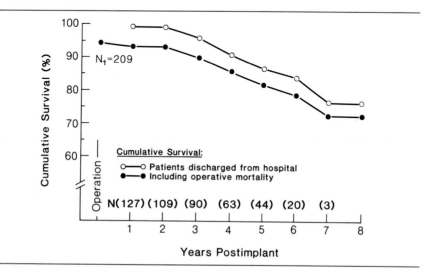

Figure 34-2. Cumulative survival following isolated mitral valve replacement in 222 patients. Operative mortality was 5.9%.

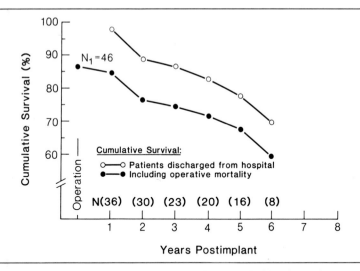

Figure 34-3. Cumulative survival among 53 patients following double valve replacement of aortic and mitral valves. Operative mortality was 13.2%.

discharged patients and 60% when hospital mortality was included (figure 34-3).

Causes of late death are summarized in table 34-9. Of the 83 late deaths, 39% were of cardiac cause but not valve-related and included primarily death from myocardial infarction and progressive congestive heart failure. Twenty-

Table 34-9. Causes of late death in 83 patients

Cause	Number	Percent
Valve-related	19	23%
Thromboembolic CVA	5	6%
Anticoagulant-related	5	6%
Prosthetic endocarditis	4	5%
Paravalvular leak	4	5%
Non-valve-related	32	39%
Cardiac cause	19	23%
Myocardial infarction	10	12%
Progressive congestive heart failure	9	11%
Noncardiac cause	13	16%
Cancer	7	8%
Pulmonary	2	2%
Renal failure	1	1%
Hepatitis	1	1%
Gastrointestinal hemorrhage	1	1%
Ruptured abdominal aortic aneurysm	1	1%

three percent of the late deaths were valve-related, with fairly equal distribution in cause from thromboembolic CVA, prosthetic endocarditis, progressive paravalvular leak (requiring reoperation), and anticoagulant-related causes. There was a 16% incidence of noncardiac causes of late death, of which cancer was the most frequent. The cause of death was unknown in 38%.

DISCUSSION AND CONCLUSION

The ST. JUDE MEDICAL cardiac prosthetic valve has been shown to be a hemodynamically effective, safe, and durable valve [1–5]. Postoperative hemo-dynamic in vivo studies have shown the valve to have superior performance, even in the smaller annular sizes, i.e., less than 21 mm [7]. Our clinical experience in 683 patients in this series corroborates these conclusions.

There were no documented cases of primary valvular failure. Valve-related complications were primarily related to thromboembolic complications or to anticoagulant-related bleeding complications. The major known causes of late death were not valve-related in 63%, with 59% of these being cardiac causes and 41% being noncardiac causes. The overall thromboembolic CVA incidence of 1.0% per patient-year compares similarly to other reports [2–5, 8, 9] and appears to be somewhat less than that for tilting disc and caged-ball prosthetic valves [10, 11].

Operative mortality was acceptably low in the series, with the exception of aortic valve replacement combined with coronary artery bypass procedures. In this group, the operative mortality was 16.5%, which caused us some surprise

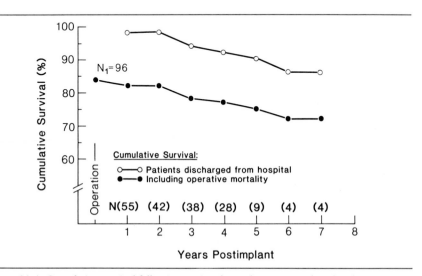

Figure 34-4. Cumulative survival following aortic valve replacement combined with coronary artery bypass in 115 patients. Operative mortality was 16.5%.

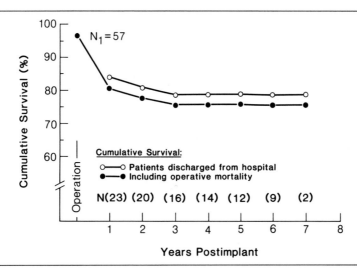

Figure 34-5. Cumulative survival following mitral valve replacement combined with coronary artery bypass in 59 patients. Operative mortality was 3.4%.

and concern. The operative mortality in the group with mitral valve replacement combined with coronary artery bypass, generally considered a higher operative risk group, was only 3.4%. However, it was noted that in this particular series, there was a significantly greater preponderance of high-risk patients in the AVR + CAB group (49% preoperative high-risk category). No other obvious cause could be found. Cumulative survival is depicted for AVR + CAB and MVR + CAB in figures 34-4 and 34-5, respectively.

Late cumulative survival and functional results were very good in all patient group categories, particularly when operative mortality is excluded and long-term survival of discharged patients is analyzed. The cumulative survival of patients with aortic valve replacement was consistently and significantly better than mitral valve replacement patients in all groups, particularly noted at follow-up beyond 5 years. It appeared from careful analyses of the patient groups that the group of patients undergoing mitral valve replacement had significantly greater hemodynamic deterioration preoperatively than the comparable groups of patients undergoing aortic valve surgery. In those mitral valve replacement patients evaluated by cardiac catheterization postoperatively, there was less evidence of reversibility of significant and severe preoperative hemodynamic defects.

In conclusion, this clinical experience has convinced us that the ST. JUDE MEDICAL cardiac prosthetic valve is an effective and durable valve, and excellent clinical results can be expected, both in terms of acceptably low operative mortality and excellent long-term functional and survival results. The ST. JUDE MEDICAL valve is currently our valve of choice.

REFERENCES

1. Mundth ED. A 57-month experience with the St. Jude Medical cardiac prosthesis at Hahnemann University Hospital. In Matloff JM (ed): *Cardiac Valve Replacement*. Martinus Nijhoff Publishing, Boston 1985; pp 167–172.
2. Arom KV, Nicoloff DM, Kersten TE, Northrup WF, Lindsay WE. Six years of experience with the St. Jude Medical valvular prosthesis. Circulation 1984; 72(II):153–158.
3. Chaux A, Czer LSC, Matloff JM, DeRobertis MA, Stewart ME, Bateman TM, Kass RM, Lee ME, Gray RJ. The St. Jude Medical bileaflet cardiac valve prosthesis. A 5 year experience. J Thorac Cardiovasc Surg 1984; 88:706–717.
4. LeClerc JL, Wellens F, Deuvaert FE, Martino A, Depaepe J, Primo G. A 60-month experience with the St. Jude Medical prosthesis at University Hospital, Brugmann. In Matloff JM (ed): *Cardiac Valve Replacement*. Martinus Nijhoff Publishing, Boston 1985; p. 195–200.
5. Lillehei CW. St. Jude Medical prosthetic heart valve: Results from a five-year multicenter experience. In Horstkotte D, Loogen F (eds): *Update in Heart Valve Replacement*. International Symposium. Steinkopff, Darmstadt 1985; pp 3–18.
6. Kaplan EL, Meier P. Nonparametric estimation from incomplete observations. Am Stat Assoc J 1958; 53:457–481.
7. Horstkotte D, Haerten K, Seipel L, et al. Central hemodynamics at rest and during exercise after mitral valve replacement with different prostheses. Circulation 1983; 68(II):(II)161–168.
8. Jamieson WR, Janusy J, Tyers FO, Gerein AN, Ricci DR, Burr LH, Miyagishima RT. Experience with standard and supra-annular Carpentier-Edwards porcine bioprosthesis. In Matloff JM (ed): *Cardiac Valve Replacement*. Martinus Nijhoff Publishing, Boston 1985; pp 45–56.
9. Gonzalez-Lavin L, Seong-Chi T, Blair C, Jung JY, Faboz AG, Lewis B, Daughters G. Aortic valve replacement with the Ionescu-Shiley bovine pericardial valve: An 81-month experience. In Matloff JM (ed): *Cardiac Valve Replacement*. Martinus Nijhoff Publishing, Boston 1985; pp 57–65.
10. Doty DB. Overview of experience with the Björk-Shiley valve. In Matloff JM (ed): *Cardiac Valve Replacement*. Martinus Nijhoff Publishing, Boston 1985; pp 41–44.
11. Pluth JR. Clinical experience with the caged-ball Starr-Edwards prosthesis. In Matloff JM (ed): *Cardiac Valve Replacement*. Martinus Nijhoff Publishing, Boston 1985; pp 37–40.

35. HEART VALVE REPLACEMENT WITH THE ST. JUDE MEDICAL® VALVE PROSTHESIS: LONG-TERM EXPERIENCE IN 743 PATIENTS RECEIVING VALVE IMPLANTS IN SWITZERLAND

D. BURCKHARDT, D. STRIEBEL, S. VOGT, A. HOFFMANN, J. ROTH,
U. ALTHAUS, J. J. GOY, H. SADEGHI, E. GRÄDEL

From November 1978 to June 1986, 743 patients received 828 ST. JUDE MEDICAL® valves (SJM) at the University Clinics of Basel, Berne, and Lausanne, Switzerland. There were 445 men and 298 women, with a mean age of 57 years (range 1–83 years), who were followed for a mean of 2.6 years (22,768 patient-months). Aortic valve replacement (AVR) was performed in 456 patients, mitral valve replacement (MVR) in 200 patients, tricuspid valve replacement (TVR) in 6 patients, double valve replacement in 77 patients, and triple valve replacement in 4 patients. In 187 patients, additional surgical interventions were performed. Operative mortality for the entire population was 1.6% and the 4-week perioperative mortality was 4.0%. During the mean follow-up period of 2.6 years, an additional 58 patients died, accounting for an annual mortality rate of 3.1%. Eighteen of these patients died of noncardiac causes, leaving an annual cardiac mortality rate of 2.1%. The thromboembolic rate was 1.25% per patient-year after AVR, 3.0% per patient-year after MVR, and 1.1% per patient-year after MuVR. In 8 of 32 patients (25%) with thromboembolic complications, symptoms were irreversible and in 14 of 32 patients (44%), the prothrombin time was not within therapeutic range. The incidence of major bleeding complications was 1.3% per patient-year. Valve dysfunction due to thrombotic obstruction occurred in 3 patients and leaflet dislocation in 1, necessitating reoperation, leading to an annual dysfunction rate of 0.2%. Twelve patients developed infectious endocarditis during the observation period (annual endocarditis incidence 0.6%). Six of these patients died, but in 4 patients, reoperation, and in 2 patients, antibiotic treatment, were successful. A paravalvular leak necessitating re-operation was present in 6 patients with AVR, 2 patients with MVR, and 2 patients with double valve replacement. In 3 patients the leak was due to infectious endocarditis. None of the patients died as a consequence of the reoperation. In 3 patients (0.4%) a mild hemolytic anemia was found, which could be corrected by iron substitution. The clinical results in our patients were excellent: of the 63% of patients who were preoperatively in (NYHA) Classes III and IV, only 6% remained in these classes after valve replacement. From the results obtained in a large number of patients, we conclude that excellent results with a low complication rate can be expected when the ST. JUDE MEDICAL prosthesis is used for valve replacement.

PART V. DISCUSSION

CHRISTOPHER T. MALONEY, MODERATOR

ANTICOAGULATION

CHRISTOPHER MALONEY: We still see significant bleeding complications following COUMADIN® therapy, not only in cases of valve replacement, but in any type of patient receiving COUMADIN therapy. Dr. Arom alluded to maintaining prothrombin time below 20, which is accepted procedure to date. Do any members of the panel keep the prothrombin time below 20 in patients having mitral valve replacement?

DENTON COOLEY: Our tendency is to more heavily anticoagulate the mitral patients than the aortic patients, especially in those who manifest atrial fibrillation as a chronic occurrence. In many patients with aortic valve replacement where anticoagulants are poorly tolerated, we have had rather encouraging results with minimal or no COUMADIN and use of aspirin and PERSANTINE®. However, I do not recommend this for the average patient, just for those who have manifested some complication.

ELDRED MUNDTH: Our target anticoagulation is generally around 1.5 times control, which would be about 18 seconds. We try to maintain the patient at 18 to 20 seconds early postoperatively, and recommend this for long-term follow-up in aortic and mitral valves.

VALVULOPLASTY

CHRISTOPHER MALONEY: In most of these presentations, we have seen a number of patients with paravalvular leaks. In the absence of endocarditis, would the panel agree that a paravalvular leak is a technical error at the time of surgery? Secondly, about two months ago, in Boston, there was a major cardiology meeting on balloon valvuloplasty, which 500 cardiologists from throughout the United States attended. Initially, they seem to have some pretty good results, but I wonder whether the cardiologists ever looked at some of the natural valves that we take out. Still, they feel strongly about this and we are going to be seeing a lot of it. What is the feeling of this panel on balloon valvuloplasty? Is it going to take over valve replacement in aged patients, or any significant replacements in all our patients? Dr. Cooley, are they doing it at your institution already?

DENTON COOLEY: Our cardiologists have become rather enthusiastic about it lately. In patients with aortic valve stenosis who are 75 years and older, our cardiologists have done some 30 procedures without a fatality. I have some skepticism about the effectiveness of balloon dilatation of the calcific aortic valve and feel it is a placebo rather than a mechanical improvement. We have had the opportunity to do some balloon dilatations with the cardiologists at the operating table under direct vision, and the results have been very disappointing. In one patient, for example, the calcific valve was torn off the aortic annulus completely. In another instance, where the valve was of the rubbery type of stenosis, as you see in some congenital valves, it had no effect whatsoever on the valve. So I think that it may have a place, but at the present time, it is not very clear. They challenged us to look at our operative results in calcific aortic stenosis in patients over 70 years of age, and I was surprised to see that we did have a mortality of 7% in that group. However, if we were to further analyze this, we might find that some of these patients were terminally ill when we operated on them. The internal review board of our hospital has declared a moratorium on mitral valvuloplasty since it has some rather disastrous complications. In the aortic valve cases, it may be a threat to the surgeon, such as the threat we see with percutaneous transluminal coronary angioplasty (PTCA).

CARLOS E. RUIZ: I am surprised at the Texas Heart Institute's results for the mitral valve; our experience is totally different. We have done close to 130 mitral valvuloplasties to date with very good results, but we have experienced some problems with this procedure in the aortic valve. We have to be very careful about how we choose the patients for aortic valvuloplasty. As Dr. Cooley said, the patients over 85 years of age with a very tight aortic valve probably should have percutaneous angioplasty, especially if they have other problems like chronic obstructive pulmonary diseases (COPD), which increase mortality in surgery. However, we are not doing the patients a favor when they are offered a valvuloplasty as a first choice for the aortic valve.

CHRISTOPHER MALONEY: There you have it from both sides. I can assure you we have not heard the end of valvuloplasty. Given the number of cardiologists throughout the country who want to try it, we are going to be standing by while they do these procedures.

VALVE FAILURE

CARLOS GOMEZ-DURAN: There has not been a single incidence of a mechanical problem with the St. Jude Medical valve. Is that correct?

DIETER BURCKHARDT: We had one young patient who dislodged a leaflet during vigorous exercise. This was 10 months after surgery in a 14-year-old boy; he was successfully reoperated in pulmonary edema.

CARLOS GOMEZ-DURAN: That is one case. The important factor is that this is a bileaflet, mechanical valve. If that sort of accident happens, and one leaflet broke while the other one stayed in, perhaps that is how the patient survived. How many hours was it between the dislodgement and the time you got the patient back into the OR and reoperated on him?

DIETER BURCKHARDT: About 4 hours.

CARLOS GOMEZ-DURAN: Are there any incidences of a disc valve becoming dislodged and the patient surviving 4 hours? Does anybody know or have personal experience of that? [No response] Dr. Burckhardt, where was the leaflet lodged?

DIETER BURCKHARDT: The surgeons did not find it and the patient didn't complain later on.

INDEX